Allergies and Hypersensitivity Disease in Animals

IAN R. TIZARD, BVMS, PhD, ACVM (Hons), DSc (Hons)

University Distinguished Professor Emeritus
Department of Veterinary Pathobiology
Texas A&M University
College Station
Texas

ELSEVIER

ELSEVIER

3251 Riverport Lane
St. Louis, Missouri 63043

Content Strategist: Jennifer Catando
Content Development Manager: Ellen Wurm-Cutter
Project Service Manager: Deepthi Unni
Content Development Specialist: Rebecca Corradetti
Project Manager: Haritha Dharmarajan
Designer: Ryan Cook

Printed in The United States of America

Last digit is the print number: 9   8   7   6   5   4   3   2   1

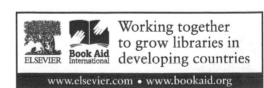

To Claire

ACKNOWLEDGMENTS

I would like to take this opportunity to express my appreciation to the many colleagues who have generously provided images of clinical cases, as well as their histopathology. I would especially like to thank Drs. Mark Johnston, Robert Kennis, Bryan Porter, Dominique Weiner, Aline Rodrigues Hoffman, and Karen Russell for their valuable contributions. Finally, this work could not have been accomplished without the encouragement and support of my wife, Claire.

**College Station,
Texas**

We live in a world in which changes are continuous and accelerating. Changes in climate, social behavior, and disease prevalence are rapid and unrelenting. Many of these changes have had unpredictable consequences; one such unanticipated change has been the huge increase in the prevalence of allergic diseases observed in Western and developing societies. The dramatic increase in human allergic disease that has occurred over the past half-century can be considered a 21st-century epidemic—or perhaps a pandemic. This allergy pandemic has been promoted by multiple factors, including environmental changes, urban air pollution, antibiotic use, dietary changes, lifestyle, and obesity. These factors have not only promoted the development of human allergic diseases but also allergies in our companion animals. As children and animals develop, their microbial environment especially, determines the manner in which their immune system matures. As a result, the massive reduction in infectious disease prevalence and parasite burden over the past hundred years has been somewhat counterbalanced by an increase in allergic diseases such as asthma, eczema, and food allergies. This increase has had a major influence on the quality of life of both humans and companion animals.

The increase in the prevalence of allergic diseases, especially in companion animals, makes this an appropriate time to draw together the science, diagnosis, and treatment of these diseases in a single volume. I have therefore sought to review the recent exciting advances and new discoveries that are beginning to "clarify" our understanding of allergic diseases. This "clarification" has, however, in some cases, shown the subject to be much more complex than previously imagined. For example, while it is clear that the microbiota influence the development of allergies in animals, the diversity of commensal bacteria within the animal body makes it appear that determining all relevant mechanisms and interactions will be a very difficult task. Nevertheless, the more we learn, the closer we will be to establish rational and effective treatments for these diseases. Inevitably, veterinarians will be at the forefront of this process.

The goal of this text is therefore to review the scientific basis of allergic diseases in domestic animals and apply them to our animals. Its intention is to advance the skills required to prevent and treat these diseases from a subjective to an objective basis.

It is perhaps here, in the study of the most common animal allergies, that we see most clearly the significant differences in disease pathogenesis between humans and the major domestic animals. The "one health" concept notwithstanding, it has proven remarkably difficult to extrapolate human allergic disease to domestic animal species. A textbook author, especially, is tasked with reconciling the conflicting data emerging from studies on humans and laboratory rodents, as well as from multiple domestic mammals. However, many species differences are real and cannot be reconciled. It is essential to bear this in mind when considering the subject of animal allergies.

It is also increasingly evident with respect to type I hypersensitivities that the IgE-mast cell-eosinophil paradigm is insufficient to explain the diversity of allergic disease endotypes in humans and domestic mammals. This is especially true when considering atopic dermatitis and allergic asthma. In addition to the role of Th2 cell-dominated responses, room must be made for inflammatory reactions mediated by other cell populations such as Th17 cells and innate lymphoid cells. Perhaps not as coequal participants, but still clinically relevant.

A related issue has been the increase not only in the diversity of cytokines but also in the recognition that many play critical roles in allergic diseases. Modern genetic techniques have also contributed to a belated appreciation of the diversity of allergic diseases. An excellent example of this complexity is revealed by the molecular dissection of the pathways and mechanisms involved in the itch-scratch cycle.

In the 1960s, Philip Gell and Robin Coombs brought order to a complex and confusing field by delineating four distinct types of hypersensitivity. However, they were fully aware that clinical situations were often much more complex and rarely involved only a single defined pathogenic pathway. In "real-world situations," multiple hypersensitivity pathways may be engaged at any specific time or in any specific tissue. Veterinary clinicians must also be aware of these complexities and use this knowledge to optimize diagnosis and subsequent treatments.

Additionally, the belated dawn of monoclonal antibody therapy has opened up a range of treatments previously unheard of. While this revolution is just beginning, it has already had a significant impact on the treatment of human allergic and inflammatory diseases and will inevitably be extended to domestic animal species as well.

The final chapter of this text deals with an important but underappreciated subject—the health of veterinarians themselves. Constant exposure to animals leads to the development of allergies and hypersensitivity diseases in both veterinarians and their staff. These are significant workplace hazards that ruin the careers of many and must not be underestimated.

In effect, the transition of veterinary allergy studies from a purely empirical subject to a quantitative science-based subject is well under way. Veterinary allergists, especially dermatologists, must be commended for their efforts in this area. Although great progress has been made, much remains to be done. I trust that this text will be a source of support and encouragement as the science of veterinary immunology advances.

TABLE OF CONTENTS

Basic Science

CHAPTER 1

The Immune System and the Defense of the Body

The immune system has evolved to fight microbial invaders. As with many such fights, the invaders may be persistent, the struggle may be intense, and collateral damage may be inevitable. Animals benefit from minimizing this collateral damage; nevertheless, invaders must be repelled even at the cost of severe damage. The immune system must do "whatever it takes" to maintain the body's integrity. Allergic responses are an essential component of these defenses, especially on the surfaces of the body, where the invaders first seek to penetrate. The skin, airways, and gastrointestinal tract are all potential invasion sites, and the local immune defenses must be armed and ready. It is these defenses that, when inappropriately activated, produce allergic diseases. Thus, a common feature of allergies is the reaction of the immune system to a perceived attack or invasion. The potential invaders do not need to be pathogens. If the system is ready, then exposure to foreign molecules (or allergens) in food, inhaled air, and on the skin might trigger the defensive cells of the body and mount aggressive defensive responses that we recognize as an allergic disease (Fig. 1.1).

Innate Immunity

Animals need to detect and eliminate microbial invaders as fast as possible. This immediate defensive response is the task of the innate immune system. The innate defenses respond rapidly, destroying invaders, while simultaneously minimizing collateral damage. Innate immune responses are triggered when cell surface pattern recognition receptors detect either microbial invasion or tissue damage. For example, cells can sense the presence of invading microbes by detecting their characteristic structural molecules. These molecules are called "pathogen-associated molecular patterns" (PAMPs). The innate immune defenses can also sense tissue damage by detecting the characteristic molecules released by damaged cells. These molecules are called "damage-associated molecular patterns" (DAMPs) or "alarmins." Specialized sentinel cells with pattern recognition receptors can detect both PAMPs and DAMPs and, once they are detected, these sentinel cells transmit signals to attract white blood cells. The white blood cells in response converge on the invaders and destroy them during inflammation. In addition, animals make many different antimicrobial proteins, such as complement, defensins, and cytokines, that can either kill invaders directly or promote their destruction by defensive cells. Some of these antimicrobial molecules are present in normal tissues, whereas others are produced in response to the presence of PAMPs or DAMPs such as damage caused by an invading bacterium. There are multiple specialized populations of white blood cells; therefore, the body can activate different populations in different situations, thus ensuring that the forces sent to repel the invaders are optimized for the task.

The innate immune system has minimal memory capability and, therefore, each infection episode is treated similarly. The intensity and duration of innate responses, such as inflammation, remain largely unchanged regardless of how often a specific invader is encountered. These responses come at a price, such as the pain and itch of inflammation. More importantly, innate immune responses act as triggers that stimulate antigen-presenting cells to initiate adaptive immune responses, eventually leading to strong, long-term protection.

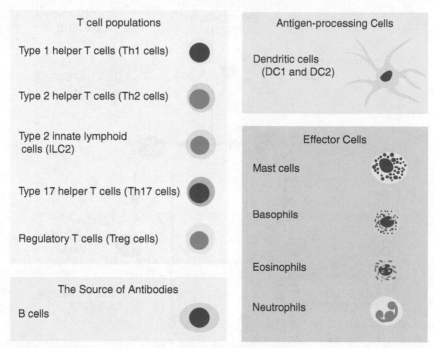

Fig. 1.1 Classification of the major cell types involved in allergic responses and a key to their identification in subsequent figures.

Several cytokines play essential roles in initiating and mediating innate responses and inflammation. These include interleukin 1 (IL-1), a cytokine produced by many different cell types. The two most important forms of IL-1 (α and β) act on type 2 helper (Th2) cells, B cells, natural killer (NK) cells, neutrophils, eosinophils, dendritic cells (DCs), fibroblasts, endothelial cells, and hepatocytes. IL-6 is also produced by many different cell types, and acts on T cells, B cells, hepatocytes, and bone marrow stromal cells. IL-8 is a proinflammatory chemokine and, similar to other chemokines, it is a relatively small (8.4 kDa) protein produced by macrophages and endothelial cells that attracts and activates neutrophils. Tumor necrosis factor-α (TNF-α) is a proinflammatory cytokine produced by macrophages, mast cells, T cells, endothelial cells, B cells, adipocytes, and fibroblasts. TNF-α is the most potent inducer of inflammation.

Adaptive Immunity

Adaptive immune responses develop when foreign antigens bind to specific receptors on lymphocytes and stimulate these cells to mount strong defensive responses. Adaptive immune responses proceed in four basic steps: Step 1, Antigen capture and processing; Step 2, Helper T cell activation; Step 3, B cell- or T cell-mediated responses that eliminate invaders, and Step 4, Generation of large populations of memory cells that respond rapidly upon subsequent exposure to an antigen (Fig. 1.2).

STEP 1: ANTIGEN CAPTURE AND PROCESSING

The initiation of any adaptive immune response requires the activation of antigen-presenting cells. These are primarily, but not exclusively, specialized DCs. Their activation is triggered by the

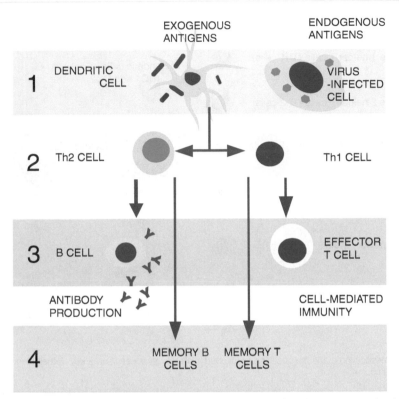

Fig. 1.2 Four steps of adaptive immunity. Step 1: appropriate processing of exogenous and endogenous antigens and differentiation of dendritic cells. Step 2: antigen presentation to the two major types of helper T cells. Step 3: either B cells or effector T cells are activated, with B cells responsible for antibody production and effector T cells responsible for killing virus-infected cells. Step 4: generation of memory T cells and B cells.

mixture of cytokines generated during the initial innate response. The activated DCs are needed to capture and process any antigens derived from the invading pathogens, especially from bacteria. DCs have a small cell body with many long cytoplasmic processes known as dendrites extending from its surface. These dendrites increase antigen capture efficiency and maximize the area of contact when they wrap themselves around lymphocytes. DCs are found throughout the body and form networks in every tissue. They are especially prominent in lymph nodes and under the skin and mucosal surfaces, which are the sites where invading microbes are most likely to be encountered.

Exogenous Antigens

Antigens fall into two distinct categories. The first category is typified by pathogenic bacteria that invade tissues and extracellular fluid. These invading bacteria mainly grow outside cells and are classified as "exogenous antigens." Exogenous antigens must first be captured by DCs, and then processed and presented to helper T cells if they are to trigger an adaptive response.

When DCs encounter foreign antigens together with "danger signals" such as DAMPs from tissue damage, PAMPs from infection, and cytokines released by the inflammatory process, they mature rapidly (Fig. 1.3). Therefore, the DCs migrate toward the source of the antigen. The activated DCs capture antigens by phagocytosis. If they ingest bacteria, they can usually kill them;

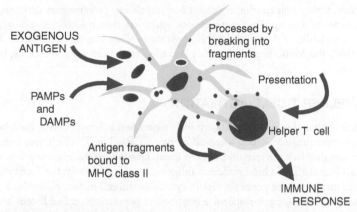

Fig. 1.3 Functions of dendritic cells (DCs). DCs capture and process exogenous antigens. Their response is stimulated by pathogen-associated molecular patterns (PAMPs) and damage-associated molecular patterns (DAMPs) acting through pattern recognition receptors. Ingested antigens are broken into small peptides, which are then bound to major histocompatibility complex (MHC) molecules and the complexes carried to the DC surface, where they are recognized by helper T cells. The cytokine mixture produced by the DCs determines whether the helper T cells become type 1 helper (Th1) or type 2 helper (Th2) cells. Th2 cells are responsible for triggering allergic responses.

however, the pH within the phagosomes of DCs is less acidic than in other phagocytic cells, and the ingested antigens are not totally degraded, with some peptides remaining intact. These ingested peptides are then bound to specialized receptors called major histocompatibility complex (MHC) class II molecules. Once an antigenic peptide binds to an MHC molecule, the MHC-peptide complex is transported to the surface of the DCs. On arrival at the surface, this MHC-peptide complex is made available for inspection by any passing T cell. The DCs embrace the T cells, whereas the T cells palpate the DCs for the presence of MHC-peptide complexes. T cells express T cell antigen receptors (TCRs) on their surface. If the TCRs can bind any of these peptides, the T cells will be triggered to respond. DCs also carry their MHC-bound peptides to nearby lymph nodes, where they can be presented to many helper T cells. The processed antigen peptides will encounter and bind to the receptors on at least one T cell. Each T cell has multiple receptors of a single specificity. TCRs only bind to peptides attached to MHC molecules, and will not recognize or respond to peptides alone.

Because helper T cells must recognize MHC-peptide complexes if they are to respond to an antigen, MHC molecules effectively determine whether an animal can mount an adaptive response. MHC class II molecules can bind some, but not all, peptides created during antigen processing; therefore, they effectively select those antigen peptides that are to be presented to the T cells. The response to antigens is thus controlled largely by the MHC genes of an animal. Therefore, MHC genes can regulate immune responses, including allergies.

Endogenous Antigens

The second category of invading organism is typified by viruses that can enter cells and force them to make new viral proteins. These viral or "endogenous antigens" are processed by the cells in which they are produced. Immune responses against endogenous antigens must be aimed at detecting and destroying any cells producing abnormal or foreign proteins. Viruses take over the protein-synthesizing machinery of infected cells and use it to make new viral proteins. Therefore, T cells must be able to recognize a virus-infected cell by detecting the viral proteins expressed on the cell surface. Living cells continually digest and recycle any proteins they produce. Therefore, these proteins are broken up into short peptides, which are then transported to a newly formed MHC class I molecule. If they fit the MHC-peptide-binding site, they will bind. Once loaded onto the MHC, the MHC-peptide complex is carried to the cell surface and displayed to any passing T cells.

STEP 2: HELPER T CELL ACTIVATION

Helper T cells are found in follicles and germinal centers within lymph nodes. Each helper T cell is covered by approximately 30,000 identical foreign TCRs. The T cells ignore normal cellular proteins because they lack the receptors to bind them. However, any foreign peptides will bind to some TCRs. Once the TCRs bind sufficient antigenic peptides correctly, the T cell will be driven to respond by turning on the genes for certain cytokines and cell surface molecules and dividing.

There are two other antigen-responsive lymphocyte populations, called B cells and cytotoxic T cells. These cannot respond properly to foreign antigens unless they first receive their instructions from the helper T cells.

The binding of an MHC-peptide complex to a TCR is insufficient by itself to trigger a helper T cell response. Therefore, when DCs present their processed antigen load to helper T cells, they must transmit additional signals. The first, as described above, is delivered when TCRs bind the antigen peptides attached to the MHC molecules. The second signal provides the T cells with additional critical co-stimulation via prolonged strong adhesion between the cells and is mediated by cell surface adhesion molecules. The third set of signals determine how naïve helper T cells will develop and the precise form the resulting immune response will take. These signals are provided by the mixture of cytokines secreted by the DCs. For example, some antigens trigger DCs to secrete IL-12, which acts on undifferentiated helper T cells causing them to develop into type 1 helper (Th1) cells and trigger a type 1 immune response. Other antigens are processed so that they cause DCs to secrete a cytokine mixture containing IL-4 and IL-6. These cytokines act on undifferentiated helper T cells to cause them to differentiate into Th2 cells, stimulating type 2 responses, especially allergies (Fig. 1.4). DCs that stimulate type 1 responses are called DC1 cells. Those that stimulate type 2 responses are called DC2 cells. (A third population of helper T cells called type 17 helper [Th17] cells are discussed in Chapter 2.)

STEP 3: B AND T CELL RESPONSES

The division of the adaptive immune system into two major branches is based on the need to recognize two distinctly different categories of foreign invaders—"exogenous "and "endogenous." Antibodies produced by a type 2 response will bind to bacteria, free virus particles, and parasites and promote their destruction. Antibodies also provide the first line of defense against organisms that may survive within cells. However, once these organisms succeed in entering cells, then antibodies are ineffective and a type 1 response mediated by cytotoxic T cells is needed to kill the infected cell, release cytokines that inhibit microbial growth, or prevent pathogen survival within the infected cells.

B Cell Responses

Helper T cells are essential for B cell activation and are required to produce high-affinity antibodies and immune memory. B cells can also capture and process antigens, present them to helper T cells, and then receive co-stimulation from the same T cells. B cells thus play two roles: they respond to antigens by making antibodies and act as antigen-presenting cells. Helper T cells stimulate these B cell responses using secreted cytokines and via interacting cell receptors.

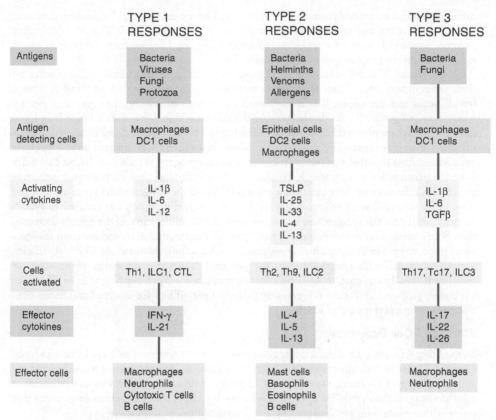

	TYPE 1 RESPONSES	TYPE 2 RESPONSES	TYPE 3 RESPONSES
Antigens	Bacteria Viruses Fungi Protozoa	Bacteria Helminths Venoms Allergens	Bacteria Fungi
Antigen detecting cells	Macrophages DC1 cells	Epithelial cells DC2 cells Macrophages	Macrophages DC1 cells
Activating cytokines	IL-1β IL-6 IL-12	TSLP IL-25 IL-33 IL-4 IL-13	IL-1β IL-6 TGFβ
Cells activated	Th1, ILC1, CTL	Th2, Th9, ILC2	Th17, Tc17, ILC3
Effector cytokines	IFN-γ IL-21	IL-4 IL-5 IL-13	IL-17 IL-22 IL-26
Effector cells	Macrophages Neutrophils Cytotoxic T cells B cells	Mast cells Basophils Eosinophils B cells	Macrophages Neutrophils

Fig. 1.4 Comparison of the three major types of adaptive immune responses. The development of each type is determined by the effects of the cytokine mixtures the responding T cells are exposed to. These results are determined by antigen-processing dendritic cells. Once the helper T cells have differentiated, they control further development by the mixture of cytokines they secrete. Type 3 responses are proinflammatory responses triggered by helper T cells that secrete interleukin-17, and are discussed in Chapter 2.

B cells are activated by helper T cells (mainly Th2 cells) within lymph nodes. When a B cell encounters an antigen that binds its receptors (B cell receptors [BCRs]), it will, with appropriate co-stimulation, respond by upregulating its BCR genes, thereby increasing the production and secretion of these receptors into body fluids, where they are called antibodies. Each B cell is covered with approximately 200,000 to 500,000 identical antigen receptors. Antibodies are simply BCRs released into body fluids, all belonging to the family of proteins called immunoglobulins (Igs).

Although the binding of an antigen to a BCR is an essential first step, this is usually insufficient to activate B cells. The complete activation of a B cell requires co-stimulatory signals from helper T cells and their cytokines. When helper T cells "help" B cells, they start the process that leads to B cell division and the development into antibody-secreting cells. The "help" also triggers somatic mutation within B cell IgG genes and results in a progressive increase in antibody-binding affinity.

When appropriately stimulated by helper T cells and co-stimulated by cytokines, B cells divide. This division is asymmetric so that one daughter cell receives a lot of antigens while the other daughter cell receives very little or none. The cell that receives a lot of antigen then differentiates into an antibody-producing plasma cell. The cell that receives less antigen continues the cycle of dividing and mutating and eventually becomes a memory cell. The cells destined to become plasma cells develop a rough endoplasmic reticulum, increase their antibody synthesis rate, and secrete large quantities of immunoglobulins.

A key feature of B cell responses is the progressive increase in the affinity of antibodies for their antigens over time. These increases in antibody affinity occur within germinal centers in lymph nodes and the spleen. B cells stimulated by antigens migrate to these germinal centers where they proliferate. B cells divide every 6–8 h so that within a few days a single B cell may develop into a clone of several thousand cells. During this phase of rapid B cell division, the BCR variable region genes (encoding the antigen-binding sites on the BCR) mutate, on average, once per division. This repeated random mutation ensures that progeny B cells have BCRs that differ from the parent cell. Once these cells have been clonally expanded, they are presented with antigens by DCs. Because of these mutations, some B cells bind the antigen with greater affinity, and others bind it with less. A selection process then occurs. If a mutation has resulted in greater receptor affinity for the antigen, this stimulates more B cell proliferation. If the affinity decreases, then B cell stimulation is also reduced. Thus, cycles of somatic mutation and selection lead to a rapid improvement in antigen binding—a process called affinity maturation. The high-affinity, antigen-selected B cells eventually leave the germinal center to form either plasma cells or memory B cells. In contrast, those B cells that have reduced antigen binding will die. Thus, the antibodies produced by B cells progressively increase their affinity for antigens and hence their effectiveness as the response proceeds.

Effector T Cell Responses

Intracellular organisms are eliminated by two processes. Either infected cells are killed rapidly by cytotoxic T cells so that the invader has no time to grow, or infected macrophages develop the ability to destroy the intracellular organisms. In general, cells infected with viruses that enter the cell cytosol or nucleus are killed by T cells, whereas organisms such as bacteria or parasites that reside within endosomes are destroyed by T cell-activated macrophages.

If endogenous antigens presented by MHC class I molecules can bind to the antigen receptors of a T cell, the T cell will respond. For example, when a virus infects a cell, some viral proteins will be expressed on the cell surface. Circulating T cells might have TCRs that bind these processed viral peptides. The T cells that respond to these endogenous antigens carry the cell surface protein called CD8, which is used to bind to the MHC class I molecules on the virus-infected cells. Once the two cells are tightly bound, their receptors interact, signals are exchanged, and the T cells kill the infected cells.

Cytotoxic T cells must be highly sensitive to the presence of viruses so that they can kill all the virus-infected cells as fast as possible. Within a few minutes of binding to a target cell, the T cell cytoplasmic granules fuse with the T cell membrane so that their toxic contents are injected into the target cell. Soon after coming into contact with a cytotoxic T cell, its target cell starts to undergo apoptosis and is dead in less than 10 min. Cytotoxic T cells can disengage and then move on to kill other target cells. Several cytotoxic cells may also join in killing a single target.

Macrophages are also activated by Th1 cell-derived gamma interferon. Once activated, these macrophages secrete proteases, cytokines such as interferons, vasoactive molecules, and complement components. Activated macrophages move more rapidly in response to chemotactic stimuli, and contain increased amounts of lysosomal enzymes and respiratory burst metabolites, and they are more avidly phagocytic than normal cells. They produce greatly increased amounts of nitric oxide synthase and kill intracellular organisms or tumor cells by generating high nitric oxide levels.

STEP 4: MEMORY CELL GENERATION

In addition to mounting an immediate defensive response, both B and T cells generate populations of memory cells. These memory cells can respond more rapidly and effectively to antigens when they re-encounter them. These memory cells confer immediate protection and generate secondary immune responses.

Memory B Cells

Primary antibody responses do not persist because the responding B and plasma cells are short-lived and die within months. However, if all these cells died, immunological memory could not develop. Some B cells must persist as memory cells, which survive within the lymph nodes and bone marrow, where they proliferate and form germinal centers. These cells persist under the influence of survival and rescue signals. If a second antigen dose is given to a primed animal, it will encounter large numbers of responsive memory B cells. Therefore, secondary immune responses are much greater than primary immune responses. Immunoglobulin class switching also occurs so that immunoglobulin G (IgG) or IgE antibodies are produced in preference to the IgM characteristic of the primary response. In addition, memory B cells secrete antibodies with a much higher affinity for antigens than primary plasma cells because of somatic mutation and affinity maturation.

Memory T Cells

Naïve CD8$^+$ T cells are long-lived cells that continuously recirculate among tissues, the bloodstream, and lymphoid organs. Once they encounter antigens, they must multiply rapidly to keep pace with the growth of the invading pathogens. The number of responding T cells may increase more than 1000-fold within a few days. They reach a peak 5−7 days after infection when pathogen-specific, cytotoxic T cells can make up 50% to 70% of the total CD8$^+$ T cell population. In contrast to the prolonged B cell responses, however, the effector phase of T cell responses is very brief, and cytotoxicity occurs only in the presence of antigens, which is logical. Excessive sustained cytotoxic activity by T cells or the overproduction of cytokines can cause severe tissue damage.

As with other lymphocytes, the asymmetric division of an effector T cell generates two daughter cells with different fates. The dividing T cell is polarized because one pole of the cell contains the antigen-binding structures. The other pole contains molecules excluded from the contact site. Thus, when the cell divides, it forms two distinctly different daughter cells. The daughter cell adjacent to the contact site is the precursor of the effector T cells. The daughter cell formed at the opposite pole is the precursor of the memory T cells. The proximal cell has increased expression of effector molecules. The distal cell has increased lipid metabolism and expression of anti-apoptotic molecules and lives much longer. Once an infection has been eliminated, up to 95% of effector T cells undergo apoptosis within 1 to 2 weeks. However, memory T cells persist for months or years, lurking in the tissues and lymphoid organs and remaining functionally silent until they re-encounter antigens. When that happens, they respond very rapidly.

Suggested Reading

Tizard IR. *Veterinary Immunology: An Introduction.* 10th ed. Elsevier; 2018.

CHAPTER 2

Type 2 Immune Responses

Helper T Cells

Over 100 years ago, the first debates occurred between scientists who claimed that immunity to infection was due to antibodies and others who maintained it was due to cells. They were, of course, both right. Their differences were resolved by recognizing two types of immune response: antibody- and cell-mediated immunities. Subsequent studies revealed that different populations of helper T cells controlled these two immune response types. The helper cells that are required for cell-mediated immunity are called type 1 helper (Th1) cells, whereas those required for antibody production are termed type 2 helper (Th2) cells. Their functional differentiation is not absolute. Both Th1 and Th2 cells can help antibody production; however, only Th1 cells can promote cell-mediated immune responses. Therefore, it has been proposed that the terms type 1 response and type 2 response be used to generalize about a specific situation.

As T cells respond to antigens, they differentiate into subpopulations that secrete different cytokine mixtures and play diverse roles in regulating innate immune responses. For example, there are three major populations of helper T cells in addition to Th1 and Th2 cells. These are called type 17 helper (Th17), follicular helper T (Tfh), and regulatory T (Treg) cells, with each distinguished by the mixture of cytokines it produces. It is this mixture of cytokines that determines the direction in which the immune response will proceed. When T cells first develop, they are functionally uncommitted and are called undifferentiated helper T (Th0) cells. When appropriately activated by dendritic cell (DC)-derived cytokines, they differentiate into Th1, Th2, Th17, Tfh, or Treg populations. Recent studies have suggested that there is a continuum of different T cell types spanning all these populations.

Dendritic Cells

To activate helper T cells, DCs generate three signals. The first signal is delivered when antigen fragments attached to major histocompatibility complex molecules on DCs are bound by T cell antigen receptors. The second signal provides these T cells with additional stimulation by tightly binding T cells and DCs for a long time. The third signal determines the direction in which the naïve helper T cells will develop.

This is provided by secreted cytokines. For example, some microbial antigens trigger DCs to secrete interleukin (IL)-12. These are called DC1 cells because the IL-12 activates Th1 cells and triggers type 1 responses. Other microbial products induce DCs to secrete IL-1 and IL-6. These two cytokines are produced by DC2 cells and stimulate type 2 responses. Other antigens may induce DC2s to secrete IL-23 and provoke the development of type 17 responses.

Pathogen-associated molecular patterns and damage-associated molecular patterns acting through different toll-like receptors (TLRs) influence the development of DC subpopulations and thus determine the specific type of immune responses induced. For example, the stimuli that promote DC1 development include double-stranded RNA acting via TLR3, bacterial lipopoly-saccharide acting via TLR4, bacterial flagellin acting via TLR5, and viral nucleic acids acting via TLR7 and TLR9. However, inflammatory mediators, such as IL-10, tumor necrosis factor-α (TNF-α), prostaglandin E_2 (PGE$_2$), histamine, substance P, extracts of parasitic worms, or the toxin of *Vibrio cholerae* promote DC2 development. DC2 responses may also be triggered by bacterial lipopolysaccharides and proteoglycans acting through TLR2, TLR6, or TLR1. Ligand binding to TLR2 promotes the production of IL-23 and initiates Th17 cell responses. A similar functional subdivision occurs in macrophages. Thus, M1 and M2 cells, when acting as antigen-presenting cells, promote different helper cell responses.

The same DCs might also promote a type 1, type 2, or type 17 response, depending on the dose and type of antigen they encounter. The response also depends on its location. For example, DCs from the intestine or airways preferentially secrete IL-10 and IL-4 and promote type 2 responses. In such cases, the intestinal microbiota provides additional DC polarizing signals.

Helper T Cells

Th1 CELLS

Type 1, or cell-mediated immune responses, are mediated by Th1 cells. Type 1 responses are responsible for immunity to bacteria, viruses, protozoa, and fungi. They generate some antibodies and strong cytotoxic T cell responses and activate macrophages. Mature Th1 cells secrete IL-2 and interferon-γ (IFN-γ). IFN-γ is the definitive Th1 cell-derived cytokine. IFN-γ activates macrophages and upregulates major histocompatibility complex expression in DC1 cells, promoting antigen presentation. IFN-γ stimulates endothelial cells, keratinocytes, and fibroblasts to secrete proinflammatory cytokines such as TNF-α and multiple chemokines. (Chemokines are a family of cytokines that control cell migration by serving as specific chemotactic molecules.) IL-12 acting on Th0 cells generates a transcription factor called STAT4 that activates the genes leading to the development of the Th1 phenotype.

Th2 CELLS

Type 2 immunity is mediated by Th2 cells (Fig. 2.1). These cells favor antibody-mediated immune responses. The antibodies generated by type 2 responses are responsible for the destruction of extracellular bacteria, viruses, and parasitic helminths, as well as allergic responses. IL-4 and IL-13 are the defining cytokines produced by Th2 cells (Figs 2.2 and 2.3). Th2 cell-derived IL-4 and IL-13 activate B cells causing their proliferation, immunoglobulin class switching, and the production of antibodies. Although IL-4 and IL-13 receptors share a common alpha chain, they have different functions. IL-13 preferentially acts in peripheral tissues and plays a major role in local allergic reactions such as atopic dermatitis. In contrast, IL-4 is predominantly produced within lymphoid organs and plays a major role in immunoglobulin E (IgE) production. Th2 cells also secrete IL-5, which is required for the production and activation of eosinophils from bone marrow stem cells. All these cytokines are involved in the development of allergic responses (Box 2.1).

Th2 Cell Subpopulations

Th2 cells are functionally heterogeneous. Thus, one subpopulation of human Th2 memory cells produces IL-17 in addition to the regular cytokines. The numbers of these Th17/Th2 cells are increased in severely allergic individuals. Humans develop a unique subset of memory cells that are closely associated with the development of allergic diseases. These are CD4$^+$ cells that are CD27$^-$ and CD45RB$^-$ but express CRT$_H$2 (a chemokine receptor), CD49d (a homing receptor), and CD161(an NK cell marker). This subset called Th2A cells, are absent from non-allergic individuals, but their numbers increase significantly in those with peanut allergies

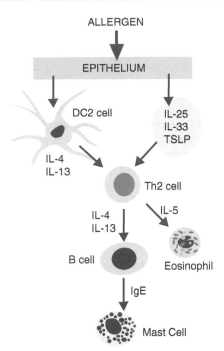

Fig. 2.1　Central role of type 2 helper (Th2) cells in the development of allergic responses. Cytokines such as interleukin 4 (IL-4), IL-5, and IL-13 produced by Th2 cells can promote B cell immunoglobulin E (IgE) production and the activation of eosinophils.

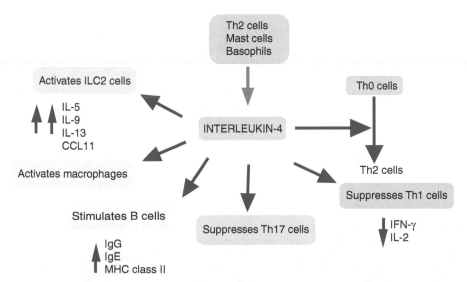

Fig. 2.2　Sources and functions of interleukin 4 (IL-4). IL-4 is mainly produced by Th2 cells. Once released, it promotes the development of more Th2 cells and type 2 innate lymphoid (ILC2) cells, while suppressing Th1 and Th17 cell responses.

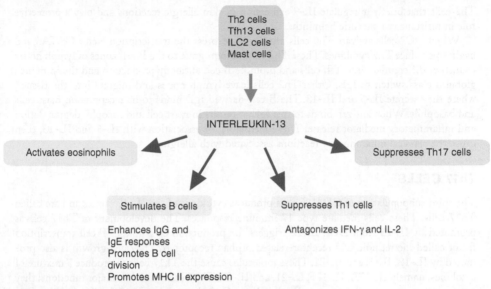

Fig. 2.3 Origins and functions of interleukin 13 (IL-13). Its primary sources are Th2 and ILC2 cells. It promotes Th2 responses while suppressing Th1 and Th17 responses.

BOX 2.1 ■ Key Cytokines Involved in Type 2 Immune Responses

Interleukin 4: Produced by activated Th2 cells, mast cells, and activated basophils. It regulates the activities of B cells, T cells, macrophages, endothelial cells, fibroblasts, and mast cells, and stimulates the growth and differentiation of B cells and promotes type 2 immune responses.

Interleukin 5: A growth factor produced by activated Th2 cells, mast cells, and eosinophils. In humans, it promotes eosinophil production.

Interleukin 9: A growth factor produced by Th2 cells activated by IL-2. It is also produced in large amounts by ILC2 cells and mucosal mast cells. It promotes the growth of helper T and mast cells, and potentiates the effects of IL-4 on IgE production.

Interleukin 13: An immunoregulatory cytokine produced by activated Th2, ILC2, Tfh13, NK, mast, and DC2 cells. It has biological activities similar to those of IL-4 because they act via a common receptor alpha chain.

---

and decrease in patients treated with appropriate immunotherapy. Thus, they play a functional role in human allergic responses, although they have yet to be described in animals.

Th9 CELLS

Th9 cells are a subpopulation of Th2 cells whose development is promoted by cytokines such as thymic stromal lymphopoietin (TSLP), IL-4, and TGFβ. They characteristically produce large amounts of IL-9, which is a mast cell growth factor that exacerbates allergic disease and promotes IL-4 driven antibody production by B cells. IL-9 can induce goblet cell metaplasia and is highly expressed in the lungs of asthmatics. Th9 cells were initially believed to be the only major source of IL-9; however, it is now clear that IL-9 is produced in larger amounts by type 2 innate lymphoid (ILC2) cells, mucosal mast cells, and eosinophils. Th9 cells are now regarded as a subset of

Th2 cells that briefly upregulate IL-9 expression in skin allergic reactions and play a protective role in resistance to parasitic helminths.

When DC2 cells activate Th0 cells, the T cells express the transcription factor GATA3 and begin to produce Th2 cytokines. These Th2 cells then migrate to the B cell zones of lymph nodes to further differentiate into Tfh cells and promote B cell antibody production and the immunoglobulin class switch to IgE. Other Th2 cells leave lymph nodes and migrate into the tissues, where they secrete IL-5 and IL-13. The B cell-derived IgE binds to its receptors on mast cells and basophils. When antigen binds to this IgE, it results in mast cell and basophil degranulation and inflammatory mediator release. These mediators, in association with IL-5 and IL-13, then cause the classical inflammatory reactions associated with allergies.

Th17 CELLS

The third subpopulation of CD4$^+$ T cells produces cytokines of the IL-17 family and are called Th17 cells. These cells mediate type 17 immune responses. The development of Th17 cells is promoted by IL-23 from DCs. IL-23 triggers the production of a unique T cell transcription factor called the retinoic acid receptor-related orphan receptor-α. Th17 cell growth is also promoted by IL-1β, IL-6, and IL-21. These molecules cause the Th17 cells to produce a mixture of cytokines, namely IL-17A, IL-17F, IL-21, and IL-22. Th17 cells have two major functions: they trigger inflammation and are potent B cell helpers. Cytokines of the IL-17 family play a key role in immunity against extracellular bacteria and assist in the clearance of fungi. Under some circumstances, Th17 cells may convert into IFN-γ-producing Th1 cells. They can differentiate into Treg cells after inflammation is resolved. The balance between Th17 and Treg cells is critical to maintaining homeostasis during immune responses and inflammation. Excessive Th17 activity can lead to the development of chronic inflammatory diseases, including some that mimic allergies.

Regulatory T Cells

No explanation of allergic mechanisms would be complete without a discussion on the role of Treg cells (Fig. 2.4). Immunity at the body surfaces, especially in the skin and the respiratory and intestinal tracts, are regulated by Treg cells. In their absence, animals will mount excessive Th2 responses and develop allergic diseases. Thus, Treg cells play a primary role in preventing allergy development. Like other T cells, the initial development of Treg cells occurs in the thymus. These cells migrate to the peripheral tissues, especially to epithelial surfaces such as the gastrointestinal tract, skin, and airways. Here, they encounter and interact with molecules generated by the local microbiota. The major function of Treg cells is to regulate local inflammation. For example, they ensure that the body does not react too aggressively against the diverse commensals that compose the microbiota. They defend against microbial invaders and promote wound and tissue repair. Treg cells suppress immune responses to food-derived antigens while simultaneously, the microbiota regulate the development and activities of the Treg cells. Alterations in the microbiota composition can reduce the availability of Treg cells and predispose an animal to the development of excessive Th2 responses and allergic diseases.

Innate Lymphoid Cells

The traditional view of type 2 immune responses has been that they are induced by the cytokines secreted by Th2 cells, i.e., IL-4, IL-5, IL-9, and IL-13. However, it is now clear that a second lymphocyte population, called ILC2 cells, can produce most of these same cytokines. ILC2 cells functionally resemble Th2 cells; however, they are usually found under body surfaces and not in

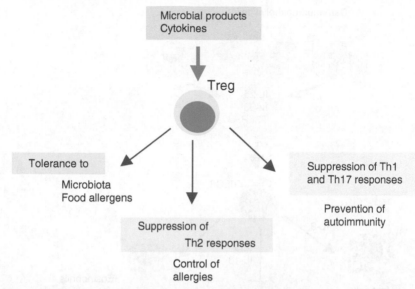

Fig. 2.4 Roles of regulatory T (Treg) cells. Depending on their target, they can induce tolerance or specifically regulate either type 1 (Th1) or type 2 (Th2) immune responses.

lymphoid organs. Thus, there are two arms of the type 2 response: an adaptive arm mediated by Th2 cells and an innate arm mediated by ILC2 cells (Fig. 2.5). Both arms interact and collaborate to mount an optimal and effective defensive response, and they can also trigger allergies.

ILC2 cells are lymphocytes found under exterior barrier surfaces such as the epithelia of the lung and skin, and especially the small intestine, where they serve as sentinel cells. They regulate the interactions between the body and external stimuli such as commensal bacteria or environmental allergens. Permanently "on guard," they enable the body to respond immediately when environmental allergens penetrate these external surfaces. ILC2 cells arise from lymphoid stem cells and use the transcription factor, retinoic acid receptor-related orphan receptor-α. Once activated, ILC2 cells produce large amounts of IL-5 and IL-13 and smaller amounts of IL-9 in response to activating signals from three cytokines, TSLP, IL-25, and IL-33, produced by damaged epithelial cells and DCs. ILC2 cells also directly regulate Th2 cells by presenting them with antigens. Thus, there is extensive Th2−ILC2 cross-talk. ILC2 cells can also develop a "memory-like" phenotype when activated by IL-33 and produce IL-17 when activated by IL-25.

In addition to initiating rapid responses to allergens, ILC2 cells are required to develop innate immunity to parasitic helminths because they are the major source of IL-13 during helminth infections. They participate in type 2 inflammatory responses such as asthma and food allergies and regulate type 2 immunity by acting on macrophages and mast cells. They control eosinophil production and can induce eosinophilia. They also induce mucus production by goblet cells, alternative activation of macrophages, and tissue repair.

Type 2 Responses

INDUCTION OF TYPE 2 RESPONSES

Allergic diseases are aberrant or inappropriate responses of a pathway that probably originated as an anti-helminth defense mechanism. However, they also play a significant defensive role.

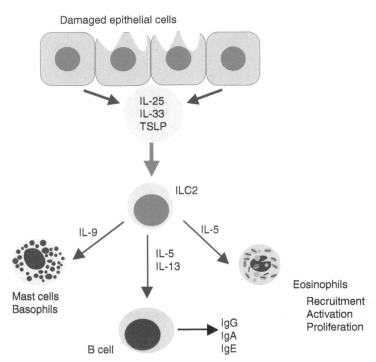

Fig. 2.5 **Roles of type 2 innate lymphoid (ILC2) cells.** These cells are activated by the three major epithelial cytokines: IL-25, IL-33, and TSLP. They release a cytokine mixture that promotes type 2 (Th2) immune responses by acting on B cells, mast cells, and eosinophils. Depending on their location, they may only produce small amounts of IL-4.

Almost all type 2 responses occur on the surfaces of the body, i.e., the skin, mucosa of airways, and the intestine. The cells involved are located in such a way that they can monitor the local environment. ILC2 cells can detect foreign invaders rapidly and respond to invasion without waiting for an adaptive response to occur. Thus, they play a key role in restricting invasion by neutralizing invaders. Many type 2 inflammatory responses attract eosinophils rather than neutrophils. Eosinophils are attracted by chemokines called eotaxins that are produced in response to IL-13 and are then maintained in tissues by the presence of IL-5.

The induction of a type 2 immune response involves interactions among DC2, Th2, and ILC2 cells. Several distinct DC2 populations can induce Th2 responses. These include CD11$^+$ and CD8α^- DCs in the spleen, FcϵR1-expressing DCs in the lung, plasmacytoid DCs in the blood, and Langerhans cells in the epidermis. Each of these DC populations can be stimulated via pattern recognition receptors such as toll-like receptors and C-type lectins. Sustained signaling through these receptors inhibits IL-12 synthesis while simultaneously enhancing IL-10 production. However, activated DC2 cells alone are not enough to trigger a significant Th2 response. This also requires IL-33, IL-25, and TSLP because these are needed for the terminal differentiation of Th2 cells.

Immune Polarization

Cytokines transmit signals that instruct the recipient cell as to how to behave. Basically, they tell a cell to turn off some genes and turn on others. Cytokines, for example, are secreted by cells when they encounter invaders. They raise the alarm by producing TNF-α, IL-1, and IFN-γ. This mixture activates DCs and tells them how to respond to the antigen. The DCs, in turn, secrete a mixture of cytokines that then activate helper T cells.

The polarization of an activated T cell does not occur until after it arrives in a lymph node and receives appropriate signals from the DCs. Thus, T cells exposed to IL-12 from DC1 cells become Th1 cells, whereas those exposed to IL-4 develop into Th2 cells. The Th2 phenotype is the default position so that if exposed to both IL-12 and IL-4, the cells become Th2 cells. It is not known whether helper cells can reverse their polarization. It is known that changes in the cytokine mixture within tissues can alter the dominant Th population. These changes in the tissue environment might activate quiescent Th0 cell populations while suppressing the previously dominant phenotypes. Polarizing cytokines can also be produced by cell types other than DCs, including B cells, mast cells, neutrophils, and macrophages. Th1 and Th2 cells also regulate each other. Thus, IFN-γ suppresses IL-4 production, whereas IL-4 and IL-10 inhibit IL-12 and IFN-γ production and Th1 cell production from Th0 precursors. Th1 cells have an absolute requirement for IL-2 if they are to proliferate and activate. However, Th2 cells do not need IL-2 if IL-4 or IL-1 are present.

Hormonal Effects

Glucocorticoids stimulate type 2 responses and inhibit type 1 responses. They directly induce IL-4 and IL-10 production and inhibit IL-2 and IFN-γ production. By suppressing IL-2 production, they prevent Th1 growth and permit Th2 expansion. However, steroids at high doses inhibit both Th1 and Th2 responses. Estrogens and progestins act as glucocorticoids and suppress Th1 responses while promoting Th2 responses. Testosterone derivatives have the reverse effect and potentiate IL-2 secretion and Th1 cell responses. Catecholamines such as epinephrine, norepinephrine, and dopamine also regulate the Th1/Th2 balance by suppressing Th1 cytokine production and upregulating Th2 cytokine production. Their inhibition of IL-2 production allows the proliferation of Th2 cells, which may affect the control of atopic diseases where β2 agonists serve as potent bronchodilators but may exacerbate allergic inflammation in the long term.

Antigen Presentation

Allergens are antigens that preferentially induce Th2 responses leading to IgE production. There is no key biochemical marker that can predict allergenicity—yet. Allergens are usually glycoproteins, lipoproteins, or proteins conjugated with drug haptens. Helper T cell polarization is influenced by the type of antigen-presenting cell involved. Thus, in their role as antigen-presenting cells, B cells promote type 2 responses even in the presence of IL-12. However, macrophages promote type 1 responses. DCs, the most important of the antigen-presenting cell populations, can promote either type of response depending on how they differentiate. These effects are also subject to feedback control. Thus, the Th2 cytokine IL-10 suppresses IL-12 production by DCs while simultaneously promoting IL-10 production and DC2 polarization. Conversely, IFN-γ stimulates DCs to secrete IL-12 so becoming DC1 cells and promoting Th1 cell activation.

Microbial Effects

The decision as to which helper T cell phenotype to employ is made early in the immune response. This is determined by signals generated via pattern recognition receptors on the DCs. For example, bacterial lipopolysaccharides from gram-negative organisms and lipoteichoic acids from gram-positives stimulate IL-12 production. CpG DNA and heat shock proteins also stimulate an IL-12 response.

Follicular Helper T Cell Effects

Helper T cells located in follicles within lymph nodes act on B cells to regulate the affinity and class of antibodies they produce. They are called Tfh cells. Mice and humans actively producing

---

BOX 2.2 ■ Role of Sodium Chloride

Salts such as sodium chloride and ions such as potassium are known to modulate T cell responses. For example, sodium chloride boosts Th17 responses whereas potassium inhibits T cell cytotoxicity. Dietary sodium chloride also promotes Th2 responses. First, it acts on memory T cells to enhance IL-4 and IL-13 production and suppress IFNγ synthesis. It also diverts differentiated T cells into the Th2 phenotype and has a similar effect on naïve T cells. Sodium chloride acts by activating NFAT5 transcription factor that regulates cytokine synthesis in high salt concentrations. Skin lesions in cases of atopic dermatitis contain elevated sodium levels compared to non-lesional atopic and normal healthy skin. Therefore, the increase in allergies associated with a Western lifestyle may also be due in part to high salt levels in processed foods. In addition to its direct effects, a high salt diet influences the composition of the microbiota in mice. These microbial changes may have profound effects on the nature of T cell-mediated immune responses.

Matthias J, Maul J, Noster R, Meinl H, et al. Sodium chloride is an ionic checkpoint for human Th2 cells and shapes the atopic skin microenvironment. *Sci Transl Med.* 2019;11(480):eaau00683. doi:10.1126/scitransmed.aau0683.

IgE rely on a subset of Tfh cells that produce IL-13 in large amounts. They are required for the production of high-affinity IgE and are essential for generating acute anaphylaxis. However, the signals that instruct B cells to make this high-affinity IgE remain unresolved. There is a unique *Il4* enhancer locus bound by the transcription factor BATF in Tfh cells that is distinct from the GATA3 required to regulate IL-4, IL-5, and IL-13 production by Th2 and ILC2 cells. Therefore, IL-4 from Tfh cells is required to induce IgE formation; however, a second Tfh13 population is required for high-affinity IgE to be produced. Two signals: one to turn on the switch and the other to turn up the dial (Box 2.2).

B Cell Responses

IgE is the antibody that mediates immediate allergic responses. The production of IgE by B cells is controlled by IL-4 and IL-13 from Th2 and ILC2 cells.

Initially, all B cells respond to antigens by expressing IgM or IgG on their surface. To produce IgE, they must undergo a class switch. During this process, their immunoglobulin variable region genes (the genes encoding the sites that bind antigens) are disconnected from the μ or γ heavy chain genes and linked directly to the gene encoding the epsilon heavy chains (Cε). B cells that undergo this class switching are located in the lymph nodes and other primary lymphoid organs, and in the submucosa of the intestinal and respiratory tracts and the gut- or airway-associated lymphoid tissues.

Immunoglobulin E

IgE is a typical Y-shaped, four-chain immunoglobulin with four constant domains in each of its ε heavy chains and a molecular weight of 190 kDa (Fig. 2.6). IgE is readily destroyed by mild heat treatment, it does not activate complement, and its ability to cross the placenta in primates is limited. It is, however, found in colostrum.

IgE does not act by simply binding and coating antigens, as do the other immunoglobulins. Instead, IgE acts as a signal-transducing molecule. When two mast cell-bound IgE molecules are cross-linked by an allergen, they trigger receptor activation leading to the release of inflammatory molecules. The resulting acute inflammation enhances local defenses and helps eliminate invaders.

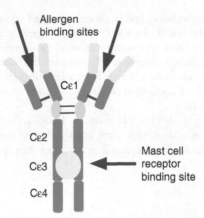

Fig. 2.6 Structure of immunoglobulin E (IgE). It binds to its receptors on mast cells via sites on the C3 domain of the ε heavy chains.

IgE is found in small quantities in serum, especially in humans but its levels vary greatly within each species (Table 2.1). In healthy humans, its concentration is age dependent; however, it only accounts for 0.0005% of the total serum immunoglobulins. In domestic animals, serum IgE levels are greatly influenced by the presence of parasites. IgE has a very short half-life of 2–3 days in humans and approximately 12 h in mice. Therefore, it has to be produced continuously to maintain its serum levels. Most of the IgE in the body is firmly bound to high-affinity FcεRI receptors on the surface of tissue mast cells. When bound to these receptors, the IgE has a half-life of 11 to 12 days. Connective tissue mast cells can extend their cytoplasmic processes between capillary endothelial cells and into the vascular lumen to "fish" for IgE that locks onto their receptors. Thus, the IgE serum concentration does not reflect its total amount in the body.

TABLE 2.1 ■ **Serum IgE Levels**

SPECIES	"NORMAL" IgE (Range)	Range in Allergic or Parasitized Animals
Human[a]	5–513 ng/mL	<240 ng/mL
Dog[b]	182±112 µg/mL (24–410)	195±108 µg/mL (85–550)
Cat[c]	46±19 µg/mL	328±124 µg/mL
Horse[d]	84±90.9 µg/mL	109±69 µg/mL
Sheep[e]	1.8±1.3 µg/mL	15–30 µg/mL
Pig[f]	2 µg/mL	~5 µg/mL

[a]Martins TB, Bandhauer ME, Bunker AM, et al. New childhood and adult reference intervals for total IgE. *J Allergy Clin Immunol.* 2013;33(2):589-591.
[b]Nimmo Wilkie JS, Yager JA, Eyre P, Parker WM. Morphometric analysis of the skin of dogs with atopic dermatitis and correlations with cutaneous and plasma histamine and total serum IgE. *Vet Pathol.* 1990; 27(3):179-186.
[c]Delgado C, Lee-Fowler TM, DeClue AE, Reinero CR. Feline-specific serum total IgE quantitation in normal, asthmatic and parasitized cats. *J Feline Med Surg.* 2010;12:991-994.
[d]Wagner B. IgE in horses: occurrence in health and disease. *Vet Immunol Immunopathol.* 2009;132:21-30.
[e]Shaw RJ, McNeill MM, Gatehouse TK, Douch PG. Quantitation of total sheep IgE concentration using anti-ovine IgE monoclonal antibodies in an enzyme immunoassay. *Vet Immunol Immunopathol.* 1997;57: 253-265.
[f]Wu JJ, Cao CM, Meng TT, Zhang Y et al. Induction of immune responses and allergic reactions in piglets by injecting glycinin. *Ital J Anim Sci.* 2016;15(1):166-173.

It is currently believed that blood IgE levels are controlled by two different processes. One is continuous low-level production in the absence of an antigenic stimulus, perhaps by long-lived plasma cells. The second is a transient increase induced by allergen exposure that is reflected in the sensitization of mast cells and basophils. IgE generated by the continuous production process has a low affinity for any individual allergen. In contrast, the IgE induced during an active response has a high affinity for the inducing allergen and, as will be described later, plays a key role in allergic diseases (Box 2.3).

Some IgG subclasses may also bind to mast cell FcεRI and mediate allergic reactions. For example, IgG4 has been associated with some cases of canine atopic dermatitis. However, the affinity of this IgG subclass for Fc receptors is much lower than that of IgE and is of much less clinical significance.

IgE AFFINITY

The strength of binding between an antibody and its cognate antigen profoundly affects its subsequent biological activity. Thus, when an antigen binds weakly (low affinity) to IgE, the resulting conformational changes in the antibody heavy chain are minimal and may be insufficient to send a strong signal to the mast cell receptors. Therefore, it may be unable to trigger a strong mast cell response. Conversely, when an antigen binds to IgE with high affinity, the IgE undergoes major conformational changes, resulting in enhanced receptor binding and leading to rapid and extensive mast cell degranulation. Thus, simply measuring IgE levels in the bloodstream does not provide information regarding the intensity or severity of any subsequent allergic response. Total IgE levels rarely correlate well with the severity of clinical disease (see Table 2.1).

IgE SIALYLATION

The biological activity of IgE depends on its sialylation level (i.e., the presence of sialic acid (also known as neuraminic acid) residues on the termini of its glycan side-chains). Thus, IgE from humans with a peanut allergy is much more heavily sialylated than IgE from non-allergic individuals. The treatment of this allergic IgE with a neuraminidase to remove its terminal sialic acid residues significantly reduces its ability to cause mast cell degranulation and anaphylaxis. The lack

---

BOX 2.3 ■ Two Subclasses of Canine IgE

Biochemical and genetic studies on canine IgE have identified two biochemically, physically, and biologically distinct IgE subclasses, IgE1 and IgE2. These are distinguished by their reactivity with monoclonal IgE antiglobulins and binding to protein A (staphylococcal immunoglobulin-binding protein). While sharing the major characteristics of IgE, including heat lability, molecular weight, mast cell binding, and reactivity with polyclonal anti-IgE, they differ in their reactivity with monoclonal antibodies and their isoelectric points. These differences are not caused by altered glycosylation. They appear to have different biological properties in that IgE2 levels are highly variable compared to IgE1 in ragweed-sensitized dogs.

Examination of the canine genome focusing on the IgE heavy chain gene locus confirms the existence of two functional IgE heavy chain genes, IGEH1 and IGEH2. The biological significance of this gene duplication remains unclear. The existence of two IgE subclasses might account for the relatively high levels of IgE in dogs compared to humans (see Table 2.1).

Peng Z, Arthur G, Rector, ES, Kierek-Jaszczul D et al. Heterogeneity of polyclonal IgE characterized by differential charge, affinity to protein A, and antigenicity. *J Allergy Clin Immunol*. 1997;100:87-95

of sialic acid does not affect IgE binding to either the antigen or the mast cell receptor, FcεRI. Instead, removing the terminal sialic acid exposes a glycan that inhibits receptor signaling to the mast cell.

This is another reason why total IgE levels in the bloodstream do not correlate well with the severity of clinical allergies and explains why some individuals might have high levels of allergen-specific IgE in their bloodstream yet show no clinical disease. These are likely low-affinity, asialylated IgE molecules.

CLASS SWITCHING

As described above, immunoglobulin gene sequences change during an immune response in an orderly series of class switches. Thus, the very first immunoglobulins produced by B cells belong to the IgM class. Class switching to IgE can occur in two ways: in a single step directly from IgM to IgE or in two sequential steps via an intermediate IgG1 stage (Fig. 2.7). Immunoglobulins progressively increase their affinity for an antigen during B cell development because of progressive somatic mutation. The B cells begin by producing low-affinity antibodies; however, repeated mutation and selection cycles eventually produce much higher-affinity antibodies. When B cells express IgE that has directly switched from IgM, they have had a minimal opportunity to undergo this mutation and selection cycle and only produce low-affinity IgE. However, B cells that undergo two-stage switching benefit from the fact that the prolonged process provides time for

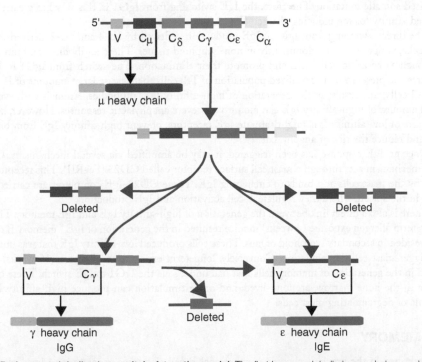

Fig. 2.7 Immunoglobulin class switch. A two tier model. The first immunoglobulin heavy chains produced by B cells are IgM antibodies. As the B cell develops under the influence of appropriate cytokines, it may either switch directly to producing IgE or alternatively switch first to IgG production and then to IgE. The second process ensures that somatic mutation has time to occur and that high-affinity IgE is generated.

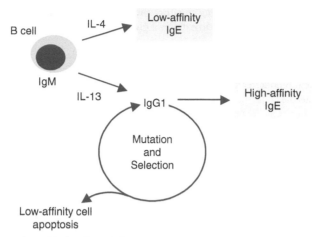

Fig. 2.8 The generation of high-affinity IgE. High-affinity IgE is only generated via the IgM-IgG1-IgE pathway where, under the influence of IL-13, somatic mutation and selection occur. B cells that switch directly from IgM to IgE production under the influence of IL-4 have had insufficient opportunities to undergo mutation and selection, and hence produce low-affinity IgE.

repeated somatic mutation. Therefore, the IgE switching from IgG1 in this way has greatly increased affinity for the inducing allergen (Fig. 2.8).

The direct switching from IgM to IgE production is driven by IL-4 and IL-21derived from Tfh cells, which occurs predominantly in non-lymphoid tissues. These antibodies can bind targets such as parasitic helminths and promote their elimination. The switch from IgG1 to IgE requires the presence of a specialized population of Tfh cells that release large amounts of IL-13 (Tfh13 cells) and results in the generation of high-affinity IgE antibodies. Animals with even a small amount of high-affinity IgE can mount very severe anaphylactic responses. However, large amounts of low-affinity IgE might saturate IgE receptors, prevent high-affinity IgE from binding, and reduce the risk of anaphylaxis.

Once an IgE response has been triggered, it may be amplified via several mechanisms. One such mechanism acts through a mast cell surface receptor called CD23 (FcεRII). This receptor is shed by the mast cells and binds to circulating IgE. These CD23-IgE complexes are carried to DCs in the spleen, where they regulate T cell activation and IgE production.

There is also a direct link between the generation of high-affinity IgE and IgE memory. Thus, short-term allergen exposure (4 weeks) in mice resulted in the generation of IgE$^+$ memory B cells that resided in secondary lymphoid organs. These cells produced low-affinity IgE that was unable to trigger mast cell degranulation. Conversely, long-term exposure to allergens (15 weeks) resulted in the generation of memory cells that had undergone the IgG1 to IgE switch. These cells reside in the bone marrow, are long-lived, and on restimulation can produce high-affinity IgE capable of degranulating mast cells.

IgE MEMORY

As described in the previous chapter, conventional B cell responses generate long-lived plasma and memory B cells. These are especially effective when boosting IgG and IgA mediated responses. Studies on IgE responses, however, suggest that IgE memory B cells are rarely produced. Thus, IgE memory appears to depend on the survival of long-lived plasma cells alone. However, even these cells only persist for a few months in the absence of antigen exposure (in mice). Their half-life is ~60 days, which is short compared to IgG1-producing cells, whose half-life is ~200 days. Even cell-bound IgE persists for only another 2 months. Nevertheless, allergies can persist for a lifetime. On re-exposure to allergens, IgG1-producing memory B cells rapidly switch to become IgE-producing plasma cells.

Suggested Reading

Annunziato F, Romagnani C, Romagnani R. The three major types of innate and adaptive cell-mediated effector immunity. *J Allergy Clin Immunol*. 2015;135(3):626-635.

Asrat S, Kaur N, Liu X, et al. Chronic allergen exposure drives accumulation of long-lived IgE plasma cells in the bone marrow, giving rise to serological memory. *Sci Immunol*. 2020;5(43):eaav8402. doi:10.1126/sciimmunol.aav8402

Eckl-Dorna J, Niederberger V. What is the source of serum allergen-specific IgE? *Curr Allergy Asthma Rep*. 2013;13(3):281-287.

El-Naccache HG, Gause WC, WC Gause. Early events triggering the initiation of a type 2 immune response. *Trends Immunol*. 2021;42(2):151-164.

Gowthaman U, Chen JS, Eisenbarth SC. Regulation of IgE by T follicular helper cells. *J Leukoc Biol*. 2020;107(3):409-418.

Gowthaman U, Chen JS, Zhang B, et al. Identification of a T follicular helper cell subset that drives anaphylactic IgE. *Science*. 2019;365(6456):eaaw6433. doi:10.1126/science.aaw6433

Guia S, Narni-Mancinelli E. Helper-like innate lymphoid cells in humans and mice. *Trends Immunol*. 2020;41(5):436-452.

He JS, Subramaniam S, Narang V, et al. IgG1 memory B cells keep the memory of IgE response. *Nat Commun*. 2017;8(1):641. doi:10.1038/s41467-017-00723-0

Maeda K, Caldez MJ, Akira S. Innate immunity in allergy. *Allergy*. 2019;74(9):1660-1674.

Perner C, Flayer CH, Zhu X, et al. Substance P release by sensory neurons triggers dendritic cell migration and initiates the type-2 immune responses to allergens. *Immunity*. 2020;53(5):1063-1077.

Shade KT, Conroy ME, Washburn N, et al. Sialylation of immunoglobulin E is a determinant of allergic pathogenicity. *Nature*. 2020;582(7811):265-270. doi:10.1038/s41586-020-2311-z

Spellberg B, Edwards JE. Type 2 immunity in infectious diseases. *Clin Infect Dis*. 2001;32(1):76-102.

Tizard IR. *Veterinary Immunology: An Introduction*. 10th ed. Elsevier; 2018.

Wagner B. IgE in horses: occurrence in health and disease. *Vet Immunol Immunopathol*. 2009;132(1):21-30.

Wambre E, Bajzik V, DeLong JH, et al. A phenotypically and functionally distinct human T_H2 cell subpopulation is associated with allergic disorders. *Sci Transl Med*. 2017;9(401):eaam9171.

Xiong H, Dolpady J, Wabl M, Curotto de Lafaille MA, Lafaille JJ. Sequential class switching is required for the generation of high affinity IgE antibodies. *J Exp Med*. 2019;209(2):353-364.

CHAPTER 3

Mast Cells

Mast cells are large, granule-filled cells found in almost all vascularized tissues. They predate all other mammalian immune system cells because they have been found in chordates that first appeared approximately 500 million years ago. Their persistence in non-mammalian vertebrates through millions of years of evolution suggests that they must be valuable cells. They are numerous cells, and it has been claimed that if they were all gathered together, they would make an organ the size of the spleen. Mast cells act as sentinel cells and release inflammatory mediators on encountering invaders. They can recognize and bind bacterial, viral, and fungal pathogen-associated molecular patterns (PAMPs) through their pattern recognition receptors (PRRs) and, in response, release proinflammatory mediators. This release normally occurs in a controlled manner and ensures that the severity and type of inflammation they trigger are appropriate to the immediate needs of the body—but not always.

Given their long evolutionary history, it is not surprising that mast cells have multiple functions that integrate and interact with many different immune processes. Mast cells play vital roles in the pathogenesis of allergic diseases. In addition, they protect animals against bacterial and parasitic infections, degrade insect and snake venoms, and contribute to anti-tumor immunity. They have been implicated in the response by the body to strokes, atherosclerosis, heart attacks, arthritis, and cystitis.

Life History

As animals develop, hematopoiesis occurs in two waves. The first wave, called "primitive" hematopoiesis, occurs around 7 days in developing mouse embryos, when the first stem cells develop in the yolk sac. During the second wave, the blood cells are produced by a process called "definitive" hematopoiesis. These later stem cells eventually travel to the bone marrow, where they function throughout adult life. The precise developmental pathways of mast cells are confusing. This is especially the case since the pathways differ between humans and mice, and cells may develop by multiple routes. Some tissue mast cells arise from early precursors derived from the yolk sac while others originate later in the bone marrow. In rodents, they probably originate from stem cells of the granulocyte/monocyte lineage and subsequently branch off from eosinophil and basophil precursors. They leave the hematopoietic organs at a very early stage of development, long before their granules develop, and then complete their maturation within the peripheral tissues.

Mast cells express a cell surface receptor called "KIT "(also called CD117) that binds a cytokine called stem cell factor (SCF). SCF (also called the KIT-ligand) is a protein of 18.5 kDa produced by fibroblasts and endothelial cells. SCF regulates the development, proliferation, survival, and activation of mast cells. It regulates mediator and cytokine release by immunoglobulin E (IgE). KIT is a transmembrane tyrosine kinase encoded by a gene called *c-kit*. The development and survival of mast cells depend on SCF signaling via KIT. Dog mast cells express KIT, and canine SCF has been sequenced. It is similar in size and structure to the human and rodent molecules. However, there are many other molecules in the mast cell microenvironment that affect their development and survival, including cytokines such as interleukin 3 (IL-3), IL-4, IL-9, IL-31, and IL-33, the chemokine CXCL 12, tumor necrosis factor (TNF)-β, and nerve growth factor.

Analysis of the genes transcribed by these cells has demonstrated that mast cells, while originating from the same stem cell population, follow a very different developmental pathway than other bone marrow-derived cells. For example, they share few gene expression patterns with basophils. Basophils are more closely related to eosinophils and other granulocytes. While long-lived in tissues, mast cell populations are replenished from circulating precursors in the blood.

The most prominent features of mast cells are their cytoplasmic granules, which form by budding off from the Golgi apparatus. Initially, these are small and uniformly sized. The granules grow and fuse with others and gradually fill with preformed inflammatory mediators. These mediators are mainly synthesized by the mast cell itself; however, cytokines such as IL-17 can also be taken up from the environment.

Structure

Mast cells are large, round cells, 15−20 μm in diameter, scattered throughout the body in connective tissue, under mucosal surfaces, and around and along blood vessels and nerves. They are easily recognizable because their cytoplasm is densely packed with large granules that stain strongly with cationic dyes such as toluidine blue (Fig. 3.1). The reaction of the blue dye with the granules causes them to stain purple. This change in color is called metachromasia. The effect is due to the way in which the proteoglycans in the granules cause polymerization of the dye molecules. The densely packed cytoplasmic granules often mask the large, bean-shaped nucleus (Figs 3.2 and 3.3). (Mast cells are so called because, when first discovered by the German scientist Paul Ehrlich in 1878, he considered them to be "well-fed" cells [German *Mastung*].)

Location

Mast cells are found in all vascular tissues, especially those exposed to the external environment such as the skin, conjunctiva, airways, lungs, and the mucosa of the intestinal tract. They are also found near blood vessels, smooth muscle cells, nerves, and mucus-producing glands. Because of their location, mast cells can regulate the local blood flow and influence cellular migration. In

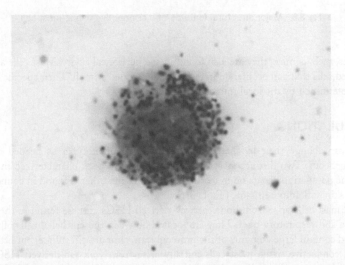

Fig. 3.1 Partially degranulated mast cell from a canine mast cell tumor. Note the variation in staining intensity of its granules both within and outside the cell. This probably reflects the different stages of mediator release. Original magnification × 100 (Courtesy Dr. Karen Russell)

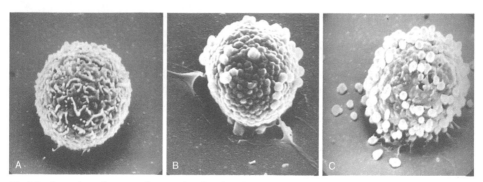

Fig. 3.2 **Scanning electron micrographs showing the mast cell degranulation process.** (A) Normal rat mast cell, (B) sensitized mast cell fixed 5 s after exposure to the antigen, and (C) sensitized mast cell fixed 60 s after exposure to the antigen. Original magnification × 3000. (From Tizard IR, Holmes WL: Degranulation of sensitized rat peritoneal mast cells in response to antigen, compound 48/80 and polymyxin B. A scanning electron microscope study, *Int Arch Allergy Appl Immunol.* 46:867-879, 1974.)

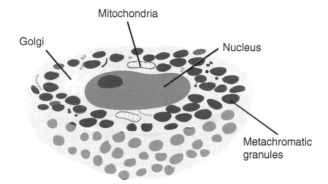

Fig. 3.3 Major structural features of a connective tissue mast cell.

some species, such as mice, they are also found in the peritoneal cavity. Mast cells are terminally differentiated cells that can proliferate in response to external stimuli. Their specific phenotype is primarily determined by the local microenvironment.

SUBPOPULATIONS

Mast cells can change their biochemical and functional phenotypes as needed and are thus very heterogeneous. Two distinct mast cell populations have been characterized in rodents and humans. One population occurs on mucosal surfaces, and the other is found in connective tissues such as the skin and adipose tissue. (Table 3.1).

Mucosal mast cells arise from bone marrow-derived HSCs and are found in the gastrointestinal mucosa and respiratory tract. They are located between the epithelial cells of the intestine and lung and contain large amounts of the proteoglycan, chondroitin sulfate, but little histamine. In contrast, connective tissue mast cells initially arise from yolk sac-derived HSCs. They are found in the skin, around blood vessels, and in the peritoneal cavity and are rich in histamine and heparin. Each mast cell may contain 3−8 pg of histamine per cell, accounting for up to 70% of the weight of the cell. Although connective tissue mast cell numbers remain relatively constant,

TABLE 3.1 ■ Comparison of the Two Major Types of Mouse Mast Cells

	Mucosal Mast Cells	Connective Tissue Mast Cells
Structure	Few, variable-sized granules	Many uniform granules
Cell size	9–10 μm diameter	19–20 μm diameter
Proteoglycan	Chondroitin sulfate	Heparin
Histamine	1–2 pg/cell	3–8 pg/cell
Life Span	<40 days	>6 months
Location	Intestinal wall, lung	Peritoneal cavity, skin

mucosal mast cells proliferate in response to the presence of intestinal worms. Mucosal mast cells play an important role in the expulsion of these worms from mice.

Connective tissue mast cells are constitutive and T cell-independent, whereas mucosal mast cells must be induced and are T cell-dependent. Induced mucosal mast cells disappear within a few weeks after intestinal worms are eliminated. These phenotypes are plastic so that, for example, connective tissue mast cells can differentiate into mucosal mast cells if transplanted into mucosal tissue. The presence of the microbiota influences the development of mast cells. For example, skin bacteria can induce a keratinocyte-derived SCF that acts as a mast cell growth factor.

Receptors

Many different receptors are expressed on mast cells, including, most importantly, the high-affinity IgE receptor, FcεR1. They also express a low-affinity IgE receptor called FcεRII, and a unique G-protein coupled receptor (GPR) called the mas-related GPR family member X2 (MRGPRX2). They also have receptors for many different cytokines, chemokines, and eicosanoids. When stimulated, these receptors trigger increases in cytosolic Ca^{++} and result in mast cell activation.

IgE RECEPTORS

There are two types of IgE receptors: high-affinity FcεRI and low-affinity FcεRII. FcεRI occurs in two forms. The predominant tetrameric form is expressed at high levels on mast cells, basophils, and neutrophils, whereas small amounts are found on dendritic cells (DCs), eosinophils, neurons, bronchial epithelial cells, and airway smooth muscle cells. This form consists of four peptide chains: one α, one β, and two disulfide-linked γ chains (αβγγ) (Fig. 3.4). The α chain is the IgE-binding subunit, which binds to the third constant domain (Cε3) on the heavy chain of IgE. The two molecules are then "locked" together by a conformational change in the Cε2 domain. The affinity of the FcεRI α chain for IgE constant domains is very high $(1 \times 10^{-10} \, M^{-1})$, so they bind almost irreversibly and thus ensure that mast cells are constantly coated with IgE. The transmembrane-spanning β chain stabilizes the complex while amplifying the α chain signals, and the paired intracellular γ chains serve as signal transducers. Each γ chain contains an immunoreceptor tyrosine-based activation motif. (This same γ chain serves as a signal transducer in other receptors such as FcγRI, FcγRIII, and γ/δ TCR)   •

The second form of FcεRI is a trimer with one α and two γ chains (αγγ). This form is expressed on antigen-presenting dendritic cells, eosinophils, neutrophils, and monocytes. When an antigen–IgE complex binds to this receptor, it is ingested, processed, and treated as an exogenous antigen. FcεRI expression on antigen-presenting cells is enhanced by IL-4 from Th2 cells. Thus, a positive feedback loop (the allergy loop) develops. The antigen-processing cells present antigen more effectively to Th2 cells. The Th2 cells then secrete IL-4 and enhance IgE production. In the absence of antigen cross-linking, IgE alone can upregulate mast cell surface expression of

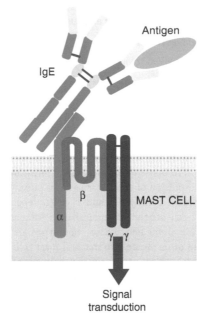

Fig. 3.4 Function of the major IgE receptor, FcεRI. The tetrameric form of the IgE receptor containing two γ chains predominates on mast cells and basophils. When cross-linked by an IgE-bound allergen molecule, the receptors aggregate and signal to the mast cell.

FcεRI and mast cell survival, making the cells resistant to apoptosis. Thus, IgE stabilizes and increases mast cell FcεRI expression, which upregulates the IgE-binding activity of the cell and mediator release via the allergy loop.

IgE uptake by mast cells is a dynamic process. Thus, perivascular mast cells acquire IgE by extending cytoplasmic processes through blood vessel walls into the bloodstream, where their high-affinity receptors capture circulating IgE.

An important feature of FcεRI receptors is their range of expression. Once expressed on the cell surface, their half-life is approximately 24 h. Some are recycled, while most are internalized and degraded. In the absence of IgE, there are approximately 8000 receptors per cell (on circulating basophils). IgE binding to these receptors stabilizes them, slows their degradation, and reduces their turnover. Therefore, their numbers can climb to an average of 250,000/cell in allergic subjects. However, receptor numbers cannot keep pace with IgE production and they are readily swamped by high levels of non–antigen-specific IgE.

FcεRII (also called CD23) is a low-affinity IgE receptor. Unlike other antibody receptors, it is a carbohydrate-binding C-type lectin that generally forms trimers. It is not restricted to mast cells but is also found on B cells, NK cells, macrophages, DCs, eosinophils, and platelets. In addition to binding IgE, soluble CD23 plays a role in regulating IgE levels. It can bind to circulating IgE-allergen complexes and transport them to the spleen where they are delivered to antigen-presenting cells and so enhance antibody responses.

CD23 may also be cleaved from mast cell surfaces by the house dust mite allergen Der p 1, increasing soluble CD23 levels and promoting the IgE response further. CD23 binds to the complement receptor CR2 (CD21). Thus, B cells expressing FcεRII can bind to CR2 on other B cells, T cells, and DCs. By linking B cells to DCs, FcεRII enhances B cell survival and promotes IgE production.

Secretory Granules

Mast cells are packed with large electron-dense granules. When activated, mast cells degranulate, rapidly releasing the granules and their contents into the extracellular fluid. These granules contain a complex mixture of potent proinflammatory molecules. Different stimuli may determine which granule subsets are exocytosed and which mediators are released. Different clinical forms of allergy may be influenced by the granule subset expelled and the mixture of vasoactive molecules released. The appropriate treatment of allergies may also differ based on the mixture of inflammatory mediators involved. The speed and extent of these responses differ among mast cells. For example, degranulation can occur within seconds after antigen binds to high-affinity IgE and cross-links its FcεRI receptors; however, it is much slower if the IgE has a low affinity for the antigen. In these cases, cross-linking and degranulation may be minimal.

GRANULE MEDIATORS

Mast cell granules are loaded with preformed mediators (Fig. 3.5). These include vasoactive amines such as histamine, serotonin, and dopamine. They also contain a mixture of lysosomal proteases including two serine proteases, a tryptase and a chymase, and one metalloprotease, carboxypeptidase A. Other granule enzymes include cathepsins, as well as granzyme B, beta-hexosaminidase, and beta-glucuronidase.

Proteoglycans (heavily glycosylated proteins) are major granule components. They have a serine-glycine-rich backbone (serglycin) with glycosamino side-chains and a very high anionic charge (Fig. 3.6). One such proteoglycan, heparin, plays an important role in packaging histamine

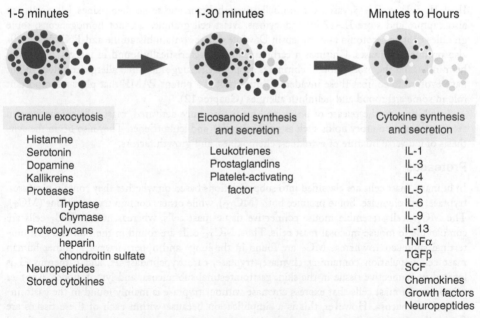

1-5 minutes	1-30 minutes	Minutes to Hours
Granule exocytosis	**Eicosanoid synthesis and secretion**	**Cytokine synthesis and secretion**
Histamine		
Serotonin	Leukotrienes	IL-1
Dopamine	Prostaglandins	IL-3
Kallikreins	Platelet-activating	IL-4
Proteases	factor	IL-5
Tryptase		IL-6
Chymase		IL-9
Proteoglycans		IL-13
heparin		TNFα
chondroitin sulfate		TGFβ
Neuropeptides		SCF
Stored cytokines		Chemokines
		Growth factors
		Neuropeptides

Fig. 3.5 Mast cell granule contents. Soluble mediators released from degranulating mast cells fall into three categories: vasoactive molecules released from exocytosed granules within minutes, lipids (eicosanoids) synthesized within minutes, and proteins such as cytokines synthesized over several minutes to hours.

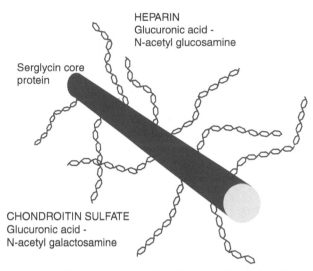

HEPARIN
Glucuronic acid -
N-acetyl glucosamine

Serglycin core
protein

CHONDROITIN SULFATE
Glucuronic acid -
N-acetyl galactosamine

Fig. 3.6 **Structure of mast cell proteoglycans.** They have a serine-glycine rich backbone (serglycin) with extensive glycosylation. The two major proteoglycans in mast cell granules are heparin and chondroitin sulfate, which differ in the structure of their carbohydrate side-chains. Heparin is a potent anticoagulant.

and proteases. Proteoglycans bind strongly to cationic molecules such as toluidine blue and the Romanowsky combination dyes and are responsible for the metachromatic staining of mast cell granules.

Mast cell granules store large quantities of growth factors and cytokines such as TNF-α, IL-4, IL-5, IL-6, IL-15, vascular endothelial growth factor, and some chemokines. Mast cells can also capture and store IL-17 by endocytosis. Mast cell granules are not homogeneous; some granules contain serotonin and cathepsin D, while others contain histamine and TNF. Mast cells also produce chitinases. Chitin is a carbohydrate characteristically found in insects, fungi, and helminths, and the production of chitinases supports the suggestion that allergic reactions might have evolved to combat these invaders. Chitin itself is a potent PAMP that plays an important role in some arthropod and helminth allergies (Chapter 12).

In addition to the release of preformed mediators, once activated, mast cells synthesize and secrete proinflammatory lipids such as prostaglandins and leukotrienes. They also begin the synthesis of a diverse mixture of cytokines, chemokines, and growth factors.

Proteases

In humans, mast cells are classified into subpopulations based on whether they contain proteases, tryptase, and chymase. Some produce both (MC_{TC}), while others contain tryptase alone (MC_T). The MC_{TC} cells resemble mouse connective tissue mast cells, whereas human MC_T cells are comparable to mouse mucosal mast cells. Thus, MC_{TC} cells are found in the skin and gastrointestinal submucosa, whereas MC_T are found in the lungs and upper airways. Another human mast cell population containing chymase, tryptase, carboxypeptidase A, and cathepsin G is located in connective tissue in the skin, gastrointestinal submucosa, and lymph nodes. Another population of mast cells that express chymase without tryptase is mainly found in the gastrointestinal submucosa. However, this is a simplification because within each of these tissues are found diverse mast cell phenotypes and subpopulations. Interestingly, tryptase is not only found in the granules but also within the nucleus of mast cells, where it induces epigenetic effects by degrading histones.

Degranulation

Mast cells degranulate and release their preformed mediators within minutes of exposure to an antigen. Although there are numerous ways by which mast cells can be induced to degranulate, the most important is mediated by antigens when they cross-link IgE molecules bound to high-affinity FcεRI receptors. Mast cells coated with receptor-bound IgE are primed to bind antigens. If a multivalent antigen binds with high affinity to several IgE molecules and cross-links at least twoFcεRI, the receptors will aggregate and this aggregation triggers degranulation.

The β and γ chains of FcεRI have an immunoreceptor tyrosine-based activation motif (ITAM) that is required for signal transduction. Immediately after IgE-antigen-IgE cross-links two FcεRI by binding to their α chains, aggregation occurs, two tyrosine kinases, Lyn and Syc are activated, and their ITAMs are phosphorylated (Fig. 3.7). This, in turn, activates phospholipase C, leading to the production of diacylglycerol and inositol triphosphate. These two mediators then trigger several downstream events, including an increase in cytosolic Ca++ and cytoskeletal rearrangements such as microtubule polymerization and actin depolymerization. The increase in Ca++ triggers protein kinase activation. The protein kinases phosphorylate myosin in the cytoskeleton, so the granules migrate to the cell surface. The granule membranes then fuse with the plasma membrane, and their contents are released into the extracellular fluid. During degranulation, the granule contents can also move along microtubules from the interior of the cell toward the plasma membrane. Thus, the granules create "degranulation channels," and their contents are released in all directions.

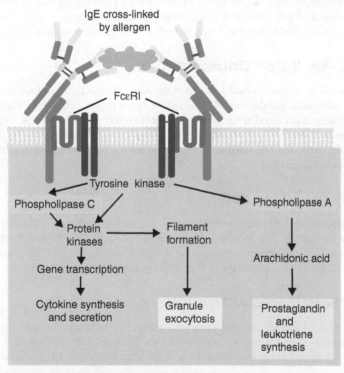

Fig. 3.7 Simplified view of mast cell signal transduction. The process is triggered by cross-linking two receptor-bound IgE molecules by an allergen. The resulting receptor aggregation leads to degranulation (granule exocytosis), leukotriene and prostaglandin synthesis, and cytokine production.

Cross-linking and aggregation of mast cell IgE−FcεRI complexes by an antigen also activates phospholipase A. This acts on membrane phospholipids to generate arachidonic acid. Cyclooxygenases and lipoxygenases then convert the arachidonic acid to leukotrienes and prostaglandins.

While IgE-mediated mast cell degranulation has been considered a simple on/off switch, this is an oversimplification. In addition to the "compound exocytosis" described above, mast cells can release their granule contents in a piecemeal fashion. In this case, small vesicles bud off from the cytoplasmic granules. These small vesicles carry their granule contents to the plasma membrane where they are shed as exosomes. These exosomes can also transport granule contents, including microRNA and major histocompatibility complex (MHC) class II molecules to distant cells. The exosomes may also contain precursors of TNF-α and proteases. These exosomes may be taken up by nearby cells. For example, they can interact with sensory nerve fibers, resulting in the release of the itch neuropeptide, substance P. They also generate tunneling nanotubes that extend from the cells like pseudopodia and then break off. These provide a rapid method of sending a signal to nearby cells. Activated mast cells can release small heparin-containing granules that are rich in TNF-α. These particles are carried in afferent lymph to draining lymph nodes, where they may trigger changes in cell behavior. The binding of heparin stabilizes the TNF-α so that it persists after delivery. Mast cells can also generate extracellular traps. Trap production is stimulated by IL-23 and IL-1β and results in the release of IL-17.

The intensity and extent of mast cell degranulation depends on the affinity of the IgE for its antigen. Weak antigen binding results in a mast cell response characterized by enhanced chemokine production but not by the release of vasoactive amines. Strong binding, in contrast, results in receptor aggregation, the formation of synapse-like clusters, and the massive release of granule contents. Therefore, mast cells show great variation in their degree of activation. These range from "resting," to low-level activation with partial degranulation, to complete activation with massive degranulation. Each level is associated with the release of a different mixture of mediators.

Non-IgE-Mediated Degranulation

Antigen binding to receptor-bound IgE is not the only stimulus that can provoke mast cell degranulation. Mast cells can degranulate in response to neuropeptides such as substance P, some toxins, complement peptides, some cytokines, chemokines, chemical agents, physical stimuli, insect and animal venoms, and viruses. Damage-associated molecular patterns, including the defensins, adenosine, and endothelins (small peptides from endothelial cells), also trigger mast cell degranulation (Fig. 3.8).

IgG-MEDIATED ACTIVATION

Mast cells express the IgG receptor FcγRII and may be activated by the binding of IgG- and IgG-antigen complexes. The relative importance of IgE- and IgG-mediated responses varies based on the species involved and the inducing stimuli. However, mouse studies have shown that IgG-mediated activation is necessary to fully develop allergic inflammation in this species.

G-PROTEIN-MEDIATED ACTIVATION

In addition to the high-affinity IgE receptor FcεRI, mast cells express numerous G-protein-coupled receptors (GPR). These are transmembrane receptors that regulate vital cellular functions. Many are related to the *mas* oncogene in mice. They are therefore called Mas-related GPR (MRGPR).

MRGPRX2 is the most important of these receptors. It is found on the plasma membrane and intracellularly in connective tissue mast cells (Fig. 3.9). Cationic peptides, including the

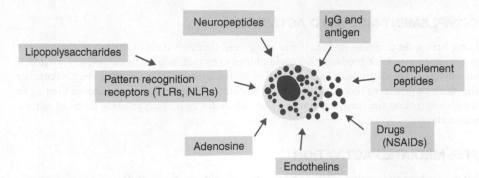

Fig. 3.8 **Non-IgE-mediated mast cell degranulation.** Diverse signals derived from other mediator-receptor interactions can also trigger mast cell degranulation.

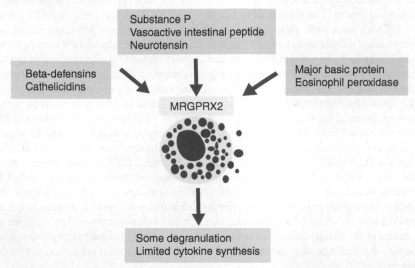

Fig. 3.9 Role of the Mas-related G-protein coupled receptor X2 (MRGPRX2) in an alternative pathway for triggering mast cell degranulation.

neuropeptides, substance P, vasointestinal peptide, and neurotensin, antimicrobial peptides such as β-defensins and cathelicidins, and eosinophil-derived molecules such as major basic protein and eosinophil peroxidase, can act through MRGPRX2 to trigger mast cell degranulation. MRGPRX2 also degranulates mast cells in response to the activating compound 48/80 (48/80 is a synthetic polymer formed by the condensation of N-methyl-p-methoxyphenethylamine by formaldehyde). MRGPRX2 is expressed at high levels on skin mast cells but not on lung or intestinal mast cells. (It is also found on eosinophils and basophils but not neutrophils). On activation, it induces calcium influx and degranulation in these cells. Activation of this receptor with ligands such as substance P causes intense itching. Some anaphylaxis-like drug reactions may be triggered via the MRGPRX2 pathway. Degranulation caused by MRGPRX2 differs from that caused by FcεRI in that it is slower than the IgE-mediated response and results in the release of smaller amounts of mediators, cytokines, and chemokines.

COMPLEMENT-MEDIATED ACTIVATION

Long before the discovery of IgE, it was recognized that activation of the serum complement system generated toxic products that could induce a reaction in animals that closely resembled anaphylaxis. These products were therefore called anaphylatoxins. They were eventually shown to be peptides called C3a and C5a. They induce mast cell degranulation on binding to their receptors on the mast cell surface. They no doubt contribute to some forms of allergic inflammation.

PRR-MEDIATED ACTIVATION

Mast cells have two critical roles. They are sentinel cells awaiting invaders and regulatory cells that control innate immunity. As sentinel cells, they express PRRs and are hard-wired to detect PAMPS from microbial invaders. However, most other cells are amateurs, whereas mast cells are professionals. Mast cells are located close to barrier surfaces where microbial invasion may be expected and are among the first cells to encounter invaders. Mast cells can also sense damage to the surrounding tissues. The mixture of signals generated by ligands binding to PRRs provides the mast cell with some basic details regarding the forthcoming threats. Most, but not all, mast cells express many toll-like receptors (TLRs) in addition to C-type lectin-like receptors, retinoic acid-inducible gene-1-like receptors (RIGs), and nucleotide-binding oligomerization domain-like receptors (NLRs). Mast cells respond to a diverse range of TLR ligands by secreting cytokines, chemokines, and lipid mediators and altering their receptor expression. Some may respond to TLR2-ligation by degranulating; however, this is controversial and likely depends on the species involved. Bacterial binding to mast cell TLRs triggers TNF-α and IL-6 production. Mast cell TLR4 is activated by bacterial lipopolysaccharides; however, this only stimulates the secretion of cytokines and chemokines rather than histamine. LPS-treated mast cells secrete IL-6 and IL-13 but not IL-4 or IL-5. Triggering of TLR3, TLR7, and TLR9 can also induce mast cell activation to some degree. Ligation of TLRs promotes mast cell responses to cross-linked IgE and enhances eicosanoid synthesis. Mast cells in different tissues may express different TLR arrays. Mast cells can use these receptors to distinguish between different pathogens and release an optimized mixture of cytokines, chemokines, and other inflammatory mediators, depending on the nature of the threat. The inflammatory mediators released by mast cells activate nearby immune cells and facilitate local neutrophil and eosinophil recruitment, activation, and bactericidal activity.

Other mast cell microbial sensors, including C-type lectin-like receptors such as the mannose receptor and dectins play a key role in antifungal defense. NLRs are intracellular receptors that are important in antiviral responses and RIGs serve as cytoplasmic receptors for viral RNA.

On degranulation, some mast cell granules like other nanoparticles, may travel through lymphatic vessels to the draining lymph nodes where they recruit passing T cells. Some granules may remain trapped in the local microenvironment and are phagocytosed by macrophages and dendritic cells. Mast cell-derived leukotrienes and prostaglandins further activate local inflammatory responses. The vascular changes triggered by mast cell mediators trigger both neutrophil and T cell migration toward invasion sites. These early responses increase local blood flow via the release of vasoactive amines. Mast cell-derived TNF-α recruits neutrophils to these inflammatory sites. Eosinophils will also be recruited if the threat involves parasites or arthropod bites. NK and NKT cells are attracted to these sites and enhance viral destruction. Mast cells can also mount a strong type 1 interferon response to viruses.

Mast cells contribute to host defenses by promoting wound healing, and they can kill bacteria in infected wounds. This antibacterial effect is mediated via IL-6, which acts on keratinocytes to stimulate the release of antibacterial defensins.

DC-MEDIATED ACTIVATION

Mast cells play an important role in promoting T cell functions in cases of allergic contact hypersensitivity (Chapter 19). Thus, contact allergens may be taken up by mast cells and presented to T cells. Migratory DCs interact with mast cells in inflamed skin. The DCs wrap their dendrites around the mast cells and during these intimate moments, the DCs transfer MHC class II molecules to the mast cell. Therefore, the mast cells can acquire the ability to present antigens to T cells.

REGULATION

Mast cells express two catecholamine receptors called the α- and β-adrenoceptors. These receptors have opposing effects. Molecules that stimulate the α-adrenoceptors (such as norepinephrine and phenylephrine) or block the β-adrenoceptors (such as propranolol) enhance mast cell degranulation. Conversely, molecules that stimulate the β-receptors or block the α-receptors inhibit mast cell degranulation. β-stimulators include isoproterenol, epinephrine, and salbutamol and are widely used in the treatment of allergies. β-receptor blockers enhance mast cell degranulation and promote allergies. Some respiratory pathogens such as *Bordetella pertussis* and *Haemophilus influenzae* can cause β-blockade. Therefore, the airways of infected animals are more likely to become inflamed because of enhanced mast cell degranulation. These infections may predispose animals to the development of respiratory allergies.

Other factors acting within their microenvironment can influence mast cell responsiveness either positively or negatively, including adenosine, sphingosine-1-phosphate, many cytokines (IL-4, IL-33, TSLP, and IFN-γ) and many chemokines. Cell–cell interactions can also influence their activities. Thus, IgE-activated mast cells can enhance T cell cytokine production and division.

Late-Phase Responses

When an antigen is injected into the skin of an allergic animal, two waves of inflammation occur. There is an immediate acute inflammatory response that occurs within 10 to 20 min because of the release of the preformed mast cell mediators. This is followed several hours later by a second wave called the late-phase reaction, which peaks at 6 to 12 h and then gradually diminishes. This late-phase reaction is characterized by redness, edema, and pruritus, and results from the release of inflammatory mediators by T cells, endothelial cells, neutrophils, and macrophages attracted by mast cell chemotactic factors. Th17 cells also play a role in this late-phase reaction.

Suggested Reading

Cildir G, Pant H, Lopez AF, Tergaonkar V. The transcriptional program, functional heterogeneity and clinical targeting of mast cells. *J Exp Med.* 2017;214(9):2491-2506.

Dudeck A, Koberle M, Goldmann O, et al. Mast cells as protectors of health. *J Allergy Clin Immunol.* 2019;144(4S):S4-S18.

Enoksson M, Lyberg K, Moller-Westerberg C, Fallon PC, Nilsson G, Lunderius- Andersson C. Mast cells as sensors of cell injury through IL-33 recognition. *J Immunol.* 2011;186(4):2523-2528.

Frossi B, Mion F, Tripodo C, Colombo MP, Pucillo CE. Rheostatic functions of mast cells in the control of innate and adaptive immune responses. *Trends Immunol.* 2017;38(9):648-656.

Gurish MF, Boyce JA. Mast cell growth, differentiation and death. *Clin Rev Allergy Immunol.* 2002;22(2): 107-118.

Halova I, Ronnberg E, Draberova L, Vliagoftis H, Nilsson G, Draber P. Changing the threshold – signals and mechanisms of mast cell priming. *Immunol Res.* 2018;282(1):73-86.

Huber M, Cato AC, Ainsooson GK, et al. Regulation of the pleiotropic effects of tissue-resident mast cells. *J Allergy Clin Immunol.* 2019;144(4S):S31-S45.

Kawarai S, Masuda K, Ohmori K, et al. Cultivation and characterization of canine skin-derived mast cells. *J Vet Med Sci.* 2010;72(2):131-140.

MacGlashan D. IgE receptor and signal transduction in mast cells and basophils. *Curr Opin Immunol.* 2008;20(6):717-723.

Maurer M, Taube C, Schroeder WJ, et al. Mast cells drive IgE-mediated disease but might be bystanders in many other inflammatory and neoplastic conditions. *J Allergy Clin Immunol.* 2019;144(4S):S19-S30.

Mukai K, Tsai M, Saito H, Galli SJ. Mast cells as sources of cytokines, chemokines and growth factors. *Immunol Res.* 2018;282(1):121-150.

Plum T, Wang X, Rettel M, J Krijgsveld, TB Feyerabend, HR Rodewald. Human mast cell proteome reveals unique lineage, putative functions, and structural basis for cell ablation. *Immunity.* 2020;52(2):404-416.

Redegeld FA, Yu Y, Kumari S, Charles N, Blank U. Non-IgE-mediated mast cell activation. *Immunol Res.* 2018;282(1):87-113.

Sandig H, Bulfone-Paus S. TLR signaling in mast cells: common and unique features. *Front Immunol.* 2012;3:185. doi: 10.3389/fimmu.2012.00185.

Siebenhaar F, Redegeld FA, Bischoff SC, Gibbs BF, Maurer M. Mast cells as drivers of disease and therapeutic targets. *Trends Immunol.* 2018;39(2):151-162.

St. John AL, Abraham SN. Innate immunity and its regulation by mast cells. *J Immunol.* 2013;190(9):4458-4463.

Stassen M, Hartmann AK, Jiminez Delgado S, Dehmel S, Braun A. Mast cells within cellular networks. *J Allergy Clin Immunol.* 2019;144(4S):S46-S54.

Varricchi G, Raap U, Rivellese F, Marone G, Gibbs BF. Human mast cells and basophils – how are they similar, how are they different? *Immunol Res.* 2018;282(1):8-34.

Voehringer D. Protective and pathological roles of mast cells and basophils. *Nat Rev Immunol.* 2013;13(5):362-375.

Wernersson S, Pejler G. Mast cell secretory granules: armed for battle. *Nat Rev Immunol.* 2014;14(7):478-494.

CHAPTER 4

Eosinophils and Basophils

Among the leukocytes circulating in the bloodstream, two cell types stand out because of the staining patterns of their granules: eosinophils and basophils. Unlike their plentiful cousins, the neutrophils, whose task it is to seek and destroy invading bacteria, eosinophils and basophils have more specialized roles. Eosinophils control parasitic helminths, while basophils are primarily directed against biting arthropods. Both cell types contribute to the development of lesions associated with allergic diseases. For example, tissues undergoing allergic inflammation often contain large numbers of eosinophils, that are attracted to mast cell degranulation sites, where they release their own complex mixture of inflammatory mediators. These include cationic proteins, cytokines, chemokines, and growth factors. When eosinophils release these proteins, they do so like mast cells via granule-mediated exocytosis. Once expelled from the cell, the granules may persist in the tissues where they release their contents into the intercellular environment.

Eosinophils

LIFE HISTORY

Eosinophils develop within the bone marrow from pluripotent hematopoietic stem cells. Cytokines such as interleukin (IL)-3, GM-CSF, and especially IL-5 act together to drive the development of the eosinophil lineage by activating transcription factors of the GATA family. Inflammatory stimuli also promote the bone marrow production of eosinophils. They are mobilized by alarmins such as IL-33 and HMGB-1 from damaged, dead, and dying cells. In humans, eosinophil progenitors are direct descendants of common myeloid stem cells that are distinct from the granulocyte/macrophage stem cells that also produce mast cells and basophils. Eosinophils develop from the granulocyte/macrophage lineage in mice and from $CD34^+$ progenitors found in the lungs and bone marrow. Eosinophils are released into the bloodstream as mature cells; however, they can be further activated by exposure to IL-5 and chemokines such as eotaxins. They spend only a short time in the bloodstream with a half-life of approximately 18 h before moving to the gastrointestinal tract and other organs where they reside for the rest of their lives. Therefore, they are minor components of the circulating leukocyte population. Eosinophils may also accumulate in the thymus at the corticomedullary junction, the lamina propria of the lower gastrointestinal tract, the ovaries, uterus, mammary gland, adipose tissues, spleen, and lymph nodes. They constitute approximately 5% of the myeloid cells in the lungs, 6% in the skin, and 1% in the heart, liver, and kidneys.

STRUCTURE

Eosinophils were first described in 1879 by Paul Ehrlich, who noted their unusual staining properties. They are polymorphonuclear cells, slightly larger than neutrophils or basophils (12–17 μm in diameter), with a large segmented nucleus and many cytoplasmic granules that stain intensely with the red dye eosin (Figs 4.1 and 4.2; Box 4.1). Eosinophil granules are approximately

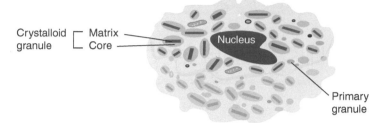

Crystalloid ⌈ Matrix
granule   ⌊ Core
Nucleus
Primary
granule

Fig. 4.1 Major structural features of an eosinophil.

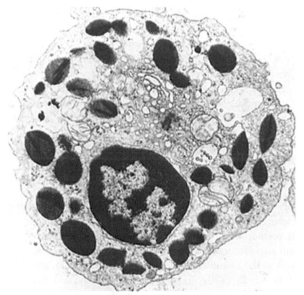

Fig. 4.2 Transmission electron micrograph of a rabbit eosinophil. Note the presence of the complex granules (Courtesy Dr. S Linthicum).

BOX 4.1 ■ Eosins

Eosins are compounds derived from the green fluorescent dye fluorescein. Since they are acidic, they react with basic amino acids such as arginine and lysine. As a result, they stain proteins yellowish pink or red. There are several forms of eosin used for staining tissues. Eosin Y is the most common form. It is a tetrabromo derivative of fluorescein. Eosin B is also used. It is a dibromo-dinitro derivative of fluorescein. When mixed with oxidized methylene blue (azure B) in a Romanowsky stain, the eosin binds to eosinophil cationic protein in the eosinophil granules to produce the characteristic staining pattern of these cells.

450–500 nm in diameter in most mammals; however, in horses, these can aggregate to form much larger structures (Fig. 4.3). Unlike basophils, eosinophils are phagocytic.

The proportion of eosinophils among the blood leukocytes varies greatly because it is affected by the presence of parasites, especially helminths. In general, the number and morphology of blood

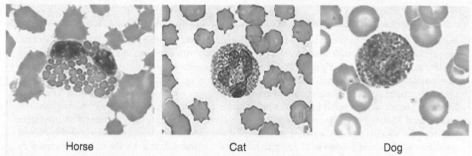

| Horse | Cat | Dog |

Fig. 4.3 **Photomicrographs of peripheral blood eosinophils from a horse (A), cat (B), and dog (C).** Each cell is approximately 12 μm in diameter. Note the large size of the equine granules. Giemsa stain. (Courtesy Dr. MC Johnson)

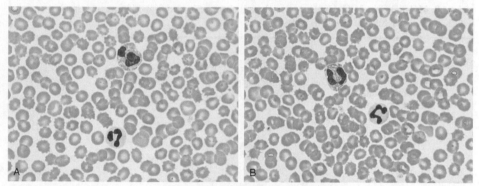

Fig. 4.4 **"Gray" eosinophils in blood smears from a golden retriever.** Note their unusual staining properties compared to the segmented neutrophils in the lower portion of the images. It is possible that these are simply prematurely degranulated cells. (Courtesy Dr. MC Johnson)

eosinophils in domestic mammals are similar. (Some canine, especially greyhound, eosinophils are different [Fig. 4.4; Box 4.2].) In beagles, there are approximately 300–500 eosinophils/μL. In unparasitized humans, there are less than 400/μL. In cats, there are from 200 to 600 eosinophils/μL, although some studies report numbers as high as 1500/μL. These higher numbers likely reflect the presence of parasites. Cat eosinophil granules may be rod-shaped. In horses, numbers range from 0 to 1000 eosinophils/μL. Their granules are large and may obscure the bilobed nucleus. In cattle, eosinophils are packed with small granules. As in other species, their numbers fluctuate and they may show a seasonal eosinophilia, reflecting changes in parasite load. In general, their absolute counts range from 100 to 1200 eosinophils/μL. These numbers and fluctuations are similar in sheep and pigs.

Granules

Eosinophils contain three distinct types of granules: large specific (crystalloid) granules, small primary granules, and small dense vesicles. They also contain lipid bodies, mitochondria, ribosomes, an endoplasmic reticulum, a small Golgi apparatus, and some glycogen granules. Similar to mast cell granules, eosinophil-specific granules contain multiple preformed mediators that are released when the cells degranulate (Fig. 4.5).

Humans, laboratory rodents, cats, and goats have specific granules with an electron dense core surrounded by a less dense matrix. They form biconvex disks with a crystalloid core consisting of

---

BOX 4.2 ■ Gray Eosinophils

Some dogs, especially greyhounds and related sighthounds such as whippets and Italian greyhounds, have unusual granules in their eosinophils. They do not stain with eosin and as a result appear pale gray or clear in blood smears (see Figure 4.4). The eosinophils appear to be vacuolated. Greyhound puppies have normally staining eosinophils, but they lose these as they age so that adult dogs have a high proportion of unstained granules. These unstained granules may cause confusion when performing differential leukocyte counts and can result in the cells being undercounted or regarded as "toxic" neutrophils. Ultrastructural studies on greyhound eosinophils reveal no unusual structural features and they stain positively for alkaline phosphatase. The presence of these apparently unusual granules probably reflects the differential staining properties of commercially available stains. It may also be an artifact caused by cells that degranulate prematurely while being sampled.

Giori L, Gironi S, Scarpa P, et al. (2011). Grey eosinophils in greyhounds: frequency in three breeds and comparison of eosinophil counts determined manually and with three hematology analyzers. *Vet Clin Pathol* 40:475-483.
Lazbik MC and Couto CG. (2005). Morphological characterization of specific granules in Greyhound eosinophils. *Vet Clin Pathol* 34:140-143.

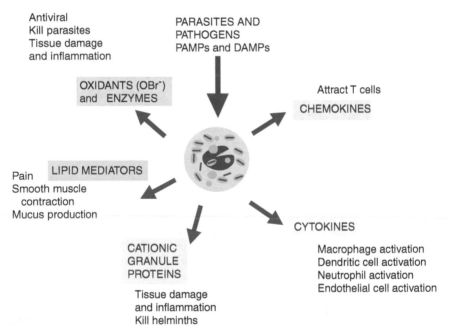

Fig. 4.5 Major molecules released by activated eosinophils. Eosinophils contain a complex mixture of molecules, many of which contribute to the development of allergic inflammation. This inflammatory response is especially effective in killing parasitic helminths in the intestine and within tissues, and is a characteristic feature of many allergic diseases.

nanocrystals containing inert deposits of major basic protein (MBP) and eosinophil peroxidase. This core is surrounded by a matrix containing two ribonucleases, eosinophil cationic protein and eosinophil-derived neurotoxin. Specific granules are also loaded with a mixture of cytokines and growth factors and multiple enzymes. Cats show great diversity in their granule size and structure. Only about 10% of canine eosinophil granules possess a distinct core. Horse eosinophil granules have a dense core varying in position within each granule and are not crystalline in nature. Cattle and mink have granules that lack a dense core and are homogeneous.

MBP is a 13.8 kDa protein that constitutes the dense core and accounts for more than half of the granule protein. When released, it can damage nearby cells by disrupting their plasma membrane. MBP stimulates histamine release from basophils and mast cells. It activates neutrophils and platelets, promotes superoxide production by alveolar macrophages, and is toxic to bacteria and helminth parasites.

Eosinophil cationic protein (ECP) is a ribonuclease of 16−21 kDa found in the specific granule matrix. ECP accounts for approximately 30% of the granule protein. When released, it damages cell membranes, promotes mast cell degranulation, and can kill bacteria, viruses, and parasites. It is also a potent neurotoxin. This protein is responsible for the high affinity of the granules for eosin.

Eosinophil-derived neurotoxin (EDN) is also a ribonuclease of 18 kDa, with almost 70% sequence homology with ECP. When injected into the brain, it damages myelinated nerve fibers, and it shows some antiviral activity against respiratory syncytial virus. It is a chemoattractant and activator of immature dendritic cells and acts as an endogenous ligand for toll-like receptor (TLR)2.

Eosinophil peroxidase (EPO) is a heme-containing peroxidase. In the presence of superoxide, it oxidizes halide ions, especially bromide, to generate hypobromous acid (HOBr). HOBr is a potent oxidizing agent that can disrupt bacterial membranes and destroy viruses, fungi, and parasites. EPO not only uses bromide in preference to chloride but also generates nitric oxide and nitrotyrosine, both potent oxidizing agents. EPO is mainly responsible for killing any ingested bacteria.

Eosinophil primary granules represent early stages in the development of specific granules and are more correctly referred to as immature granules. As the cell develops, these primary granules coalesce, and their cores crystallize, becoming specific granules. They contain arylsulfatase, peroxidase, acid phosphatase, catalase, some ECP, and lysophospholipase. Charcot-Leyden crystal protein, found in human eosinophils, is a lysopalmitoylphospholipase stored in the primary granules and the cytoplasm, comprising 7%−10% of the total eosinophil protein. It crystallizes in tissues at eosinophil infiltration sites. Eosinophil lipid bodies store arachidonic acid and are sites for the synthesis of eicosanoids. Eosinophils also synthesize platelet-activating factor (PAF).

FUNCTIONS

Eosinophils are phagocytic cells and can ingest both gram-positive and gram-negative bacteria and yeasts. However, they are significantly less efficient at phagocytosis than neutrophils. For example, they cannot phagocytose antibody-coated red cells. At least 35 cytokines have been identified as coming from eosinophils. Like other cells, eosinophils express many diverse receptors on their plasma membrane. These receptors bind growth factors, other cells, cytokines, and chemokines. Among the most important are the IL-5 receptor, the chemokine receptor (CCR3), lectins, and multiple pattern recognition receptors (Fig. 4.6).

Activation

Eosinophils are predominantly tissue-resident cells, and the great majority of the eosinophils in the body are located within the intestinal wall. Both type 2 helper (Th2) cells and mast cells produce IL-5 and the chemokines known as eotaxins that stimulate the release of eosinophils from the bone marrow.

The three epithelial cytokines, thymic stromal lymphopoietin (TSLP), IL-25 and IL-33, as well as IL-23, can promote eosinophilia by inducing IL-5 production. By itself, IL-33 activates eosinophils and stimulates their adhesion, degranulation, chemotaxis, and surface protein expression.

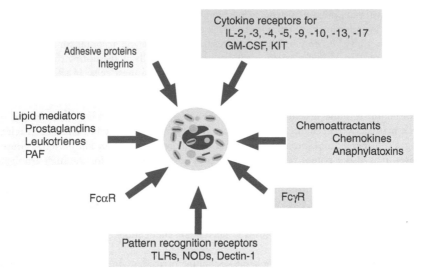

Fig. 4.6   Most important cell surface receptors expressed on eosinophils.

Th2 cells mobilize eosinophils and promote immunoglobulin E (IgE) responses. These eosinophils are attracted to mast cell degranulation sites by eotaxins, histamine and its breakdown product imidiazoleacetic acid (see Fig. 5.1), leukotriene B_4, 5-hydroxytryptamine, and platelet-activating factor. Eosinophils are especially attracted by CXCL8 (IL-8) complexed to IgA. These activated eosinophils have increased bactericidal activity because of the enhanced generation of oxidants and enzymes such as acid phosphatase. The mobilization and activation of eosinophils enhances their ability to damage and kill parasites and supports the belief that the major function of these IgE-mediated eosinophilic response is the control and elimination of helminth parasites.

Interleukin 5. IL-5, produced primarily by Th2 cells, plays a major role in controlling eosinophil production, development, and release from the bone marrow (Fig. 4.7). IL-5 is produced in smaller amounts by mast cells, NK cells, type 2 innate lymphoid (ILC2) cells, NKT cells, and eosinophils themselves. Once bound to its receptor, IL-5 activates eosinophils via a series of phosphorylation steps and eventually promotes their survival and proliferation. IL-5 functions synergistically with the other Th2 cytokines, IL-4 and IL-13, and with the three eotaxins (CCL11 [eotaxin], CCL24 [eotaxin 2], and CCL26 [eotaxin 3]). When allergic skin disease develops, CCL11 is produced first followed by CCL24 and CCL26. Together, they attract eosinophils to

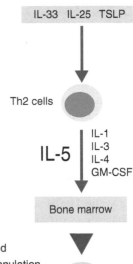

Fig. 4.7   Central role of interleukin 5 (IL-5) in the activation of eosinophils. IL-5 is derived from type 2 helper (Th2) cells under the influence of the epithelial cytokines. It acts on bone marrow stem cells to promote the production and function of eosinophils. However, many other cytokines also contribute to this process.

inflammatory sites. Other chemokines such as CCL5, CCL7, and CCL12 can also cause eosinophil activation.

The IL-5 receptor α subunit (IL-5Rα) is expressed in both eosinophils and basophils. The receptor itself is a heterodimer where the α subunit is paired with a signaling β-subunit shared with the IL-3 and GM-CSF receptors.

Other Activators. As they develop, eosinophils express receptors for IL-18. IL-18 is related to IL-1. It is produced by macrophages as a pro-cytokine and then activated by subsequent enzymatic cleavage. It activates eosinophils and promotes eosinophil accumulation and inflammation in the airways. IL-18 overexpression can enhance eosinophil-mediated inflammation.

Eosinophils express many different pattern recognition receptors, including TLRs1−5, TLR7, TLR9, NOD1, NOD2, and dectin 1 (see Fig. 4.6). When these bind their ligands, they trigger an oxidative burst, increase cell adhesiveness, and release IL-1, IL-6, IL-31, tumor necrosis factor-α, GM-CSF, and their cytotoxic granule contents. TLR activation also promotes eosinophil mobilization and survival.

Degranulation

Although eosinophils can phagocytose small particles, they are much more suited to the extracellular destruction of large parasites because they can degranulate into the surrounding tissues. Once free in the extracellular fluid, the intact eosinophil granules can function as independent structures. These free granules express membrane receptors for interferon-γ, and eotaxins that, when triggered, stimulate granules to secrete their contents. Thus, eosinophil granules function autonomously to contribute to the defenses against helminths.

Eosinophils can also undergo piecemeal degranulation. Their granule contents decrease, and their lipid bodies increase in size. A specialized "docking complex" forms on their plasma membrane. These docking complexes, called "sombrero vesicles," are formed by exocytosing granules (They resemble a Mexican hat under an electron microscope). Granules migrate to the plasma membrane, where they fuse with the docking complex and release their mediators into the extracellular space. Piecemeal degranulation occurs in response to cytokines such as interferon-γ and CCL11. Degranulation also occurs in response to IgE-coated parasites, many chemokines, PAF, and C5a.

Eosinophils and Lymphocytes

Eosinophils respond to IL-5 produced by T cells. However, T cells also respond to eosinophils. While not professional antigen-presenting cells, eosinophils express major histocompatibility complex class II molecules and the costimulatory molecules CD80 and CD86. Therefore, eosinophils can process antigens and effectively use these processed antigens to stimulate T cells. The T cells respond by proliferating and secreting their cytokines. Eosinophils can promote allergic inflammation by regulating the production of chemokines such as CCL17 and CCL22 that attract Th2 cells. Eosinophils also promote humoral immune responses by priming B cells for antibody production. Bone marrow eosinophils colocalize with plasma cells and secrete the cytokine APRIL (activation and proliferation-induced ligand) and IL-6 that support plasma cell survival. Eosinophils are required for the homing of long-lived plasma cells to the bone marrow and their long-term survival. An absence of eosinophils prevents efficient B cell class switching to IgA within Peyer's patches. In effect, eosinophils generate and maintain mucosal IgA plasma cells. The production by eosinophils of multiple Th2 cytokines and indoleamine dioxygenase inhibits local Th1 responses and ensures that a "Th2 environment" is maintained.

Eosinophils and Mast Cells

While their tissue distribution is different, eosinophils and mast cells come together at sites of allergic inflammation to form what has been called an "allergic effector unit." Within this unit,

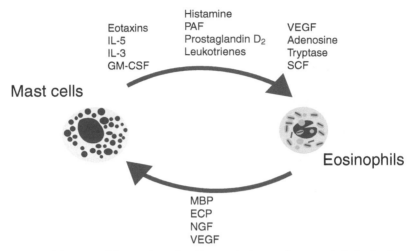

Fig. 4.8 Eosinophil–mast cell interactions. Cytokines and other mediators act in both directions. These interacting cell pairs have been termed an "allergic effector unit."

each cell communicates with the other. For example, mast cells influence eosinophil functions through IL-5, stem cell factor, histamine, PAF, prostaglandin D_2, leukotrienes, and vascular endothelial growth factors (Fig. 4.8). Histamine induces eosinophil chemotaxis via their H4 receptors. Adenosine from mast cells acts on eosinophils to potentiate mediator release. Mast cell tryptase stimulates eosinophil activation and degranulation via the activation of protease activated receptor 2. Stem cell factor induces the release of EPO and leukotriene C_4 from eosinophils.

Conversely, eosinophils influence mast cell functions by releasing ECP, MBP, nerve growth factor, and vascular endothelial growth factors. ECP induces the mast cell release of histamine and tryptase by acting through the Mas-related G-protein coupled receptor X2 (MRGPRX2) (Chapter 3). MBP activates mast cells and promotes histamine release through its actions on integrin-β1. These bidirectional interactions are important contributors to local allergic inflammation.

Eosinophils and Parasites

Invading helminth parasites attract eosinophils by releasing excretory and secretory products. Damaged epithelial cells will release IL-33, IL-25, and TSLP that also attract eosinophils. The resulting inflammation generates IL-5 and other cytokines from Th2 cells. IL-5 and GM-CSF from Th17 cells can also mobilize bone marrow eosinophils, releasing large numbers into the circulation. When eosinophils are exposed to helminth proteins, they increase their expression of MHC class II molecules, process these antigens and promote Th2 responses and IgE production.

Eosinophils employ their Fc receptors to bind to antibody-coated parasites. Once attached, they can release their granule contents directly onto the worm cuticle (Fig. 4.9). These contents include HOBr, nitric oxide, lysophospholipase, and phospholipase D. MBP, the crystalline core of the eosinophil-specific granules, can damage the cuticles of schistosomula, *Fasciola*, and *Trichinella*. ECP and EDN are also lethal for helminths.

Many nematodes are damaged or killed by eosinophil toxic products, supporting the idea that eosinophils serve a protective function. Nevertheless, this may not apply to all parasitic worms. Reagents such as anti-IL5 that block the development of eosinophilia paint a more nuanced

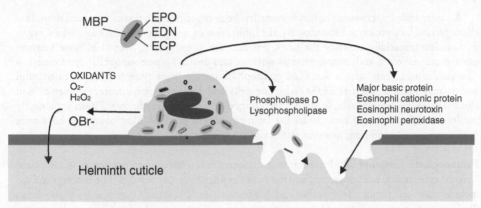

Fig. 4.9 Some of the molecules released from eosinophils and their granules that can cause lethal damage to the cuticle of parasitic helminths.

picture. For example, an absence of eosinophils had no apparent effect on the response of mice to *Schistosoma mansoni*. In contrast, eosinophil depletion resulted in prolonged survival of *Strongyloides stercoralis* and *Angiostrongylus cantonensis* larvae. Both *Teladorsagia circumcincta* and *Haemonchus contortus* produce chemoattractants for eosinophils, whereas the free-living nematode *Caenorhabditis elegans* does not. Therefore, some nematodes may actively encourage eosinophil recruitment, and the presence of eosinophils in some situations might ameliorate the tissue damage caused by helminth larvae.

Eosinophils and Infectious Agents

The cationic eosinophil granule proteins MBP and ECP have antibacterial properties, whereas EDN has some antiviral activity. ECP has an affinity for bacterial lipopolysaccharides and peptidoglycans and can agglutinate gram-negative bacteria. Eosinophils are phagocytic and can release extracellular traps, composed of mitochondrial DNA combined with MBP and ECP.

EOSINOPHIL PATHOLOGY

Eosinophil-specific granules contain toxic substances that can kill nearby cells. For example, MBP and EPO can kill airway epithelial and cardiac muscle cells. Other granule components, such as the two ribonucleases EDN and ECP, may also play a role in tissue remodeling. The diverse mixture of chemokines, cytokines, enzymes, and oxidants released by eosinophils contributes to lesion development.

Eosinophilia

Eosinophilia is defined as a blood eosinophil count greater than $5000/\mu L$. This might be a primary eosinophilia as in the case of proliferative disorders driven by IL-5 or hematopoietic malignancies. Secondary eosinophilia is much more common. This may be triggered by worms in the intestine, migrating helminth larvae, or heartworms. This is the likely cause of eosinophilic bronchopneumopathy in dogs. Chronic eosinophilia is associated with prolonged inflammation in visceral organs, especially the skin, gastrointestinal tract, and lungs. Other causes may include flea allergy, adverse drug reactions, bronchial asthma, eosinophilic granuloma complex, eosinophilic enteritis, mast cell tumors, and lymphomas.

An idiopathic hypereosinophilic syndrome has been described in humans, cats, and dogs. It is characterized by a prolonged eosinophilia, the infiltration of many organs with eosinophils, organ dysfunction (especially affecting the heart, but also the lungs, spleen, liver, skin, bone marrow, gastrointestinal tract, and central nervous system), and death. Hypereosinophilic syndrome is a rare condition in cats with a sustained eosinophilia lasting more than 6 months. Eosinophil counts may reach as high as $39,000/\mu L$. The cells and IgE levels are apparently normal, and clinical signs are non-specific, including vomiting, diarrhea, and weight loss. Death presumably results from the release of toxic molecules from eosinophil granules. Corticosteroids have been used to treat this condition; however, with minimal success.

Paraneoplastic Eosinophilia. Paraneoplastic diseases are the systemic consequences of neoplasia. In some cases of cancer in dogs, cats, and horses, an eosinophilia may develop. The cancers involved include mast cell tumors, lymphomas and lymphosarcomas, basal cell carcinomas, leiomyomas, fibrosarcomas, myxosarcomas, and mammary carcinomas. These eosinophilias might result from the production of IL-5 or eotaxin 1, either directly by tumor cells or indirectly by tumor-infiltrating Th2 cells. In some cases, a basophilia may simultaneously occur. As with all eosinophilias, other causes must be excluded, including parasites and food allergies, before diagnosing it as paraneoplastic. One indicator of its paraneoplastic origin is that the eosinophil count rises and falls in association with tumor growth and remission. Myelogenous eosinophilic leukemia occurs in animals but, in contrast to paraneoplastic eosinophils, the tumor cells are generally immature and structurally abnormal.

Eosinopenia

Low eosinophil numbers might have minimal clinical significance as they are within the normal range in healthy animals. Glucocorticoids cause eosinopenia, and catecholamines reduce eosinophil numbers by acting through β-adrenergic receptors.

Eosinophilic Granuloma Complex

The eosinophilic granuloma complex consists of a group of skin lesions in dogs and cats (Figs 4.10 and 4.11). They have one feature in common, the presence of large numbers of eosinophils in the lesions. Although their cause is unknown, these lesions are most commonly associated with flea and mosquito hypersensitivity and food or environmental allergies. It has also been suggested that

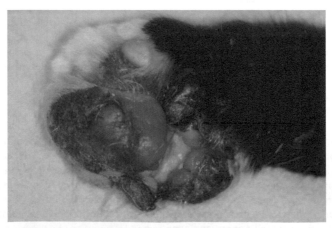

Fig. 4.10 Eosinophilic granuloma on the footpad of a cat (Courtesy Dr. Robert Kennis).

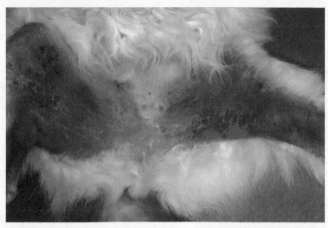

Fig. 4.11 Eosinophilic plaque in the inguinal region of a cat (Courtesy Dr. Robert Kennis).

the major cat allergen Fel d 1 (Chapter 21) might act as an autoantigen and thus be responsible for chronic inflammatory reactions. When purified eosinophil granule proteins are injected into guinea pig or rabbit skin, they disrupt skin integrity and cause inflammation. ECP usually produces ulcers, whereas EDN generates cellular exudates. Purified eosinophil peroxidase and the chemokine MBP-1 produce induration and erythema. The escape of these proteins might explain the development of eosinophil-associated skin diseases.

The eosinophilic granuloma complex consists of three distinct lesions: eosinophilic granulomas, eosinophilic plaques, and indolent ulcers. Cats may suffer from one, two, or even all three of these simultaneously. They have a similar pathogenesis and histological appearance as eosinophils accumulate and release their granule contents. All are associated with intense pruritus, inflammation, and swelling. Fleas and mosquitos often trigger these reactions, and affected animals should be carefully checked for ectoparasites.

Eosinophilic granulomas are the most frequently diagnosed of the three conditions, consisting of firm swellings that biopsy shows to consist of immune cells, macrophages, and fibroblasts infiltrated with eosinophils. The granulomas are raised, somewhat linear, well defined, and mildly erythematous. Some may present as scattered individual crusted papules. There is, however, much variation in their shape and size. Granulomas may develop in any location; however, they are commonly observed on the rear legs, on the feet, and around the mouth. They are not usually pruritic.

Eosinophilic plaques present as red, flat, inflamed swellings, usually on the ventral abdomen or inner thighs. They are histologically similar to feline miliary dermatitis.

Linear eosinophilic ulcers (sometimes called indolent or rodent ulcers) are commonly located in the oral cavity or on the lips. These are open weeping sores or ulcers with raised edges that develop on the upper lip of cats adjacent to the canine teeth. They are often bilateral and may involve the hard palate. Avoidance of any identified allergens may result in clinical improvement, and corticosteroid treatment is usually of benefit. The linear form and indolent ulcers may be difficult to treat. These eosinophilic lesions often resolve spontaneously but, while present, may be highly pruritic. Self-inflicted trauma may then prevent healing and cause secondary infections. Steroid treatment is usually successful unless secondary infections have developed.

An atypical eosinophilic dermatitis may develop in cats because of a mosquito allergy. It develops on hairless areas susceptible to mosquito attack and presents as scattered individual, intensely pruritic, crusted papules. The lesions may be masked by self-inflicted trauma and secondary bacterial infection. Histologically, they are associated with a local mast cell and eosinophil infiltration, and an eosinophilia.

Eosinophilic Myositis

This is an inflammatory disease primarily affecting the mastication muscles. It mainly affects large breed dogs. It may also affect their eye muscles. This is probably an autoimmune disease directed against M2 muscle fibers. Eosinophils are present in some cases. Their significance is unclear but may reflect the presence of intramuscular parasites.

Eosinophilic Panosteitis

Panosteitis is a disease of rapidly growing young dogs between 3 and 18 months of age. It is most often seen in German shepherds but can occur in other large breeds. Affected animals have a history of shifting lameness. Lesions may develop in any of the long bones, e.g., the humerus, radius, ulna, femur, and tibia. The radiographic lesions show an increased density in the medullary cavity that resolves within 2−3 months. About half the cases develop eosinophilia, and eosinophils accumulate in the marrow of the affected bones. Its cause remains unknown.

Eosinophilic Gastroenteritis

When investigating any disease associated with excessive eosinophils, it is important first to eliminate the presence of parasites. This is especially relevant to the gastrointestinal tract and idiopathic inflammatory bowel diseases. In dogs, the clinical signs of eosinophilic gastroenteritis such as vomiting, hematemesis, inappetence, weight loss, abdominal pain, melena, and bloody diarrhea are similar to other types of gastroenteritis, although the prognosis is poorer. It most commonly occurs in Boxers, Doberman pinschers, German shepherds, Rottweilers, and Shar-peis. It probably results from allergic responses to foods or gastrointestinal parasites. The inflammation may occur anywhere along the gastrointestinal tract, from the esophagus to the large intestine. In dogs and humans, eosinophilic esophagitis has been associated with a food allergy. Eosinophilic gastritis is commonly caused by food allergies in humans but may result from parasitic infestations in dogs. For example, an eosinophilic enteritis may result from canine hookworm infestation.

Eosinophilic enteritis is also a common form of inflammatory bowel disease. Affected dogs may not show eosinophilia; therefore, biopsies from different regions of the gut may be required for a definitive diagnosis. Eosinophilic infiltrations in different regions of the gastrointestinal tract have been reported. Eosinophilic colitis is rare in dogs and humans and a colonoscopy and biopsy are required for diagnosis. Treatment involves ensuring that parasites are eliminated and that a food allergy is not responsible for the disease. Immunosuppressive drugs may be used once other causes of disease have been disproven.

In cats, the situation is similar, with eosinophilic gastroenteritis regarded as a form of idiopathic inflammatory bowel disease. Eosinophils may predominate in the lesions or be present in smaller numbers in lymphoplasmacytic enteritis. Ultrasonographic examination may reveal greatly thickened intestinal walls.

Eosinophilic Dermatitis (Wells-Like Syndrome)

This is an uncommon condition in which skin lesions develop in dogs with preexisting gastrointestinal disease, such as vomiting or diarrhea. The acute skin lesions consist of a red macular rash with papules or plaques or a generalized erythema most evident on the abdomen. Biopsies show that this is an acute eosinophilic dermatitis with edema. It is, in effect, an eosinophilic cellulitis. It differs from typical atopic dermatitis in its abrupt onset and histopathology. Pruritus is not usually a feature, nor does it involve the limbs. The tissues may contain collagen flame figures (foci of dermal collagen fibers encrusted with eosinophil granules). Flame figures are also seen in feline eosinophilic granulomas. Systemic corticosteroids such as prednisolone and H1 and H2 histamine receptor antagonists may be used for treatment. The gastrointestinal symptoms are treated symptomatically, including antiemetics and antibiotics. They usually resolve before the skin lesions, with the latter resolving within 3 weeks and not recurring. The cause of this syndrome is unknown. but it is suspected that it may be an adverse drug reaction.

Eosinophilic Cystitis

This has been reported in both dogs and cats in which it presents as painful frequent urination. The bladder wall is infiltrated with eosinophils. The disease does not respond to antibiotic treatment and it is likely caused by a food allergy. In such cases, identification of the offending allergen via the use of elimination diets might be appropriate.

Basophils

Continuing his studies on the staining of blood leukocytes with aniline dyes, Paul Ehrlich discovered basophils in 1878. Basophils, the least common type of blood leukocyte, are functionally and phenotypically similar to mast cells, although their origins and gene expression profiles are very different. Basophils originate in the bone marrow, circulate as mature cells within the bloodstream, and can be recruited to inflammatory sites in tissues. While classified as polymorphonuclear granulocytes, unlike neutrophils and eosinophils, basophils are not phagocytic. Unlike mast cells that are long-lived and may divide, basophils are short-lived, non-dividers. They probably die by apoptosis in tissues after participating in inflammatory reactions. In general, basophils constitute less than 1% of mammalian blood leukocytes. They are fairly large, being 14—16 μm in diameter (Fig. 4.12). Basophils are rare cells in the blood of all domestic mammals. In dogs, they contain relatively few small basophilic granules; cat basophils have many very small granules; in horses, the basophils are packed with densely staining granules that may obscure the cell nucleus; and basophils in cattle, sheep and pigs are similar.

Basophils contribute to the defenses of the body against arthropods, such as ticks and helminths. They play an important role in IgE-mediated skin inflammation and are implicated in the late-phase response in allergic asthma. Basophils are abundant in reptiles and account for more than 59% of the blood leukocytes in the snapping turtle (*Chelydra serpentina*). However, these may not be true basophils, simply neutrophils that stain strongly with basic dyes. These cells have not been functionally described, but they release histamine when appropriately stimulated.

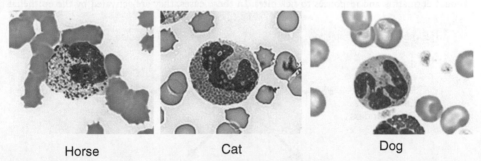

Horse   Cat   Dog

Fig. 4.12 Photomicrographs of peripheral blood basophils from a horse (A), cat (B), and dog (C). These cells are approximately 15 μm in diameter; all were photographed at the same magnification. Giemsa stain. (Courtesy Dr. MC Johnson)

LIFE HISTORY

Like mast cells, basophils originate from stem cells of the granulocyte/macrophage lineage. They branch off from eosinophil precursors, and subsequently from basophil/mast cell precursors. Stem cell factor acting through KIT does not promote their production, but IL-3 does. IL-3 is an essential cytokine for basophil survival. Basophil production is also influenced by blood IgE levels. They mature as they circulate in the bloodstream and have a lifespan of only 60–70 h. Basophils are smaller than mast cells with multilobular nuclei and fewer, smaller cytoplasmic granules. Basophil cytoplasmic granules stain metachromatically with alanine dyes, such as Wright, Giemsa, May-Grünwald-Giemsa, and Leishman. These granules contain histamine and some proteases. They are not normally found outside the bloodstream and only enter tissues under the influence of some T cell-derived chemokines.

ACTIVATION

The IgE Pathway

Similar to mast cells, basophils express FcεR1, and cross-linking this receptor by antigen-bound IgE induces basophil activation and degranulation. Basophil granules contain a mixture of active molecules similar, but not identical to, those in mast cells, including histamine, proteases, cytokines, and lipid mediators (Fig. 4.13). When activated, basophils produce IL-4, IL-6, IL-13, and TSLP and they synthesize leukotrienes. Basophils also release PAF in response to IgG1-mediated stimulation. IL-3 promotes the reactivity of activated basophils so that, in its presence, they produce more IL-4 and IL-13. Basophils produce relatively high levels of IL-4 and, as a result, are major differentiation promoters for Th2 and ILC2 cells.

Although mast cells induce acute inflammation, basophils mediate more long-term allergic states such as chronic allergic dermatitis and the late-phase allergic reaction. As with mast cells, the intensity of the basophil degranulation response is likely determined by the affinity of IgE for its allergen.

Basophils can initiate allergen- and helminth-driven type 2 immune responses by functioning as antigen-presenting cells. Basophils can capture antigens via FcR-bound antibodies. They endocytose, process, and present soluble antigens but not particulate antigens. Basophils play a protective role in helminth, tick, and bacterial infections. They degrade toxins in venoms and contribute to tumor rejection. Basophils play an important role in the early phase of delayed hypersensitivity responses (Chapter 19).

The TSLP Pathway

Basophils play an important role in IgE-independent allergic inflammation, including allergic contact dermatitis and responses to tick bites. In these cases, they are activated by the epithelial

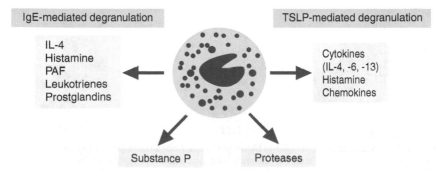

Fig. 4.13 Products released by basophils on activation by the IgE pathway or the thymic stromal lymphopoietin (TSLP)-mediated pathway.

alarmin, TSLP. TSLP promotes basophil expression of IL-3, IL-4, IL-6, IL-18, and IL-33 receptors, and chemokine receptors. Thus, IL-3 can directly stimulate the release of cytokines from TSLP-elicited basophils. IL-3 promotes basophil accumulation in lymph nodes, whereas TSLP promotes recruitment to the skin. However, the basophil TSLP pathway is, in part, dependent on IL-3 activities. TSLP-elicited basophils show a different pattern of gene expression compared to IL-3-induced basophils. Because its receptors are expressed on basophil precursors in the bone marrow, TSLP also regulates basophil production.

TSLP-elicited basophils produce greater amounts of IL-4 and IL-6 and increased expression of IL-18 and IL-33 receptors and multiple chemokines. TSLP-induced basophils play a role in atopic dermatitis, food allergies, and protection against helminth parasites. They also play a key role in anaphylaxis in mice, although their importance in other species remains unclear. Cutaneous basophil and ILC2 responses are dependent on the presence of TSLP. Therefore, both basophils and ILC2s accumulate and form clusters in inflamed skin. This basophil accumulation precedes the ILC2 influx. Basophils are the major source of IL-4 in inflamed skin, and it is IL-4 that causes the influx of ILC2s. (ILC2s express the IL-4R and proliferate in response to IL-4).

Suggested Reading

Bastan I, Rendahl AK, Seelig D, et al. Assessment of eosinophils in gastrointestinal inflammatory disease of dogs. *J Vet Intern Med*. 2018;32(6):1911-1917.

Bloom PB. Canine and feline eosinophilic skin diseases. *Vet Clin North Am Small Anim Pract*. 2006;36(1): 141-160.

Fondati A, Carreras E, Fondevila D, Ferrer L, Cuchillo CM, Nogues V. Characterization of biological activities of feline eosinophil granule proteins. *Am J Vet Res*. 2004;65(7):957-963.

Fulkerson PC, Rothenberg ME. Targeting eosinophils in allergy, inflammation and beyond. *Nat Rev Drug Discov*. 2013;12(2):117-129.

Iazbik MC, Couto CG. Morphologic characterization of specific granules in Greyhound eosinophils. *Vet Clin Pathol*. 2005;34(2):140-143.

Karasuyama H, Yamanishi Y. Basophils have emerged as a key player in immunity. *Curr Opin Immunol*. 2014;31:1-7.

Kawakami Y, Galli SJ. Regulation of mast cell and basophil function and survival by IgE. *Nat Rev Immunol*. 2002;2(10):773-785.

Marchetti V, Benetti C, Citi S, Taccini V. Paraneoplastic hypereosinophilia in a dog with intestinal T-cell lymphoma. *Vet Clin Pathol*. 2005;34(3):259-263.

Mauldin EA. Canine acute eosinophilic dermatitis with edema (Wells-like Syndrome). *Vet Clin North Am Small Anim Pract*. 2019;49(1):47-51.

Melo RCN, Weller PF. Contemporary understanding of the secretory granules in human eosinophils. *J Leukoc Biol*. 2018;104(1):85-93.

Nakashima C, Otsuka A, Kabashima K. Recent advancement in the mechanism of basophil activation. *J Dermatol Sci*. 2018;91(1):3-8.

Ramirez GA, Yacoub MR, Ripa M, et al. Eosinophils from physiology to disease: a comprehensive review. *BioMed Res Int*. 2018;2018:9095275, doi: 10.1155/2018/9095275.

Rosenberg HF, Dyer KD, Foster PS. Eosinophils: changing perspectives in health and disease. *Nat Rev Immunol*. 2013;13(1):9-20.

Sattasathuchana P, Steiner JM. Canine eosinophilic gastrointestinal disorders. *Anim Health Res Rev*. 2014;15(1):76-86.

Takeuchi Y, Matsuura S, Fujino Y, et al. Hypereosinophilic syndrome in two cats. *J Vet Med Sci*. 2008;70(10):1085-1089.

Wedi B, Gehring M, Kapp A. The pseudoallergen receptor MRGPRX2 on peripheral blood basophils and eosinophils: expression and function. *Allergy*. 2020;75(9):2229-2242.

Weller PF, Spencer LA. Functions of tissue resident eosinophils. *Nat Rev Immunol*. 2017;17(12):746-759.

Weller PF, Wang H, Melo RCN. The Charcot-Leyden crystal protein revisited – a lysopalmitoylphospholipase and more. *J Leukoc Biol*. 2020;108(1):105-112.

CHAPTER 5

The Mediators of Inflammation and Allergy

Many different cell types participate in allergic inflammation and produce a wide array of molecules contributing to these reactions. The primary sources of these molecules are mast cells, eosinophils, and basophils. However, many others such as epithelial and endothelial cells, lymphocytes, and other leukocytes also contribute. Inflammatory mediators originate from multiple sources. Some are derived from inactive precursors in plasma, whereas others are derived from sentinel cells such as macrophages and mast cells, from leukocytes such as neutrophils, basophils, and platelets, or are released by damaged tissues. Sensory nerves produce neurotransmitters that also cause inflammation, itch, and pain.

Acute inflammation develops within minutes after tissues are damaged. The damaged tissue generates three types of signals. First, broken cells release molecules (or damage-associated molecular patterns) that trigger the release of cytokines, chemokines, and enzymes from sentinel cells. These are also called alarmins. Second, invading microbes provide molecules (pathogen-associated molecular patterns [PAMPs]) that trigger additional sentinel cell responses. Third, tissue damage causes sensory nerves to release neuropeptides, resulting in pain or itch. This complex mixture of molecules attracts white blood cells and acts on blood vessels, resulting in increased local blood flow leading to redness and swelling.

Inflammatory Mediators

The major signs of inflammation, redness and swelling, result from changes in small blood vessels brought about by vasoactive molecules. Immediately after injury, blood flow through the small capillaries at the damaged site briefly decreases, allowing circulating leukocytes to bind to the blood vessel walls. Shortly after, the small blood vessels in the damaged area dilate, and blood flow to the injured tissue increases greatly. As these changes in blood flow occur, cellular responses are also occurring. These act on adjacent blood vessels to cause increased endothelial stickiness and permit circulating neutrophils and monocytes to adhere to vessel walls and then emigrate into tissues. If blood vessels are damaged, platelets may also bind to injured endothelium and release their vasoactive and clotting molecules. Inflamed tissues swell because of the leakage of fluid from blood vessels, which occurs in two stages. First, there is an immediate increase caused by vasoactive molecules produced by sentinel cells, damaged tissues, and nerves. The second stage occurs several hours after the onset of inflammation, when the leukocytes are beginning to emigrate. Endothelial and perivascular cells contract and pull apart, allowing fluid to escape through the intercellular spaces. After the invaders are eliminated, the inflammation subsides and blood flow returns to normal.

VASOACTIVE AMINES

Histamine

One of the most important mediators of allergic inflammation is histamine. Histamine is a small amine of only 111 kDa derived from the amino acid L-histidine by decarboxylation (Fig. 5.1).

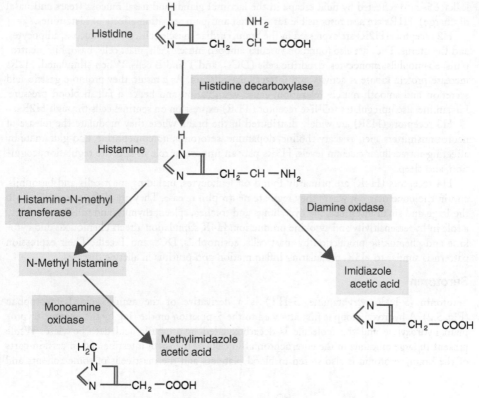

Fig. 5.1 The production, structure, and metabolism of histamine.

This reaction is mediated by the enzyme L-histidine decarboxylase. Histidine decarboxylase is expressed by many cell types, including neurons within the central nervous system, parietal cells in the gastrointestinal tract and, most importantly, mast cells and basophils. It is also present in small amounts in monocytes and lymphocytes. Once synthesized, histamine is stored in mast cell and basophil granules and released when these cells are appropriately stimulated. Histamine is also present in the brain, where it acts as a neurotransmitter. Histamine can be degraded either by methylation of its imidazole ring by histamine N-methyltransferase or oxidative deamination of its amino group by diamine oxidase.

Histamine exerts its effects by acting through four different cell receptors. These are designated H1, H2, H3, and H4 and are numbered in the order of their discovery. These histamine receptors transmit signals through G-proteins coupled to intracellular second messengers.

H1 receptors (H1R) are expressed on brain cells, sensory nerves, airway smooth muscle cells, the skin, gastrointestinal tract, genitourinary tract, adrenal medulla, immune cells, and heart and vascular endothelial cells. Signaling through H1R causes an increase in intracellular Ca^{++}. As a result, smooth muscle cells in the airways and gastrointestinal tract contract causing bronchoconstriction. H1R activation in vascular endothelial cells stimulates them to convert L-arginine to nitric oxide, a potent vasodilator and so causes a fall in blood pressure. The increase in intracellular Ca^{++} also stimulates the production of prostaglandins, which cause blood vessel endothelial cells to pull apart, leading to fluid escape and tissue edema, and resulting in urticaria (hives). The leakage is also reflected by fluid escape in the lacrimal glands and nasal mucosa (tears and nasal discharge). H1Rs are also responsible for the itch and pain sensation effects of histamines.

H2 receptors (H2R) are expressed in the brain, cardiac muscle cells, gastric mucosa, adipocytes, and the uterus. They are also found on vascular smooth muscle cells, mast cells, basophils, neutrophils, eosinophils, monocytes, dendritic cells (DCs), and T and B cells. When stimulated, H2Rs increase protein kinase A activity and intracellular calcium. As a result, they promote gastric acid secretion and smooth muscle relaxation, cause vasodilation and hence a fall in blood pressure. Histamine also upregulates toll-like receptor (TLR) expression on sentinel cells through H2Rs.

H3 receptors (H3R) are widely distributed in the brain, where they modulate the release of neurotransmitters such as acetylcholine, dopamine, serotonin, norepinephrine, and glutamate by affecting intracellular calcium levels. H3Rs play an important role in appetite regulation, cognition, and sleep.

H4 receptors (H4R) are primarily found on leukocytes, including mast cells and basophils, and in the bone marrow, where they regulate neutrophil release. They are also expressed in both the large and small intestines, the liver, lungs and trachea, spleen, thymus, and tonsils. They play a role in hypersensitivity and cytokine production. H4R stimulation affects chemotaxis and cytokine and chemokine production by mast cells, eosinophils, DCs, and T cells. Their expression pattern is similar to H3R, modulating inflammation and pruritus in allergic diseases.

Serotonin

Serotonin (5-hydroxytryptamine, 5-HT) is a derivative of the amino acid L-tryptophan (Fig. 5.2). A hydroxyl group is first attached to the 5-position on the ring by the enzyme tryptophan hydroxylase and the molecule is decarboxylated by aromatic acid decarboxylase. While present in large amounts in the enterochromaffin cells of the small intestine and in certain parts of the brain, serotonin is also stored in blood platelets and the mast cells of some rodents and

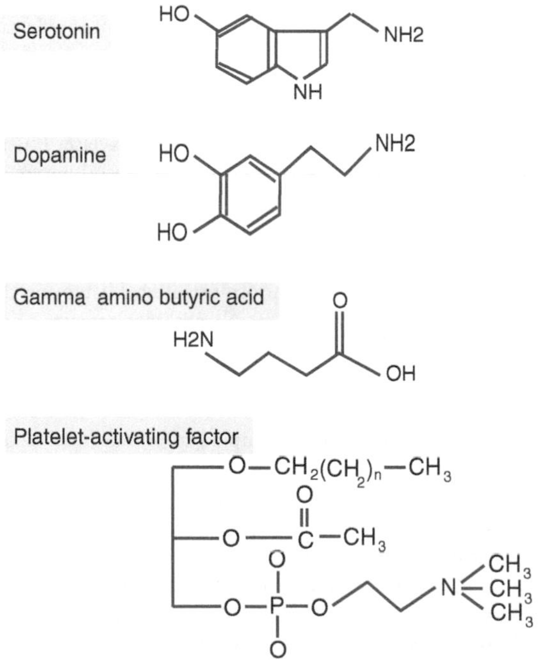

Fig. 5.2 The structure of some of the major vasoactive molecules generated during acute inflammation.

large domestic herbivores. Serotonin causes vasoconstriction that increases blood pressure (except in cattle, where it is a vasodilator), and it has little effect on vascular permeability, except in rodents where it induces acute inflammation.

Dopamine

Dopamine is a contraction of 3,4-dihydroxyphenethylamine. Dopamine can be synthesized, stored, and secreted by mast cells. It is stored within mast cell granules bound to the proteoglycan. Tyrosine hydroxylase expression, a key component of the dopamine synthesis pathway, increases as mast cells mature. While the function of dopamine in allergies is unclear, it can bind to receptors on lymphocytes and suppress their proliferation. It impairs neutrophil function, activates macrophages, and stimulates natural killer (NK) cell activity. Dopamine may also act directly on neurons and serve as a neurotransmitter. Dopamine is a major mediator in cattle and is released in large amounts during bovine anaphylaxis. Both serotonin and dopamine are ligands of the aryl hydrocarbon receptor (Chapter 9).

Gamma-Aminobutyric Acid (GABA)

GABA is a neurotransmitter released by stimulated neurons. Immune cells possess receptors for this neurotransmitter and it regulates their production of cytokines. GABA acts on airway epithelium in response to activation by allergens, contributing to the pathogenesis of asthma.

VASOACTIVE PEPTIDES

Complement Components

When the complement system is activated, several of its components are subjected to proteolytic digestion and small peptides are cleaved off from their peptide chains. Two of these small peptides, C3a and C5a, have significant proinflammatory activity and are called anaphylatoxins. (A third small complement peptide, C4a is also classed as an anaphylatoxin but has limited biological activity.) Both peptides have a molecular weight of approximately 9 kDa. C3a contains 77 amino acids and C5a contains 74. They share only 36% sequence homology, and C5a is glycosylated.

Anaphylatoxins are potent inflammatory mediators that influence innate immunity by mediating chemotaxis, regulating vascular dilation and permeability, and killing bacteria. They cause smooth muscle contraction, induce wheal-and-flare reactions on intradermal injection, and activate platelets. They can induce a respiratory burst in macrophages, neutrophils, and eosinophils. Anaphylatoxins bind to receptors on mast cells and promote degranulation and the release of histamine and leukotrienes. They stimulate the release of eosinophil cationic protein and promote eosinophil migration. They modulate the release of interleukin 6 (IL-6) and tumor necrosis factor-α (TNF-α) from B cells and monocytes. They are also potent attractants for monocytes, neutrophils, activated B and T cells, basophils, and mast cells. Anaphylatoxins regulate tissue regeneration and fibrosis, and brain development.

Kinins

As described in Chapter 3, much of the mast cell granule content consists of the highly sulfated proteoglycan heparin, which is released when mast cells degranulate. Thus, heparin provides a readily available negatively charged surface to which blood clotting factor XII can bind and become activated. This contact activation induces a conformational change, permitting factor XII to act as a protease and activate other high-molecular-weight proteases called kallikreins. Once activated, the kallikreins act on kininogens to release small vasoactive peptides called kinins (Fig. 5.3). Kinins increase vascular permeability, and stimulate smooth muscle contraction and trigger pain receptors. They may also have defensin-like antimicrobial activity. The most

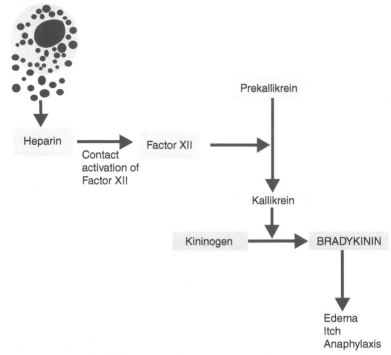

Fig. 5.3 The generation of bradykinin as a result of contact activation of Factor XII by the proteoglycan heparin derived from mast cell granules.

important of these kinins is bradykinin, which contains nine amino acids with the sequence: Arg-Pro-Pro-Gly-Phe-Ser-Pro-Phe-Arg. It acts through its G-protein coupled receptors, B1R and B2R, to activate signaling pathways leading to increases in vascular permeability and vasodilation, resulting in hypotension and tissue edema. Bradykinin also causes pain and fever. Bradykinin is short-lived and is rapidly degraded by kininases; however, it triggers the production of superoxide radicals and nitric oxide and stimulates the release of histamine, arachidonic acid, prostaglandin E_2 (PGE$_2$), IL-1, and TNF-α. Bradykinin is involved in the activation of neutrophils, DCs, and macrophages. Other kinins that might play a role in allergies include lysylbradykinin (also called kallidin) and methionyl-lysyl-bradykinin.

Neuropeptides

Many peptides secreted by neurons and glial cells have a profound influence on inflammation and immunity. They all act on target cells via G-protein-linked receptors.

One of the most important of these peptides is substance P (SP). SP is a member of the tachykinin family that acts both as a neurotransmitter and as a mediator of allergic inflammation. The tachykinins are a family of related neuropeptides that have significant proinflammatory effects by acting on target cells through neurokinin receptors. These receptors are found on cutaneous sensory neurons and glia, vascular endothelial cells, fibroblasts, mast cells, and leukocytes. SP is a peptide of 11 amino acids with the sequence Arg-Pro-Lys-Pro-Gln-Gln-Phe-Phe-Gly-Leu-Met. It is a key mediator of neurogenic inflammation.

SP is released from sensory nerve terminals in the skin, joints, and muscles in response to stressors. It is also produced by inflammatory cells, including macrophages, eosinophils, lymphocytes, and DCs. SP induces degranulation and the release of histamine and serotonin by human and rat mast cells. It also activates eosinophils, triggering their degranulation and production of superoxide, and enhancing their chemotactic responses to platelet-activating factor (PAF) and leukotriene B_4 (LTB$_4$). SP activates the arachidonate pathway to trigger prostaglandin synthesis, and it evokes the release of other neurotransmitters such as histamine, acetylcholine, and GABA from spinal ganglia. It promotes wound healing. It is a potent vasodilator and bronchoconstrictor and plays an important role in pain and itch perception. Other related neuropeptides such as neurokinin K and calcitonin gene-related peptide (CGRP) produced by sensory nerves also cause pain, trigger vasodilation, and increase vascular permeability (Chapter 6).

VASOACTIVE LIPIDS

Eicosanoids

When tissues are damaged or sentinel cells activated, inflammasomes are generated. These protein complexes activate phospholipases that act on cell wall phospholipids to release arachidonic acid, a 20-carbon unsaturated fatty acid (Fig. 5.4). Within 5–30 min, the enzyme 5-lipoxygenase converts this arachidonic acid to biologically active lipids called leukotrienes. Alternatively,

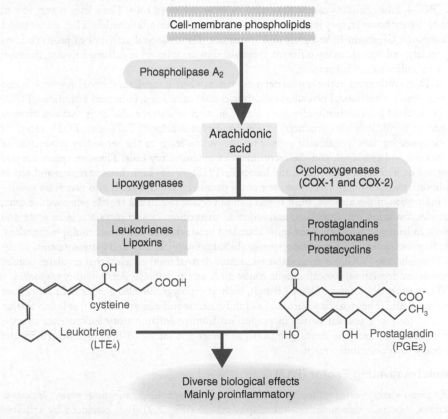

Fig. 5.4 **The production of leukotrienes and prostaglandins by the actions of lipoxygenase and cyclooxygenase on arachidonic acid.** Both prostaglandins and leukotrienes may have proinflammatory or antiinflammatory activity depending on their chemical structure. Note that the leukotrienes are linked to the amino acid cysteine.

another enzyme, prostaglandin endoperoxide synthase, commonly called cyclooxygenase (COX), converts arachidonic acid to a different family of vasoactive lipids called prostaglandins. There are two isoforms of this enzyme, COX-1 and COX-2. COX-1 mediates the production of low levels of prostaglandins in normal tissues, whereas COX-2 causes an increase in prostaglandin production in inflamed tissues. COX-2 is the target of many non-steroidal anti-inflammatory drugs. The collective term for all these complex lipids is eicosanoids.

Four leukotrienes promote leukocyte recruitment, survival, and activation. The most important of these, LTB_4, is a neutrophil attractant and activator produced by neutrophils, macrophages, and mast cells. LTB_4 also stimulates eosinophil chemotaxis and random motility. Leukotrienes C_4, D_4, and E_4, in contrast, increase vascular permeability and cause slow smooth muscle contraction. All three contain the amino acid cysteine conjugated to the lipid backbone, and are called cysteinyl leukotrienes. They are produced by mast cells, eosinophils, and basophils. While IL-13 upregulates the production of LTD_4, stimulation of its receptor, LTD_4 upregulates IL-13 production. This feedback loop is a major contributor to allergic inflammation. Collectively, the mixture of the three leukotrienes constitutes slow-reacting substance of anaphylaxis (SRS-A), which is a thousand times more potent than histamine but causes slower muscle contraction and has a longer duration of action, hence its name.

There are four major proinflammatory prostaglandins: PGE_2, $PGF_2\alpha$, PGD_2, and prostacyclin (PGI_2). Prostaglandins can be generated by most nucleated cells. Their level is very low in normal tissues; however, they increase significantly during acute inflammation. They act on target cells through G-protein-linked prostanoid receptors. The biological activities of prostaglandins vary widely, and because many different prostaglandins are released in inflamed tissues, their net effect on inflammation is complex.

PGD_2 is synthesized in the central nervous system, where it regulates sleep. However, it is also the predominant prostanoid produced by activated mast cells. Thus, in human asthmatics, PGD_2 can be detected in bronchoalveolar fluid within minutes of allergen challenge and can increase at least 150-fold. It is also produced by DCs and type 2 helper (Th2) cells. PGD_2 receptors are expressed on airway epithelial cells. Their activation leads to the secondary production of chemokines and cytokines, and the recruitment of inflammatory cells. These receptors are also expressed on Th2 cells, eosinophils, and basophils. PGD_2 causes bronchoconstriction and acts as a pulmonary and coronary vasoconstrictor and a peripheral vasodilator. It also promotes eosinophil infiltration of the airways. $PGF_2\alpha$ plays an important role in the female reproductive tract, regulating ovulation and luteolysis, and inducing parturition. It also plays a role in acute and chronic inflammation. PGE_2 is the most abundant prostaglandin and serves multiple functions, including the regulation of immune responses, blood pressure, fertility, and gastrointestinal integrity. Thromboxane (TXA_2) is an unstable eicosanoid derived from platelets that regulates platelet adhesion and regulation, smooth muscle contraction, and endothelial inflammatory responses.

When neutrophils enter inflamed tissues, their 15-lipoxygenase also generates lipoxins from arachidonic acid. These oxidized eicosanoids inhibit neutrophil migration. Thus, as inflammation proceeds, there is a gradual switch in production from proinflammatory leukotrienes to anti-inflammatory lipoxins. The increase in PGE_2 in tissues also inhibits 5-lipoxygenase activity and eventually suppresses inflammation.

Platelet-Activating Factor (PAF)

PAF, acetyl-glyceryl-ether-phosphorylcholine, is a phospholipid affecting many leukocyte functions, especially inflammation and anaphylaxis (see Fig. 5.2). It is produced by activated neutrophils, mast cells, basophils, eosinophils, platelets, and endothelial cells. PAF is a potent bronchoconstrictor that decreases cardiac blood flow and contractility and increases pulmonary resistance. PAF makes endothelial cells even stickier, and thus enhances neutrophil adhesion and emigration from the bloodstream. PAF aggregates platelets and stimulates them to release their vasoactive molecules and synthesize thromboxane. It similarly acts on neutrophils, promoting neutrophil aggregation, degranulation, chemotaxis, and the release of oxidants. Many of the cells that can produce PAF also respond to it in an autocrine manner. Its release from mast cells and basophils can be triggered by antibodies against immunoglobulin E (IgE), implying a relationship to allergic sensitization. Intradermal injection of PAF will induce a wheal-and-flare reaction and pruritus, probably because of secondary histamine release. PAF plays a key role as a mediator of severe anaphylaxis in some species. It is incredibly potent, and its activity can be detected at concentrations as low as 10^{-12}M. PAF is approximately 10,000 times more effective than histamine in increasing vascular permeability.

PROTEASES

Tryptases and chymases play an important role in allergic inflammation. Four genes encode different mast cell tryptases – α, β, γ, and δ. The most important of these is tryptase δ, which is stored in mast cell granules as a pro-tryptase. It is released in bursts from degranulating mast cells, and after activation, it forms tetramers, which create a central cavity lined by the four enzymatically active sites. The released tryptases contribute to the development of urticaria, angioedema, and bronchospasm. Basophils contain much less tryptase than mast cells.

Mastin is a tryptic protease produced by canine mast cells. Similar to tryptases, it can form active tetramers with a central pore where the active sites are located. It was originally found in canine mastocytomas and was called mastocytoma protease. Mastin-like enzymes have been identified in pigs and mice.

Cytokines

While hundreds of cytokines control almost all aspects of cellular functions, some are more important than others. These include the three cytokines TNF-α, IL-1, and IL-6 that initiate innate immune responses and the resulting inflammation. They also include the three major epithelial cell cytokines, IL-33, IL-25, and thymic stromal lymphopoietin (TSLP) that enhance and regulate allergic inflammation. Two other cytokines that contribute significantly to allergic inflammation, IL-9 and IL-31, are also discussed here. Finally, many smaller proteins called chemokines attract appropriate cells to inflammatory sites and promote their response.

INITIATING CYTOKINES

When exposed to infectious agents or PAMPs via pattern recognition receptors, sentinel cell signaling pathways activate the genes that cause the synthesis and secretion of three major cytokines. These are TNF-α, IL-1, and IL-6. TNF-α is produced very early in inflammation and is followed by waves of IL-1 and IL-6. Activated sentinel cells also secrete a mixture of chemokines, which attract leukocytes to microbial invasion sites. Simultaneously, the activated cells synthesize enzymes such as nitric oxide synthase 2 (NOS2) that, in turn, generates nitric oxide, a powerful and lethal oxidant. They also make the enzyme COX-2 that generates prostaglandins. When these molecules reach the brain and liver, they cause fever and sickness behavior, and promote an acute-phase response. If the sentinel cells detect the presence of damaged or foreign DNA or RNA, such as that from viruses, they will also secrete the antiviral interferons IFN-α and IFN-β.

Tumor Necrosis Factor-α (TNF-α)

TNF-α is a protein of 17 Da produced by endothelial cells, T cells, B cells, and fibroblasts in response to TLR stimulation (Fig. 5.5). It is initially membrane-bound but is subsequently cleaved from the cell surface by a protease called TNF-α convertase. TNF-α acts through two

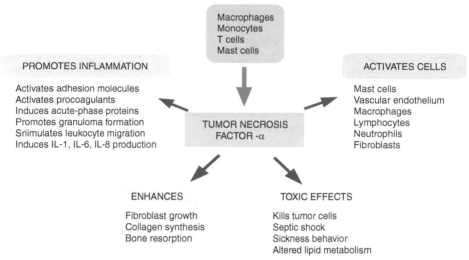

Fig. 5.5 The sources and functions of TNF-α.

receptors: TNFR1 is found on many different cells, where it can bind both soluble and membrane-bound TNF-α; and TNFR2 is restricted to immune system cells and responds only to membrane-bound TNF-α.

Soluble TNF-α triggers the release of chemokines and cytokines from nearby cells and promotes the adherence, migration, attraction, and activation of leukocytes. Subsequently, TNF-α facilitates the transition from innate to adaptive immunity. TNF-α production is stimulated through the TLRs and by neurotransmitters such as neurokinin-1.

TNF-α is an essential mediator of inflammation because, in combination with IL-1, it triggers changes in small blood vessels. A local increase in TNF-α causes the classic signs of inflammation, including heat, swelling, pain, and redness. Circulating TNF-α can depress cardiac output, induce microvascular thrombosis, and cause capillary leakage. TNF-α acts on neutrophils to enhance their ability to kill microbes. It attracts neutrophils to sites of tissue damage and increases their adherence to vascular endothelium. TNF-α stimulates macrophage phagocytosis and oxidant production; amplifies and prolongs inflammation by promoting macrophage synthesis of important enzymes such as NOS2 and COX-2; and activates mast cells. TNF-α induces macrophages to increase its own synthesis, together with that of IL-1. TNF-α can kill some tumor and virus-infected cells. In high doses, TNF-α can cause septic shock.

Interleukin 1 (IL-1)

When stimulated through CD14 and TLR4, sentinel cells also synthesize cytokines of the IL-1 family. These are mainly produced by monocytes, macrophages, and DCs, with smaller amounts from B, NK, epithelial cells, and fibroblasts. The most important members of the family are IL-1α and IL-1β (Fig. 5.6). IL-1β is produced as a large precursor protein that is cleaved by caspase-1 to form the active 17kDa molecule. Ten- to 50-fold more IL-1β is produced than IL-1α, and whereas IL-1β is secreted, IL-1α remains attached to the cell surface. Therefore, IL-1α only acts on cells that come into direct contact with macrophages. Transcription of IL-1β messenger RNA occurs within 15 min of ligand binding. It reaches a peak 3 to 4 h later and levels off for several hours before decreasing.

Like TNF-α, IL-1β initiates and amplifies inflammation. For example, it acts on vascular endothelial cells to make them bind neutrophils. IL-1 also acts on macrophages to stimulate their

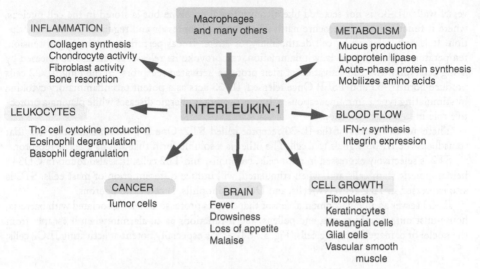

Fig. 5.6 The sources and functions of interleukin-1.

synthesis of NOS2 and COX-2. During severe infections, IL-1β circulates in the bloodstream where, in association with TNF-α, it is responsible for sickness behavior, acting on the brain to cause fever, lethargy, and malaise. It acts on muscle cells to mobilize amino acids, causing pain and fatigue, and liver cells to induce the production of acute-phase proteins that assist in the defense of the body. IL-1 is a member of a large family of cytokines that regulate innate immune responses. Other important family members include IL-1RA, IL-18, IL-33, IL-36, IL-37, and IL-38, which signal through closely related receptors. Some, like IL-36, have a proinflammatory effect, while others, such as IL-37, have anti-inflammatory effects.

Interleukin 6 (IL-6)

IL-6 is a glycoprotein of 21 kDa produced by macrophages and T and mast cells. Its production is triggered by bacterial endotoxins and by IL-1 and TNF-α. IL-6 promotes inflammation, especially in response to tissue damage and severe infections, and it is a major mediator of fever, the acute-phase response, and septic shock. IL-6 receptors are found on T cells, neutrophils, macrophages, hepatocytes, and neurons. IL-6 plays an anti-inflammatory role by inhibiting TNF-α and IL-1 activities and promoting the production of the suppressive cytokine IL-10. IL-6 might also regulate the transition from a neutrophil-dominated process early in inflammation to a macrophage-dominated process later.

MASTER CYTOKINES

As stated previously, three cytokines produced by damaged epithelial cells play a critical role in triggering and regulating allergic inflammation. These are IL-33, IL-25, and TSLP. All three promote Th2 and type 2 innate lymphoid (ILC2) cell activation and cytokine production.

Interleukin 33 (IL-33)

IL-33 is a protein of 30 kDa belonging to the IL-1 family and is found in many different cell types, especially those acting as epithelial barriers. These include keratinocytes, bronchial epithelial cells, and enterocytes. Because of its presence in endothelial cells, it is also found in blood vessel walls. IL-33 is not secreted like a conventional cytokine but is stored in the cell nucleus, where it functions as a heterochromatin transcriptional repressor and regulates DNA transcription. It is only released by cell death, injury, or stress. Local perturbations in oxygen tension, temperature, pH, and especially inflammation, can provoke its release. It can also be released by living cells following the activation of their protease-activated receptors. In the lung, ILC2 cells produce both IL-33 and TSLP. Once released, IL-33 acts as a potent proinflammatory cytokine by stimulating type 2 immune responses. It thus promotes allergic diseases while playing a protective role in helminth infections.

There are two forms of the IL-33 receptor called ST2. One is a transmembrane form that transduces the IL-33 signals to a cell. The other is a soluble form that acts as a decoy receptor.

ST2 is selectively expressed in mast cells, basophils, and Th2 cells. It is also found in CD34$^+$ hematopoietic stem cells and, when stimulated, will induce differentiation of mast cells. ST2 is also expressed in Treg cells, NK cells, and DCs, eosinophils, B cells, and neurons.

IL-33 serves as an environmental sensor that detects protease activity associated with bacteria, house dust mites, mold spores, and pollens, and it functions as an alarmin when it escapes from the nuclei of damaged or dying cells (Fig. 5.7). IL-33 is especially potent at activating ILC2 cells;

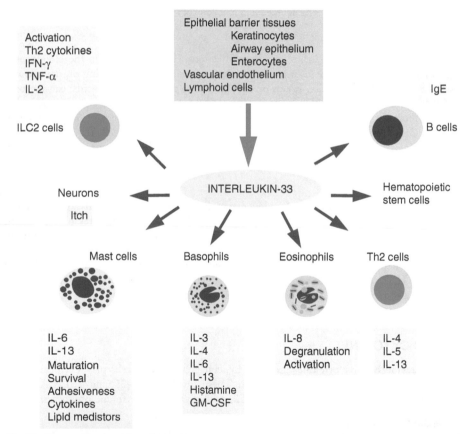

Fig. 5.7 The sources and functions of interleukin-33. IL-33 is released by dying cells as well as epithelial cells in response to PAMPs. It stimulates the production of inflammatory cytokines and chemokines from many different cell types. It stimulates the production and activation of eosinophils. It acts on sensory neurons to induce itch. It is therefore a major contributor to the development of allergic disease.

however, it also activates DC2, Th2, Tfh, Treg and mast cells. Therefore, IL-33 release by protease-activated epithelial cells results in the development of type 2 allergic inflammation. IL-33 is a key inducer of the type 2 cytokines, IL-4, IL-5, and IL-13. (IL-33 together with IL-25 and TSLP all promote Th2 responses, but IL-33 is by far the most potent.) When IL-33 is incubated with extracts from molds, house dust mites, and pollens, or by neutrophil and mast cell proteases, it is broken into short, potent peptides. These peptides promote type 2 activity by stimulating mast cell and ILC2 cell production of IL-5, IL-6, and IL-13, and thus triggering eosinophil production.

IL-33 promotes IgE-mediated degranulation of mast cells as well as IgE production, eosinophilia, and goblet cell proliferation. Additionally, it induces mast cell production of leukotrienes and cytokines and can trigger acute allergic attacks in the absence of allergens. Similarly, it can stimulate basophils to release their Th2 cytokines. IL-33 binds to sensory neurons, triggering intense pruritus and scratching behavior. IL-33 levels are elevated in the blood of humans suffering anaphylactic shock, in helminth infections, in atopic human tissues, and in the lungs of those with severe asthma. When IL-33 and the neuropeptide SP are administered together, they synergize and cause a massive, 1000-fold increase in TNF-α production by mast cells. IL-33 is thus a key mediator of atopic disease.

Thymic Stromal Lymphopoietin (TSLP)

TSLP was originally detected in culture fluid from a thymus cell line. It is a 15 kDa member of the IL-2 family that is a key regulator of type 2 inflammation at mucosal barriers (Fig. 5.8). It is expressed by cells on body surfaces, including bronchial and colonic epithelial cells, mast cells,

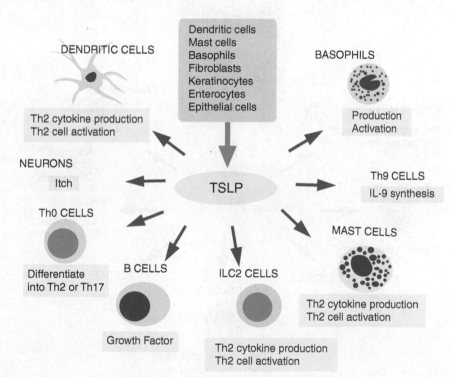

Fig. 5.8 **The sources and functions of thymic stromal lymphopoietin (TSLP).** Note that this cytokine is also a major itch mediator.

keratinocytes, tuft cells, and lung fibroblasts. Its highest expression is found in bronchial smooth muscle cells and keratinocytes. TSLP production is upregulated in inflamed skin, especially when associated with epidermal barrier dysfunction. TSLP is produced by keratinocytes and mast cells in response to antimicrobial peptides such as β-defensins and cathelicidins. Its release is also stimulated by contact with allergens (especially those with protease activity), infections, and some chemicals. TSLP receptors are expressed on DC2, T, B, and mast cells, eosinophils, basophils, airway epithelial and innate lymphoid cells.

TSLP may be considered a master regulator that triggers and maintains allergic inflammation at barrier surfaces. Its activities overlap significantly with the other two master cytokines, IL-33 and IL-25. Like IL-33, TSLP activates DC2 cells and stimulates their production of type 2 cytokines, which promote IgE production. The activated DC2 cells also secrete chemokines that attract neutrophils and eosinophils. TSLP causes DC2 cells to release the chemokines CCL17 and CCL22 that specifically attract Th2 cells. TSLP stimulates basophil production in the bone marrow, and over 70% of activated basophils express TSLP receptors. TSLP is also a potent mediator of itching because its receptors are expressed on the dorsal root ganglia neurons and sensory nerve endings that mediate itch. Thus, when keratinocytes release TSLP, these act on nearby neurons to cause severe itching.

Interleukin 25 (IL-25)

The third master cytokine, IL-25, is an 18 kDa member of the IL-17 family (Fig. 5.9). Its major sources are Th2, epithelial, tuft, and innate lymphoid cells. It is also produced by alveolar macrophages, DCs, mast cells, basophils, eosinophils, keratinocytes, and mucosal epithelial cells. Its

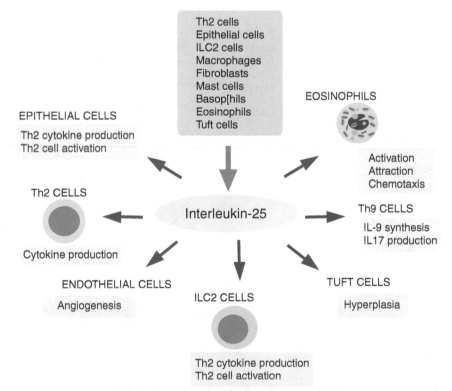

Fig. 5.9 The sources and functions of interleukin-25.

release is triggered by exposure to proteases such as tryptase. Mast cells produce IL-25 after cross-linking of their FcεRI, IgE receptors Basophils also produce IL-25 after IgE receptor cross-linking. Unlike IL-33 that is stored in the nucleus, IL-25 is expressed in the cell cytosol. IL-25 receptors are expressed in Th2 cells, fibroblasts, epithelial cells, endothelial cells, and eosinophils.

IL-25 induces DC responses that initiate and sustain type 2 responses. Unlike other members of the IL-17 family that attract neutrophils, IL-25 attracts eosinophils, induces an eosinophilia, and promotes IgE production. It is a major activator of ILC2 cells. Eosinophils produce IL-25 after treatment with IL-5 and granulocyte/macrophage colony stimulating factor (GM-CSF). Repeated intranasal application of IL-25 results in the production of IL-5 and IL-13 and the induction of airway hypersensitivity. When lung epithelial cells are exposed to allergens such as *Aspergillus* or ragweed pollen, IL-25 production is upregulated, suggesting that it might also initiate respiratory allergic responses. IL-25 promotes angiogenesis and activates Th2 and ILC2 cells and induces IL-9 production. Other targets of IL-25 are fibroblasts and epithelial cells, which it induces to secrete eotaxins. These can recruit both eosinophils and Th2 cells.

Tuft Cells. Among the less-common cells that line the small intestine are tuft cells, so called because they have a small tuft of apical microvilli that extends into the intestinal lumen. These cells play a key role in initiating type 2 immune responses to parasitic helminths. Tuft cells sense the "taste" of intestinal helminths. In response, they produce large amounts of IL-25, which recruits eosinophils and activates Th2 and ILC2 cells. IL-13 and IL-4 from the activated ILC2 cells then stimulate further tuft cell proliferation and IL-25 production. In the presence of helminths, IL-25 promotes hyperplasia of tuft cells and mucus-producing goblet cells. IL-13 acts together with IL-4 to promote allergic inflammation, and increase gut motility and mucus production. This combination of local hypersensitivity and increased motility and mucus secretion can expel many helminth parasites (Fig. 5.10).

If parasitic worms cause tissue damage, this will trigger the release of all three Th2-stimulating cytokines, TSLP, IL-25 and IL-33, from enterocytes. These cytokines target DC2 and ILC2 cells. For example, TSLP activates DCs, IL-25 stimulates the production of type 2 cytokines by ILC2 cells and facilitates differentiation of Th2 cells. IL-33 acts on Th2 cells, ILC2 cells, basophils, and mast cells to drive IL-4, IL-5, and IL-13 production.

In response to this flood of cytokines, T cells release their own effector cytokines. For example, T cells in the intestinal epithelium produce IL-4 and IL-25. Similarly, Th2 cells produce more IL-4 in a positive feedback loop, generating other Th2 cytokines and IL-25. The IL-4 activates the transcription factor STAT6, which upregulates GATA3 and causes differentiation into Th2 cells and suppresses Th1 responses. IL-6 acts with TGF-β to induce Th17 responses. IL-13 repairs epithelia, enhances mucus production, and together with IL-9, recruits and activates mucosal mast cells. Both IL-4 and IL-13 activate enterocytes, smooth muscle cells, and macrophages. Increased enterocyte proliferation and turnover may cause parasite disengagement. These cytokines also increase intestinal permeability and fluid secretion. The Th2 cytokines stimulate Paneth cells, and a consequent increase in intestinal defensins may damage helminths. The cytokines also stimulate goblet cells to produce a resistin-like molecule that interferes with worm feeding.

OTHER IMPORTANT CYTOKINES

Interleukin 9 (IL-9)

IL-9 is a glycoprotein of approximately 40 kDa produced by Th2 cells. A subset of Th2 cells that can be stimulated by IL-4 and TGFβ to produce large quantities of IL-9 has been called Th9 cells (Fig. 5.11). Th9 cells are generated by a combination of IL-4 and TGFβ. IL-25 and TSLP treatment of these cells also induces IL-9 release and enhances allergic responses. Other cells that can produce IL-9 include ILC2 cells and a subset of mucosal mast cells.

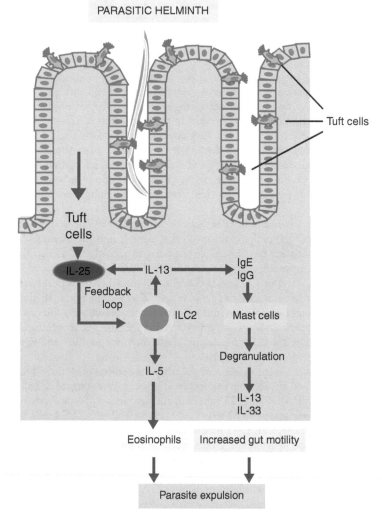

Fig. 5.10 **The role of Tuft cells in sensing and responding to the presence of parasitic helminths in the intestine.** They generate IL-25 that in turn activates ILC2 cells in the submucosa. These cells then release cytokines, triggering a strong Th2 response, eosinophil infiltration, and eventually, worm expulsion.

IL-9 promotes the differentiation of Th2 and ILC2 cells, Th1 cells where it reduces differentiation, mast cells where it promotes mediator release, and eosinophils where it promotes their development and survival. The main function of IL-9-producing cells is probably to defend against helminths. However, they are found in the blood of allergic patients, where their numbers correlate with IgE levels and enhance allergic inflammation by promoting mast cell activation. Th9 cells exacerbate chronic allergic inflammation in the lungs and are strongly linked to the development of asthma. They play important roles in the development of atopic dermatitis, allergic contact dermatitis, and food allergies.

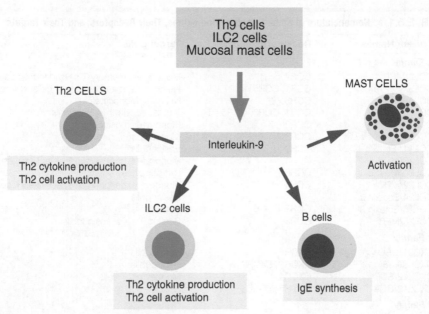

Fig. 5.11 The sources and functions of interleukin-9.

Interleukin 31 (IL-31)

IL-31 is a protein of 18 kDa and a member of the IL-6 family. It is produced by activated Th2 cells, mast cells, macrophages, basophils, and DCs. Its receptors are expressed on keratinocytes and other epithelial cells, eosinophils, activated macrophages, and especially on dorsal root ganglia neurons and peripheral neurons. When activated, they signal to cells via the Janus kinase pathway. IL-31 is a potent inducer of itch and skin inflammation, and plays a key role in the pathogenesis of atopic dermatitis. It also stimulates the production of T cell-attracting chemokines that further promote Th2 cell immigration and inflammation. IL-31 is released by Th2 cells partially in response to histamine acting via H2 receptors (see Fig. 6.4). IL-31 activity can be blocked by the monoclonal antibody, lokivetmab (Chapter 17).

Chemokines

Chemokines are a large family of 8–10kDa proteins. They coordinate the migration of leukocytes and dictate the course of many inflammatory and immune responses via their chemotactic activities (Table 5.1). In addition to being chemotactic, chemokines activate immune cells. Chemokines are produced by sentinel cells, including macrophages and mast cells. They are classified into subfamilies based on their amino acid sequences. For example, the CXC chemokines have two cysteine (C) residues separated by another amino acid (X), whereas the CC chemokines have two adjacent cysteine residues. Chemokine nomenclature is based on each molecule or receptor receiving a numerical designation. In addition, ligands have the suffix "L" [e.g., CXCL8], whereas receptors have the suffix "R" [e.g., CXCR1].)

TABLE 5.1 ■ Nomenclature of Some Selected Chemokines, Their Receptors, and Their Targets

Current Names	Receptor	Target Cells
α Family		
CCL2/MCP-1	CCR2	Monocytes, memory T cells, dendritic cells
CCL3/MIP-1a	CCR1, CCR5	Neutrophils, macrophages, T cells, NK cells
CCL4/MIP-1b	CCR5	NK cells, Monocytes
CCL5/RANTES	CCR1, CCR3, CCR5	T cells, eosinophils, basophils
CCL7/MCP-3	CCR3	Monocytes, eosinophils
CCL8	CCR3	Monocytes
CCL11/ Eotaxin 1	CCR3	Eosinophils
CCL13/MCP-4	CCR3	Monocytes, eosinophils, T cells, basophils
CCL20/MIP-3a	CCR6	Lymphocytes
CCL22/MDC	CCR4	Monocytes, dendritic cells, activated T cells
CCL24/Eotaxin 2		Eosinophils
CCL26/Eotaxin 3	CCR3	Eosinophils
CCL28/MEC	CCR3	Resting T cells, eosinophils
β Family		
CXCL1/GRO1	CXCR2	Neutrophils
CXCL8/IL-8	CXCR1, CXCR2	Neutrophils
CXCL12/SDF	CXCR4	Monocytes, T cells
CXCL13/BCA-1	CXCR5	B cells
γ Family		
XCL1/Lymphotactin	XCR1	T cells
δ Family		
CX3CL1/Fractalkine	CX3CR1	T cells, monocytes

The classification of chemokines is based on the location and spacing of their cysteine (C) residues and their separation by other (X) amino acids. L (Ligand), R (receptor).

Inflammatory chemokines are upregulated in inflammation and are mainly involved in leukocyte recruitment. Others promote new blood vessel growth. Some are found in normal tissues, where they regulate cellular migration and homing, and many have overlapping functions.

One of the most important chemokines is CXCL8 (also called interleukin 8). CXCL8 attracts and activates neutrophils, triggering granule release and stimulating their respiratory burst. Another important chemokine is CXCL2, which is secreted by macrophages and attracts neutrophils.

CC chemokines act predominantly on macrophages and DCs. Thus, CCL3 and CCL4 are produced by macrophages and mast cells. CCL4 attracts CD4$^+$ T cells, whereas CCL3 attracts B cells, eosinophils, and cytotoxic T cells. CCL2 is produced by macrophages, T cells, fibroblasts, keratinocytes, and endothelial cells. It attracts and activates monocytes, stimulating their respiratory burst and lysosomal enzyme release. CCL5 is produced by T cells and macrophages. It attracts monocytes, eosinophils, and some T cells. It activates eosinophils and stimulates histamine release from basophils.

Most chemokines are produced in infected or damaged tissues and attract other cells to sites of inflammation or microbial invasion. The chemokine mixture produced by damaged or infected tissues likely regulates the precise composition of incoming inflammatory cell populations. In this way, the body can adjust these cellular responses to optimize the destruction of different microbial invaders. Many chemokines, such as CXCL4, CCL20, and CCL5, are structurally similar to the antimicrobial defensins and have antibacterial activity.

Suggested Reading

Bach MK. Mediators of anaphylaxis and inflammation. *Annu Rev Microbiol.* 1982;36:371-413.

Caughey GH. Tryptase genetics and anaphylaxis. *J Allergy Clin Immunol.* 2006;117(6):1411-1414.

Cayrol C, Duval A, Schmitt P, et al. Environmental allergens induce allergic inflammation through proteolytic maturation of IL-33. *Nat Immunol.* 2018;19(4):375-385.

Haraldsen G, Balogh J, Pollheimer J, Sponheim J, Kuchler AM. Interleukin-33 – cytokine of dual function or novel alarmin? *Trends Immunol.* 2009;30(5):227-233.

Harrison S, Geppetti P. Substance P. *Int J Biochem Cell Biol.* 2001;33(6):555-576.

Klos A, Tenner AJ, Johswich KO, Ager RR, Reis ES, Kohl J. The role of anaphylatoxins in health and disease. *Mol Immunol.* 2009;46(14):2753-2766. doi:10.1016/j.molimm.2009.04.027.

Oschatz C, Maas C, Lecher B, et al. Mast cells increase vascular permeability by heparin-initiated bradykinin formation in vivo. *Immunity.* 2011;34(2):258-268.

Peine M, Marek RM, Lohning M. IL-33 in T cell differentiation, function, and immune homeostasis. *Trends Immunol.* 2016;37(5):321-331.

Peters LJ, Kovacic JP. Histamine: metabolism, physiology, and pathophysiology with applications in veterinary medicine. *J Vet Emerg Crit Care.* 2009;19(4):311-328.

Regoli D, Gobeil F. Kinins and peptide receptors. *Biol Chem.* 2016;397(4):297-304.

Ricciotti E, Fitzgerald GA. Prostaglandins and inflammation. *Arterioscler Thromb Vasc Biol.* 2011;31(5):986-1000.

Sala-Cunill A, Bjorkqvist J, Senter R, et al. Plasma contact system activation drives anaphylaxis in severe mast cell-mediated allergic reactions. *J Allergy Clin Immunol.* 2015;135(4):1031-1043.

Schneider C, O'Leary CE, Locksley RM. Regulation of immune responses by tuft cells. *Nat Rev Immunol.* 2019;19(9):584-593. doi:10.1038/s41577-019-0176-x.

Tsuge K, Inazumi T, Shimamoto A, Sugimoto Y. Molecular mechanisms underlying prostaglandin E2-exacerbated inflammation and immune diseases. *Int Immunol.* 2019;31(9):597-606. doi:10.1093/intimm/dxz021.

CHAPTER 6

The Itch-Scratch Cycle

In addition to its role as a protective barrier, the skin is innervated by a dense network of somatosensory neurons. The function of these neurons is to convert sensory stimuli into perceptions such as temperature, touch, pain, and itch by transmitting signals from the skin to the central nervous system. These sensory neurons share functions with innate immune responses in that they detect and respond to environmental stimuli. In addition, the nervous system and the immune system communicate. Soluble mediators from immune system cells activate neurons while simultaneously, neurotransmitters cause the local activation of immune system cells. The itch sensation mediated by cutaneous nerves is a prime example of this. Itch sensation occurs in all mammals, where it serves to trigger scratching, a protective response against irritating ectoparasites and toxins. Itch is caused by the actions of a complex mixture of chemical mediators released by diverse skin cells. These itch mediators bind to receptors on neurons (pruriceptors) that signal to specific areas of the brain. The itch sensation, in turn, triggers a reflex scratching response that delivers rapid but often temporary relief. Scratching activates pain sensory fibers that block the itch sensation. Ideally, it also removes the itch stimulus.

There are many causes of chronic itching, including the presence of ectoparasites, secondary infections, other irritants, lack of humidity or excessive water loss resulting in dry skin (xerosis), and reduced desquamation.

An itch is, however, a defining feature of atopic dermatitis (AD). Relentless, severe itching and scratching are among the most important and distressing features of AD in humans and animals (Box 6.1). Chronic itch is potentially debilitating, and the skin damage resulting from aggressive scratching may result in local infections. Associated morbidities resulting from chronic itch include sleep disruption, agitation, anxiety, self-mutilation, and altered eating habits (Box 6.2). Severe itch and the resulting chronic scratching are the primary reasons why owners bring their pets to veterinarians to treat dermatologic diseases.

Itching and scratching are interdependent symptoms that generate what is, in effect, an itch-scratch cycle. Until recently, itch was believed to be a mild form of pain. However, it is now recognized that it is a related but completely different sensation acting through a subpopulation of specialized nerve fibers. Itch and pain neurons are distinctly different cells in cats and mice. (This is not entirely the case in humans, where it is suggested that the lack of a protective fur coat may have resulted in alterations in itch pathways.)

While itch may be classified based on its source, the itch discussed in this chapter originates within the skin and is termed a pruriceptive itch. There is no single cause of itch. Mechanisms of itch are complex and the list of possible pruritogens is long. In addition, each pruritogen acts via its own specific receptor on different target neurons. Histamine has been the most widely studied and best recognized of these pruritogens; however, it is clearly not the only mediator involved. Other major pruritogens include serotonin, mast cell proteases, cytokines, and many different neuropeptides. For clinical purposes, itch can be considered to consist of two distinct forms depending on whether it responds to antihistamine treatment (histaminergic itch) or not (non-histaminergic itch). These two itch signaling pathways are

---

BOX 6.1 ■ Itching for All Eternity

The great Florentine poet Dante Alighieri wrote his masterwork, *The Divine Comedy,* in 1320. In this poem, he described the torments of hell. These included many imaginative and terrible ways that sinners were punished for eternity. Down in the eighth circle of hell, one of the lowest levels, he found the "falsifiers of metals" being eternally punished. They were covered in scabs from head to toe and suffered from persistent severe itching for which there was no cure.

BOX 6.2 ■ Itch-Related Stress

Constant itching is highly distressing to both humans and animals. Humans with chronic itch due to eczema report psychological problems arising as a result. Survey data indicate that similar, severe chronic psychological stress occurs in itchy dogs. When compared to non-itching dogs, the affected animals are clearly distracted and show increased hyperactivity, excitability, and attention seeking, and decreased trainability. The constant itch may result in excessive grooming. In addition, they engage in increased problem behaviors such as mounting, chewing, coprophagia, begging, and stealing food.

---

entirely independent of each other. Each pathway employs its own receptors and nerve fibers, which are connected to different neural tracts within the brain (Fig. 6.1).

Itch Sensation

In contrast to pain that is typically confined to deeper structures, itch is unique in that it only occurs in the superficial skin, some mucous membranes, and the cornea. No other organs experience the itch sensation. The sensation originates when itch-specific nerve fibers in the epidermis and at the dermal epidermal junction are stimulated. These itch nerve fibers extend into the stratum granulosum to form a complex network. The nerve fibers terminate around blood vessels, hair follicles, and sweat glands in the dermis and epidermis. The cell bodies of these sensory neurons are located within the ganglia of the spinal cord. Each has two branches. One branch innervates the skin, whereas the other synapses are in the dorsal horn of the spinal cord. Their cell bodies are located either in the trigeminal ganglion if the nerve innervates the face or the dorsal root ganglia if the nerve innervates other sites. Itch originates in receptors on sensory nerve fibers in the epidermis and upper dermis. The signals are transmitted to the

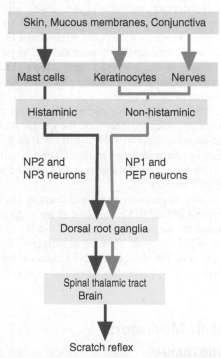

Fig. 6.1 Animals possess two distinct itch pathways. One is triggered by histamine while the other is activated by diverse other mediators. The two pathways remain separate until they reach the brain where they converge on the main itch center.

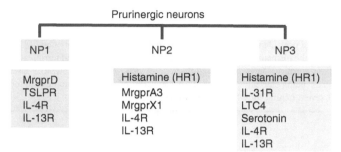

Fig. 6.2   There are three types of non-peptidergic neurons in the somatosensory system of mice. Each expresses a mixture of receptors for known pruritogens. NP2 and NP3 cells express histamine H1 receptors and mediate histaminergic itch. The three types also express significant amounts of different Mas-related G-protein receptors (MRGPR). The receptor for interleukin 31 (IL-31) is highly expressed in NP3 neurons.

dorsal root ganglion and thence to the brain via the spinal thalamic tract pathway, where they provoke sensory perception and an itch sensation.

Sensory nerve fibers are classified into three major groups: Aβ, Aδ, and C, depending on their myelination, diameter, and conduction velocity. Most itch signals are transmitted by small, un-myelinated slow-conducting C-fibers. These C-fibers have highly branched terminals and each may innervate large areas of skin. Thinly myelinated Aδ fibers also play a role in some forms of itch. Both of these nerve fiber types also transmit pain. However, after the discovery of itch-specific receptors such as the Mas-related G-protein receptors (MRGPRs), it is now clear that there are specialized itch neuronal pathways and that neuronal hypersensitivity resulting from increases in skin innervation or reduced signaling thresholds or a combination of both, contribute to the development of chronic itch. Thus, itchy animals may become increasingly sensitive to itch stimuli as time passes.

Single-cell genomic studies indicate that there are four families of itch neurons that differ in their receptors and, therefore, the specific purinergic mediators required to activate them. Three of these families (NP1, NP2, and NP3) do not produce neuropeptides; therefore, they are classi-fied as non-peptidergic neurons. The fourth family releases a mixture of neuropeptides such as calcitonin gene-related peptide (CGRP) and substance P (SP). These are classified as peptidergic (PEP) neurons.

NP1 neurons are non-histaminergic, i.e., they are not triggered by histamine. Instead, they express MRGPRD receptors that are triggered by ligands such as β-alanine. They also express receptors for interleukin 4 (IL-4) and IL-13. A second family, the NP2 neurons, express hista-mine H1 receptors. They are also triggered by ligands such as chloroquine acting via MRGPRA receptors. The third family, NP3 neurons, express low levels of histamine H1 receptors but high levels of IL-31 receptors. They also express the receptors for leukotrienes (LTC4) and serotonin (Fig. 6.2).

Itch Mediators

HISTAMINE

Mast cells contain large amounts of histamine that is released into tissues when they degranulate; therefore, it was assumed that this was the primary source of allergic itch. Histamine causes va-sodilatation, pain, and itching on intradermal injection. However, tissue histamine levels do not always correlate with itch severity, and plasma histamine levels do not differ significantly between normal and atopic dogs. Despite its apparent importance, H1 antihistamines work in some, but not all, acute urticaria cases and are ineffective in treating chronic itch or the itch associated with canine AD. Injection of the histamine release agent 48/80 intradermally in dogs results in the development of a wheal-and-flare reaction but not pruritus. Therefore, not all itching is a response to histamine released by mast cells.

The itch induced by mast cell histamine is mediated via H1 receptors on NP2 and, to a lesser extent, NP3 sensory nerves. A histamine-mediated itch can be inhibited by H1 receptor antagonists that block both the itch and the accompanying wheal-and-flare reaction.

However, H4 receptors are also involved in histaminergic itch. H4 inhibitors can block the itch but not the vascular changes that accompany it. Inhibitors of H4R can also block the itch in a contact dermatitis model (a type IV hypersensitivity mediated by T cells). In some cases, blockage of H1R and H4R together is more effective in reducing itch than either alone.

Non-Histaminergic Itch

Non-histaminergic itch is mediated via pathways involving MRGPRs on NP1 neurons and serotonin receptors on PEP neurons.

CYTOKINES

Many cytokines play a role in generating the itch sensation (Fig. 6.3). In general, the cytokines released during type 1 or type 17 immune responses such as IL-1β, IL-6, tumor necrosis factor-α (TNF-α), and IL-17A mediate pain. In contrast, the cytokines released during type 2 immune responses such as IL-4, IL-13, IL-31, IL-33, and thymic stromal lymphopoietin (TSLP) mediate

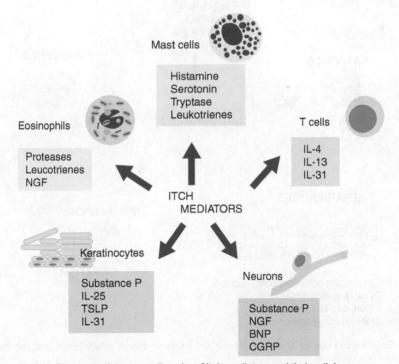

Fig. 6.3 Summary of the great diversity of itch mediators and their cellular sources.

itch. (If, as believed, type 2 responses have evolved to protect the body surfaces from environmental threats, and scratching is considered a protective reflex that physically removes irritants, then the linkage between enhanced type 2 responses and itch makes perfect sense, i.e., both are defensive responses.)

Some cytokines, such as IL-4 and IL-13, are poor pruritogens themselves; however, they sensitize neurons to the effects of other cytokines such as TSLP. Both IL-4 and IL-13 act on sensory nerves and promote IL-31 production. As described previously, IL-33 is released from damaged keratinocytes because of vigorous skin scratching. This activates type 2 innate lymphoid cells, promotes the production of IL-31, and plays a key role in maintaining the itch-scratch cycle.

Interleukin 31 (IL-31)

The most important cytokine itch mediator in dogs is IL-31, acting through its receptor IL-31R expressed on NP3 neurons (Fig. 6.4). IL-31 levels in tissues increase significantly in pruritic diseases, including AD and allergic contact dermatitis. Scabies (sarcoptic mange) is also characterized by severe and persistent itching. Examination of scabies lesions shows increased IL-31

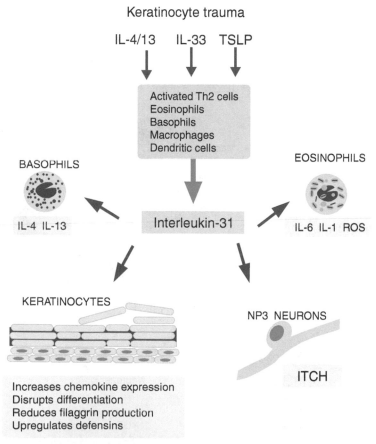

Fig. 6.4 Sources and targets of IL-31. Note that IL-31 acts on diverse cellular targets and itch mediation is only one of its functions.

and TSLP levels. The percentage of dog neurons responding to IL-31 was reported to be twice that in mice or humans. Dogs mount a strong pruritic response when challenged by IL-31 but not when challenged with histamine or serotonin. In humans with AD or allergic contact dermatitis, the IL-31 mRNA level is also higher in skin lesions than in normal skin. Increased IL-31 levels have also been detected in humans with chronic spontaneous urticaria and some patients with mastocytosis.

IL-31 is produced by activated type 2 helper cells. Its production is stimulated by IL-4 and IL-13. Microbial products such as Staphylococcal toxins and superantigens also promote IL-31 release. Peripheral blood mononuclear cells from dogs exposed to allergens (house dust mites) plus Staphylococcal enterotoxin B produce high IL-31 levels. Thus, the combination of allergens and the presence of certain bacteria might stimulate T cells, keratinocytes, and neurons to trigger the inflammation and pruritus of AD by releasing large quantities of IL-31.

Eosinophils are also a major source of IL-31, in addition to mast cells, basophils, macrophages, and dendritic cells. Thus, the recruitment of basophils and eosinophils into an AD lesion plays a key role in developing IL-31-mediated itch. IL-31 signals via receptors expressed on keratinocytes, other epithelial cells, eosinophils, basophils, dendritic cells, and activated macrophages. As discussed elsewhere, it signals through its receptor to target cells via the janus kinase (JAK) family of tyrosine kinases.

IL-31 acts through its receptors on sensory NP3 C-fibers in dorsal root ganglia. NP3 cells in dorsal root ganglia cells express IL-13R and IL-31R, with both required for IL-31 to generate itch signals. Despite using the same family of neurons, histamine-induced and IL-31-induced itch are distinctly different in humans. For example, histamine induces itching rapidly (<5 min), whereas IL-31 takes over an hour to induce itching following injection. In addition to inducing a slowly developing itch, IL-31 also promotes the branching and elongation of sensory nerve fibers in the epidermis.

Drugs that interfere with IL-31 signaling are effective in controlling this itch. A monoclonal antibody against IL-31, lokivetmab, is highly effective in reducing pruritus in dogs. It binds to IL-31 and prevents it from binding to the IL-31 receptor. Drugs such as oclacitinib maleate that block JAK signaling are also effective in reducing itch (Chapter 17).

IL-31 has immunoregulatory activities in that it promotes type 2 immunity. For example, it acts on keratinocytes to induce the production of chemokines and increases basal cell proliferation in mice, resulting in a thickening of this skin layer. However, it also increases transdermal water loss by suppressing filaggrin production by keratinocytes.

Thymic Stromal Lymphopoietin (TSLP)

The epithelial-derived cytokine, TSLP, is an important mediator of itch. Stimulation of their protease-activated cell receptors triggers keratinocytes to produce TSLP. TSLP is also produced by dendritic cells, mast cells, basophils, and fibroblasts. It activates cutaneous NP1 neurons by acting via their TSLP receptors to activate an intracellular calcium-signaling pathway and an irritant receptor called TRPA1. Therefore, TSLP from damaged keratinocytes can communicate directly with TSLP-sensitive neurons to trigger an itch response.

NEUROPEPTIDES

Many peptides released by activated sensory PEP neurons are involved in generating the itch sensation. These include SP, nerve growth factor (NGF), vasoactive intestinal peptide, brain-derived neuropeptide, gastrin-releasing peptide, CGRP, and natriuretic peptide b (Nppb). The most important are SP, CGRP, and NGF.

Substance P (SP) is released by sensory neurons in the skin and binds to neurokinin receptors on mast cells, keratinocytes, and cutaneous nerve endings, inducing itch sensations. Although it activates mast cells and triggers their histamine release, SP-induced itch does not depend on histamine (the itch persists even when the histamine is blocked), but it does depend on mast cells. SP also triggers the release of itch mediators from keratinocytes and endothelial cells and some immune cells.

NGF is a peptide that modulates nervous system development. Its presence in the skin correlates well with itchiness in mice but not in humans. It likely promotes some of the neural overgrowth occurring in AD lesional skin and makes it hypersensitive. For example, NGF is produced by mast cells and its injection causes mast cells to accumulate around nerve fibers. Eosinophils are also a major source of NGF. NGF release is stimulated by mast cell-derived histamine. NGF upregulates the expression of other neuropeptides such as SP and CGRP.

CGRP is produced by dorsal root ganglion sensory neurons during infections. Its receptor is found in many immune cells. It inhibits TNF-α production by macrophages, and modulates the ability of neutrophils to ingest and destroy bacteria. It also acts on mast cells via the MRGPRB2 receptor to promote their release of inflammatory mediators and on dendritic cells to induce IL-23 formation and hence a Th17 response.

Mast cell mediators, such as serotonin, LTC4, and sphingosine-1-phosphate directly stimulate NP3 neurons to trigger itch. These NP3 neurons characteristically express Nppb. If Nppb production is knocked out experimentally, itch responses to many pruritogens, including histamine, chloroquine, and serotonin, are blocked. Thus, Nppb is required for itch perception in general.

Cells Involved

KERATINOCYTES

Keratinocytes act as sentinel itch sensors. When appropriately stimulated, they initiate the itch sensation and transmit it to sensory nerves. They can release multiple itch mediators, including cytokines, proteases, SP, and NGF (Fig. 6.5). They also express relevant receptors, including that for IL-31. Thus, keratinocytes can activate nerves by secreting factors that mediate itch while they too can be activated by itch mediators.

MAST CELLS

Activation/Degranulation

The activation of mast cells can occur either through IgE-receptors or MRGPRX2. These two types of activation have different consequences for sensory neurons (Fig. 6.6). For example, the intradermal inoculation of the MRGPRX2 ligand PAMP-20 (a hypotensive peptide derived from proadrenomedullin) into mice induced significant scratching that was not inhibited by antihistamines. In contrast, itch induced by the injection of anti-IgE antibodies could be blocked by H1 and H4 antihistamines.

While both types of mast cell degranulation induce a calcium influx in the dorsal root ganglion cells, the neurons involved and their kinetics differ. Most neurons reacting to anti-IgE responded to histamine only. Only ~30% of the neurons responding to PAMP-20 also responded to histamine. NP3 neurons responding to PAMP-20 also respond to serotonin and related molecules. (Serotonin induces mild to moderate itch in rodents.) Therefore, there is a subpopulation within the NP3 neuron family where different types of mast cell responses may generate different neural responses and itch.

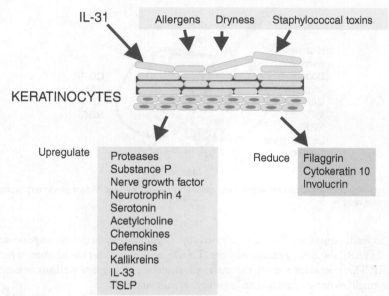

Fig. 6.5 Keratinocytes release multiple mediators that can act on neurons to trigger itch. They also release molecules that can reduce skin barrier functions.

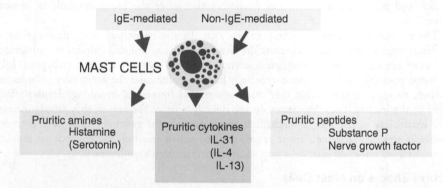

Fig. 6.6 Some of the pruritogens released by mast cells. Serotonin is not pruritic in all species.

Mast Cell-Nerve Connection

The physical link between nerves and mast cells was long recognized by anatomists but it is also clear that they are functionally linked. Thus, mast cell-nerve communication is a major component of neurogenic inflammation (Fig. 6.7). Mast cells are found in large numbers associated with small-caliber sensory myelinated Aδ and unmyelinated C-fibers. Most mast cells are located within the paracrine signaling distance of a sensory nerve fiber. Other nerves can come into direct contact with mast cells and form neuroimmune synapses.

Mast Cell Effects on Neurons

When mast cells degranulate, their mediators transmit signals to nearby neurons. This signaling contributes to the development of itching, pain, and inflammation. Histamine contributes

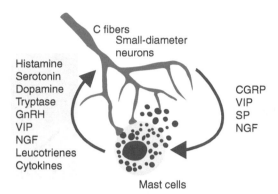

Fig. 6.7 **Two-way conversations between mast cells and nearby nerves.** Note that some neurons directly innervate mast cells.

directly to pain sensation. Tryptase released by degranulation activates protease-activated receptor-2 (PAR_2) on sensory neuron endings. This, in turn, stimulates the neurons to release SP and CGRP. These peptides activate the mast cell, stimulating yet more mediator release. Thus, this cycle amplifies nerve activation and neurogenic inflammation.

The result of this mast cell to neuron signaling contributes to the itch sensation. Mast cell-derived histamine leads to the histamine receptor-dependent activation of purinergic sensory nerves. In response, sensory nerves release their neuropeptides, resulting in neurogenic inflammation and itch sensation. Mast cell mediators also lower the firing threshold of sensory nerves.

These interactions occur not only in the skin. In the respiratory tract, non-myelinated (C-fiber) vagal afferent nerves innervate the airways and lungs. Inhaled irritants or endogenous mediators can cause bronchoconstriction, airway hypersensitivity, cough, and tachypnea. IgE-mediated mast cell mediator release, especially histamine, increases the excitability of bronchial C-fibers to such an extent that they may be activated by normal breathing. Similar effects occur in the trachea. These mediators do not directly activate the nerves; they simply increase their excitability in response to mechanical stimulation. In the gastrointestinal tract, mast cell mediators activate enteric neurons to cause increased mucus secretion and enhance gut motility. Overactivity of intestinal mast cells may result in irritable bowel syndrome.

Neural Effects on Mast Cells

The interaction between neurons and mast cells is a two-way conversation. Mast cells possess receptors for neurotransmitters; therefore, their activities may be readily modulated by neural signals. These neurotransmitters include acetylcholine, SP, vasoactive intestinal peptide, and CGRP. Psychological stress can also affect mast cell degranulation, which is mediated by SP and corticotrophin releasing hormone. Therefore, stress exacerbates some allergic diseases.

SP is a major participant in these neuronal-mast cell conversations. SP can trigger mast cell degranulation via the MRGPR pathway and induce the differential release of mast cell cytokines such as TNF-α and IL-6 and lipids such as prostaglandins and leukotrienes in the absence of complete degranulation. At low concentrations, SP may simply prime mast cells by lowering their threshold for mediator release.

The important skin cell receptors that detect itch signals include the MRGPR family of receptors. Some of these detect noxious chemicals and temperature. Others detect itch signals. A related receptor family consists of protease-activated receptors. Their activation induces non-histaminergic itch, probably mediated by PEP neurons. Proteases that can trigger this include cathepsin, tryptase, dust mite allergens, and some Staphylococcal proteases. Expression of at least one of these receptors (PAR$_2$) on keratinocytes is upregulated in both the lesional and non-lesional skin of AD patients.

Another family of cell surface receptors that can trigger purinergic nerves is the transient receptor potential proteins. Their function is to transmit positive ions across the cell membrane. Two such receptors, TRPV1 and TRPV4, expressed on C nerve fibers are activated by histamine and prostaglandins. TRPV1 serves as a receptor for capsaicin. TRPV1-expressing C-fibers transmit pain and heat sensations, and can include Nppb neurons. The inflammatory flare that accompanies a histaminergic itch results from the TRPV1-mediated release of SP and CGRP. Its expression is upregulated in AD skin lesions. Other transient receptor potential receptors are expressed in keratinocytes, fibroblasts, and sensory C-fibers. For example, TRPA1 is a transmitter of histamine-independent itch via NP2 neurons.

BASOPHILS

Basophils can secrete a wide variety of itch mediators, including histamine, cytokines, and chemokines such as TSLP, IL-4, IL-13, and IL-31. They also produce proteases, prostaglandins, and platelet-activating factor that will contribute to the process. Recent evidence suggests that acute itch flares are mediated by LTC4 from basophils independent of mast cell activity.

EOSINOPHILS

Eosinophilic granulomas may be intensely pruritic. When activated by the presence of a contact allergen, eosinophils can release large amounts of IL-31 that act on skin NP3 neurons to promote neurite growth, enhance SP production, and promote itch.

NEURONS

The development of chronic, persistent pruritus depends on the release of itch mediators and an increased density of cutaneous sensory nerve fibers that extend into the epidermis in lesional skin. Thus, patients with chronic pruritus associated with AD have increased cutaneous innervation. The diameter of these fibers is increased in AD cases because there is an increased number of axons within individual nerve fibers. Several different mediators control this neuronal growth and branching process. For example, IL-31 acts on NP3 sensory neurons in the skin to induce a unique transcriptional program that activates genes, leading to small-diameter nerve elongation and increased branching. A subset of small-diameter sensory neurons expresses the IL-31 receptor subunit, IL-31RA. It is these neurons that are stimulated to branch and elongate within the affected skin.

NGF also acts in the skin environment to promote neuronal branching, acting on a different subset of small-diameter neurons than IL-31 (PEP neurons). Lesional skin may develop increased sensory nerve density in the dermis and epidermis due to mast cell production of NGF. A major growth factor also implicated in increased neuronal branching of PEP neurons is brain-derived neurotrophic factor (BDNF).

The main source of these NGFs appears to be degranulating eosinophils located close to the dorsal root ganglia nerve fiber terminals. (Intact eosinophils are usually not a prominent feature of atopic skin lesions, but their granule proteins are present.) Thus, they generate BDNF and IL-31 in response to SP. This release and the resulting neuronal outgrowth and axonal branching are further promoted by platelet-activating factor from keratinocytes and mast cells.

Scratching

Relentless, repetitive scratching is a feature of many chronic inflammatory skin diseases, especially AD (Fig. 6.8). It results from itching, an evolutionarily conserved process that occurs in all mammals and birds. Itching persists because it serves as a protective mechanism that warns of harmful stimuli on the skin surface. The resulting scratching can effectively repel or remove adherent insects and other ectoparasites. However, scratching can also disrupt the epithelial barrier and result in secondary infection. The brain region that processes such danger signals as heat and pain also receives input from the spinal itch neurons. The itch signal is stressful and accompanied by changes in the limbic system. Both pain and itch elicit specific reflex responses. Thus, pain signals trigger a withdrawal reflex. Conversely, itch signals trigger the scratch reflex, in effect triggering local cell damage (Box 6.3). Scratching is a very rapid and efficient method of removing skin irritants; therefore, it is unremarkable that the nervous system triggers this in response

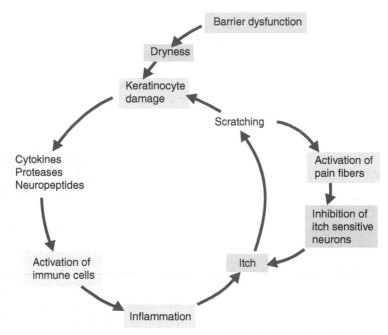

Fig. 6.8 **Why scratching helps.** The major pathways linking the itch and scratch pathways.

BOX 6.3 ■ Measurement of Pruritus

Pruritus is a subjective sensation that cannot be objectively quantitated. Humans sense it, while pet owners observe the consequential scratching or other itch-associated behaviors. Scratching can be measured by the use of activity monitors; however, these are not widely available and have yet to be fully validated. Nevertheless, an objective assessment of pruritus is required if treatment results are to be assessed. Several different pruritus scales have been developed in an effort to provide a quantitative basis for such assessment. The most commonly used are based on a scale of 0 to 5 initially developed at the University of Edinburgh (Table 6.1). Many variations of this scale have been developed subsequently in an effort to validate it and improve its repeatability and reliability. A visual analog scale is often added in attempts to improve precision (Fig. 6.9).

TABLE 6.1 ■ **A Scoring System for Pruritus:**

Score	Description
0	A normal dog. The dog does not itch more than it did before the disease appeared. Itching is not a problem.
1	Occasional episodes of itching (A small increase in itching relative to the situation prior to disease development).
2	More frequent episodes of itching, but this stops when the dog is sleeping, eating, playing, or exercising, or is otherwise distracted.
3	Regular episodes of itching are seen when the animal is awake. The dog occasionally wakes up in order to scratch, but this stops if the dog is sleeping, eating, playing, or exercising, or is otherwise distracted.
4	Prolonged episodes of itching are observed when the dog is awake. The dog regularly wakes up to scratch or even scratches in its sleep. Itching also occurs when the dog is playing, eating, exercising, or is otherwise distracted.
5	Almost continuous itching that does not stop when the dog is distracted, and the dog needs to be physically restrained from scratching.

It is assumed that behaviors such as scratching, biting and nibbling, licking, chewing, and rubbing are collectively, directly correlated to the intensity of the itching sensation.
(Colombo S, Hill PB, Shaw DJ, Thoday KL. Effectiveness of low dose immunotherapy in the treatment of canine atopic dermatitis: a prospective, double-blinded, clinical study. *Vet Dermatol.* 2005;16:162-170)

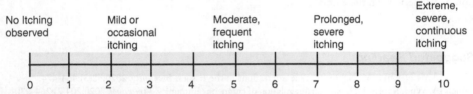

Fig. 6.9　A simple example of a pruritus visual analog scale. The animal owner is asked to mark on the scale their opinion of the severity of their animal's itching. "On a scale of one to ten, how severe is your dog's scratching, chewing, licking, or rubbing? Ten is most severe, while one indicates that you have seen no evidence of itching. Mark the value that best reflects the severity of your dog's itching."

to an itch. The pain of scratching or vigorously rubbing the site effectively relieves the itch sensation. Scratching activates spinal interneurons that inhibit itch-sensitive neurons and block the transmission of itch signals to the brain. In effect, scratching induces pain, which is preferable to an itch. Scratching is also sometimes pleasurable, probably because of the release of serotonin during scratching. Thus, scratching blocks itch signals (negative reinforcement) while providing pleasure (positive reinforcement). This arrangement may become disrupted in chronic itch. Multiple itch signals may desensitize or overwhelm the inhibitory neurons so that the skin may become hypersensitive. Therefore, the pain of scratching becomes less effective in suppressing itch.

In addition to the mechanisms described above, scratching significantly reduces the effectiveness of IL-13 as an itch promoter. IL-13 plays a key role in generating an itch. Keratinocytes express two receptors for IL-13. One is a heterodimer consisting of IL-4Rα and IL-13Rα1, while the other is a monomer consisting of IL-13αR2. The former is a functional receptor while the latter is a non-functional decoy receptor. The decoy receptor binds IL-31 with high affinity;

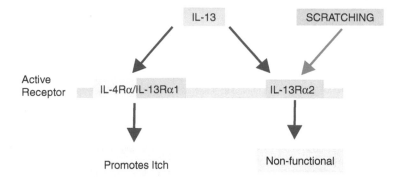

Fig. 6.10   Role of scratching in upregulating the IL-13 decoy receptor and suppressing the itch sensation.

however, it lacks a functional cytoplasmic domain. Scratch injuries significantly and selectively upregulate the expression of the decoy receptor IL-13Rα2. Therefore, scratching reduces the itch sensation by increasing the expression of the decoy, leading to a rapid depletion of the available extracellular IL-13 and decreased signaling by its functional receptors (Fig. 6.10).

Scratching is only effective if the affected site can be readily accessed by the paw or hand. The scratch reflex is indeed powerful, and animals often distort their bodies in strange ways to gain access to the itch site. This access issue likely plays an important role in determining the distribution of AD lesions on the animal body.

Suggested Reading

Chu C, Artis D, Chiu IM. Neuro-immune interactions in the tissues. *Immunity*. 2020;52(3):464-474.

Cohen JA, Wu J, Kaplan DH. Neuronal regulation of cutaneous immunity. *J Immunol*. 2020;204(2):264-270.

Feld M, Garcia R, Buddenkotte J, et al. The pruritus and Th2-associated cytokine, IL-31 promotes growth of sensory nerves. *J Allergy Clin Immunol*. 2016;138(2):500-508.

Forsyth P. Mast cells in neuroimmune interactions. *Trends Neurosci*. 2019;42(1):43-55.

Furue M, Yamamura K, Kido-Nakahara M, Nakahara T, Fukui Y. Emerging role of interleukin-31 and interleukin-31 receptor in pruritus in atopic dermatitis. *Allergy*. 2018;73(1):29-36.

Green D, Dong X. The cell biology of acute itch. *J Cell Biol*. 2016;213(2):155-161.

Gupta K, Harvima IT. Mast cell neural interactions contribute to pain and itch. *Immunol Res*. 2018;282(1):168-187.

Guseva D, Rudrich U, Kotnik N, et al. Neuronal branching of sensory neurons is associated with BNDF positive eosinophils in atopic dermatitis. *Clin Exp Allergy*. 2020;50(5):577-584. doi:10.1111/CEA.13560.

Hill PB, Lau P, Rybnicek J. Development of an owner-assessed scale to measure the severity of pruritus in dogs. *Vet Dermatol*. 2007;18(5):301-308.

Mack MR, Kim BS. The itch-scratch cycle. A neuroimmune perspective. *Trends Immunol*. 2018;39(12):980-991.

Mollanazar NK, Smith PK, Yosipovitch G. Mediators of chronic pruritus in atopic dermatitis: getting the itch out. *Clin Rev Allerg Immunol*. 2016;51(3):263-292.

Nakashima C, Ishida Y, Kitoh A, Otsuka A, Kabashima K. Interaction of peripheral nerves and mast cells, eosinophils, and basophils in the development of pruritus. *Exp Dermatol*. 2019;28(12):1405-1411.

Nakashima K, Otsuka A, Kabashima K. Interleukin-31 and interleukin-31 receptor: new therapeutic targets for atopic dermatitis. *Exp Dermatol*. 2018;27(4):327-331.

Saleem MD, Oussedik E, D'Amber V, Feldman SR. Interleukin-31 pathway and its role in atopic dermatitis: a systematic review. *J Dermatol Treat*. 2017;28(7):591-599.

Sanders KM, Fast K, Yosipovitch G. Why we scratch: function and dysfunction. *Exp Dermatol.* 2019;28(12):1482-1484.

Siiskonen H, Harvima I. Mast cells and sensory nerves contribute to neurogenic inflammation and pruritus in chronic skin inflammation. *Front Cell Neurosci.* 2019;13:422. doi:10.3389/fncel.2019.00422.

Solinski HJ, Kriegbaum MC, Tseng PY, Barik A, Chesler AT, Hoon MA. Nppb neurons are sensors for mast cell-induced itch. *Cell Rep.* 2019;26:3561-3573.

Steinhoff M, Buddenkotte J, Lerner EA. Role of mast cells and basophils in pruritus. *Immunol Res.* 2018;282(1):248-264.

Ulzii U, Kido-Nakahara M, Nakahara T, et al. Scratching counteracts IL-13 signaling by upregulating the decoy receptor IL-13Rα2 in keratinocytes. *Int J Mol Sci.* 2019;20(13):3324-3335.

Usoskin D, Furlan A, Islam S, et al. Unbiased classification of sensory neuron types by large-scale single-cell RNA sequencing. *Nat Neurosci.* 2015;18(1):145-153. doi:10.1038/nn.3881.

Wang F, Kim BS. Itch: a paradigm of neuroimmune crosstalk. *Immunity.* 2020;52(5):753-766.

Wang F, Trier AM, Li F, et al. A basophil-neuronal axis promotes itch. *Cell.* 2021;184(2):1-19.

Wheeler JJ, Lascelles DX, Olivry T, Mishra S. Itch-associated neuropeptides and their receptor expression in dog dorsal root ganglia and spinal cord. *Acta Derm Venereol.* 2019;99(12):1131-1135.

CHAPTER 7

The Hygiene Hypothesis

Given the numbers, diversity, and significance of the commensal organisms living on body surfaces, it is important for these organisms to live together harmoniously. Nothing is gained if the immune system aggressively attacks its microbiota. To ensure that this attack does not happen, the microbiota are selectively immunosuppressive. Thus, on healthy, normal surfaces, the microbiota prevent immune attack by promoting immunoregulatory pathways such as the induction of regulatory T (Treg) cells. If, however, these microbial populations change and dysbiosis results, then this suppressive effect may be reduced. Released from constraints, the immune system can then respond by increasing its inflammatory and immune responses. In practical terms, as dysbiosis develops, regulation is reduced, the immune systems become activated, and allergies can develop.

The Hygiene Hypothesis

The prevalence of allergic diseases in human populations has increased significantly in developed societies over the past 50 years. For example, the prevalence of allergic dermatitis in British children is estimated to have increased from 5.1% in 1946 to 7.3% in 1958, 12.2% in 1970, 15%–20% in 1994, and 20%–30% in 2006. Similarly, the prevalence of allergic asthma has increased 4-fold since the 1950s. While most obvious in humans, this increase has also affected companion animals. In seeking an explanation for these increases, research initially centered on the "Western lifestyle." For example, at the time of the fall of the Soviet Union, allergies were very much more prevalent in West Germany than in the less-developed East. After German reunification, the prevalence of allergic disease in the East gradually increased to match the Western level. Initially, research focused on the environmental and economic differences between the two communities. Eventually, however, it came to focus on diets and the associated changes in the intestinal microbiota. By the 1980s, it became clear that children who had grown up in an environment where they were exposed to diverse microbes and infections, such as those from large families or those brought up on farms or with pets, were much less likely to develop asthma in later life. A "Western lifestyle" involving clean food and drinking water, lack of exposure to animals, the disappearance of chronic infectious diseases, exposure to pollutants such as diesel fumes, and the promiscuous use of antibiotics has resulted in significant disruption and dysbiosis in our commensal microbiota and that of our companion animals. Other contributing factors include more time spent indoors, a lack of physical activity, and obesity due to a diet low in fiber and high in sugars and fats. An urban environment predisposes both dogs and their owners to allergic diseases. Allergic dogs are more likely to have allergic owners than healthy dogs because they share some components of their microbiota and environment (Table 7.1).

The original hygiene hypothesis suggested that excessively hygienic behavior and contacts were the triggers for allergies. This theory was supported by the "farm effect" on asthma and allergies and by the emergence of the type 1 helper (Th1)/type 2 helper (Th2) paradigm. The farm effect results in those living on farms with livestock developing fewer allergies. Farms are a significant source of

TABLE 7.1 ■ Possible Explanations for the Current Allergy Epidemic

Urbanization with decreased exposure to the rural/farm microbiota.
Changes in the enteric microbiota as a result of diet.
Changes in dietary habits as a result of an increase in calories or a loss of some nutrients.
Obesity.
Fewer serious infectious diseases in childhood.
Exposure to urban pollutants such as diesel fumes.
Increased time spent indoors with exposure to indoor allergens.
Reduced breast feeding.
Increased societal stress.
Excessive antibiotic use.

environmental bacterial and fungal exposure and have high endotoxin levels. The farm effect has been attributed in large part, to drinking unprocessed milk and exposure to cattle and straw.

The hygiene hypothesis has undergone several revisions as our ideas regarding the microbiota have evolved. A current version is "the microbial deprivation signal hypothesis" that suggests that an absence of some specific organisms and their signals will trigger allergies. All such theories highlight our evolutionary adaptations to the presence of huge numbers of microorganisms living on body surfaces. The surfaces of the body are stable, nutrient-rich ecosystems where microbes thrive. Each surface is populated by enormous numbers of commensal bacteria, archea, fungi, and viruses—the microbiota. Bacteria in huge numbers live on the skin, in the respiratory tract, in parts of the genitourinary tract, and sometimes within the body but mainly within the gastrointestinal tract. Their composition and density depend on environmental conditions such as nutrient availability, humidity, pH, oxygen tension, and temperature. It has been estimated that in an animal body, at least half of all the cells are microbial. Because of their life-long, intimate association with body surfaces, the microbiota can be considered an integral part of the body—"a virtual organ." Thus, they play a key role in the regulation of immune responses. Animals and their microbiota together form "superorganisms" that share nutrition and exchange energy and metabolites, and whose interactions are regulated by immune mechanisms.

Therefore, the hygiene hypothesis suggests that the recent increases in the prevalence of allergic diseases are the direct result of changes in Western lifestyles and diets over the last half-century. Consequently, changes have occurred in the body's intestinal microbiota (Fig.7.1). These changes have resulted in a predisposition toward type 2 responses and are believed responsible, in part, for the observed increases in the prevalence of allergic and inflammatory diseases.

The Intestinal Microbiota

The intestinal microbiota consists of billions of different bacteria, archea, fungi, and viruses. There may be as many as 10^{14} microbial cells living in the healthy mammalian intestine. The most obvious of these are trillions of bacteria belonging to hundreds of different species. In dogs and cats, these bacterial populations are dominated by Firmicutes and Bacteroidetes, with fewer numbers of Actinobacteria and Proteobacteria. There are also many lesser phyla such as the Spirochaetes, Fusobacteria, Tenericutes, and Verrucomicrobia. The canine small intestine harbors more than 200 bacterial species, whereas the canine colon may be home to as many as 1000 different species.

The microbiota of each individual is unique, and its composition is determined by diet, antibiotic exposure, and genetic and environmental factors. The Firmicutes mainly consist of gram-positive bacteria, many of which are spore forming. Important members include the Clostridia, some *Streptococci*, and *Staphylococci*. The Actinobacteria are also gram-positive

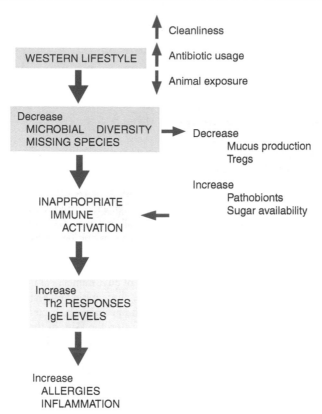

Fig. 7.1 The hygiene hypothesis. A lack of microbial diversity in the intestinal microbiota and the resulting dysbiosis alters the regulatory signals reaching T helper cells. Because of a decline in Treg cells, some individuals develop an immune system where Th2 responses predominate and result in the development of allergic disease.

bacteria whose DNA has a different nucleotide content than the Firmicutes. The Bacteroidetes are gram-negative bacteria that ferment indigestible plant carbohydrates to produce short-chain fatty acids (SCFAs). The Proteobacteria include gram-negative enterobacteria such as *Escherichia coli* and Klebsiella.

Firmicutes, especially Clostridia, are the main bacterial phylum in the horse. Other phyla found in the equine large intestine include Spirochaetes, Fibrobacteres, Ruminococcus, and Bacteroidetes.

Microbial Immunosuppression

Evolutionary pressures have ensured that the body must strike a balance between protecting itself from microbial invasion while simultaneously maintaining an environment where beneficial commensal microorganisms can survive and thrive. This balancing act needs to be managed by constant cross-talk. Therefore, the immune system depends on signals originating in the microbiota to establish and maintain an appropriate activity level. If the microbiota is disrupted and the situation becomes unbalanced, then unwanted responses such as inflammation and allergies follow. Conversely, the immune system can produce IgA and antibacterial molecules that influence the composition and behavior of the microbiota. These interactions thus occur in both directions.

The significance of the microbiota is readily seen when germ-free mice are reared under aseptic conditions. In germ-free or antibiotic-treated mice lacking a diverse microbiota, the animals develop increased type 2 immune responses, elevated levels of interleukin 4 (IL-4), increased basophil numbers, and high levels of immunoglobulin E (IgE). As a result, these mice are very much skewed toward a Th2 phenotype. They can develop severe allergies to food or airborne antigens. This Th2 skewing can be prevented by colonizing the mice with a normal mixed microbiota or selected bacteria from conventional animals. However, this colonization must be performed within 3 weeks of birth to be fully effective.

The intestinal immune system must be able to ignore the commensal microbiota and the ingested food antigens while still responding to potential pathogens. Therefore, the key to successful accommodation with the microbiota depends on the regulation of immune responses in the gut wall. Intestinal helper T cell phenotypes are "plastic," and Th0 precursor cells can differentiate into other types of helper T cells. This differentiation is regulated by signals from two major sources, the microbiota and other tissue cells such as endothelial cells. In effect, the microbiota manage these helper T cell populations with the help of cytokines. Local immune stability is achieved by adjusting T cell populations to maintain a balance between each of the proinflammatory helper T cell types (Th1, Th2, and Th17) and anti-inflammatory Treg cells (Fig. 7.2).

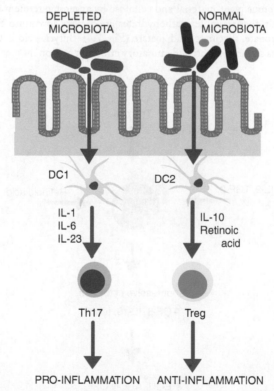

DEPLETED MICROBIOTA

NORMAL MICROBIOTA

DC1

DC2

IL-1
IL-6
IL-23

IL-10
Retinoic acid

Th17

Treg

PRO-INFLAMMATION   ANTI-INFLAMMATION

Fig. 7.2 Countervailing activities of Treg and Th17 cells require a balanced microbiota to maintain health.

MICROBIAL SUPPRESSIVE FACTORS

An appropriately balanced microbiota generates metabolites that influence T cell functions and immune regulation. In general, these metabolites are anti-inflammatory and immunosuppressive because they promote Treg functions. However, others can promote Th17 responses and have a countervailing effect.

Treg Stimulation

A healthy microbiota is a powerful promoter of Treg cell function (Fig. 7.3). One feature of the Treg cells produced under the influence of the microbiota is their use of a novel transcription factor called RORγt. RORγt$^+$ Treg cells are profoundly reduced in germ-free or antibiotic-treated mice. The microbiota can regulate the Treg/Th17/Th2 balance by altering RORγt levels. Under other circumstances, Treg cells may convert to Th2 cells and promote a switch to IgA production. Approximately 75% of the IgA directed against the microbiota is produced via a pathway controlled by Treg cells.

Mucosal inflammation is actively suppressed by the production of large numbers of IL-10-producing Treg cells. Under stable conditions, the production of Treg cells is favored, whereas that of effector T cells is suppressed. However, in the absence of Treg cells, uncontrolled effector T cell responses may be directed against microbial antigens and so trigger inflammatory bowel disease. IL-10-deficient mice develop chronic, unremitting colitis driven by IL-23 and the Th17 pathway.

Animals digest fibrous plant material and cellulose by anaerobic fermentation in the caecum and colon. As a result, these complex carbohydrates are broken down into SCFAs such as formate, butyrate, propionate, succinate, and acetate (Fig. 7.4). Butyric acid is the most important of these because it has significant anti-inflammatory effects. It acts on mast cells to inhibit FcεR1

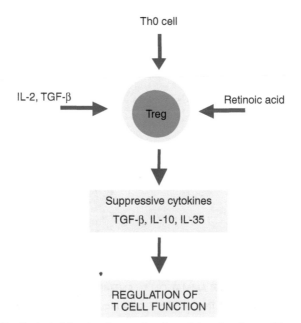

Fig. 7.3 Control of the development and regulatory functions of Treg cells.

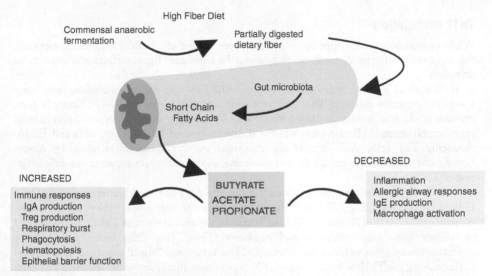

Fig. 7.4 Short-chain fatty acids, especially butyrate, are critically important in promoting Treg functions and maintaining a balanced immune response. These fatty acids are derived from the digestion of complex carbohydrates in a high fiber diet.

signaling and hence degranulation. It boosts Treg cell numbers both in the intestine and elsewhere in the body. Butyrate also enhances intestinal barrier function by stimulating enterocyte growth and increasing goblet cell differentiation and mucus production.

Likewise, the production of propionate by intestinal bacteria suppresses lung dendritic cell (DC) function, inhibits Th2 responses, and protects from allergic airway disease. SCFAs act by inhibiting histone deacetylases. As a result, acetylation of the FoxP3 transcription factor occurs and this in turn enhances Treg differentiation. SCFAs also inhibit NF-κB signaling.

Because of the production of SCFAs, high fiber diets play a key role in regulating inflammation in the intestine and lung. Humans who consume large amounts of fiber have a lower prevalence of colitis and inflammatory bowel disease. Conversely, diets low in fiber increase pathogen susceptibility in mice. (It has been suggested that the beneficial influence of cattle exposure on asthma may be mediated by volatile SCFAs such as propionate exhaled by ruminants.)

Several polyamines such as putrescine, spermine, and spermidine are synthesized from arginine by gut bacteria. These also have immunoregulatory activities. For example, spermine suppresses the production of proinflammatory cytokines such as tumor necrosis factor-α, IL-1, IL-6, and some chemokines by mononuclear cells. These polyamines also suppress NF-κB activation.

Some specific bacteria are also immunosuppressive. Clostridia, *Lactobacillus,* and *Bifidobacterium* can stimulate DCs to secrete immunosuppressive molecules such as IDO, TGF-β, and IL-10. Some Clostridial clusters specifically stimulate Treg cell and IL-10 production in the gut. Clostridia enhance the release of immunosuppressive cytokines such as TGF-β from enterocytes. In addition to Clostridia, the capsular polysaccharide-A of *Bacteroides fragilis* triggers IL-10 production. Some commensal bacteria can actively suppress intestinal inflammation. For example, *Lactobacillus* and *Bacteroides* inhibit the innate signaling pathways triggered by TLRs and NLRs. A common commensal, *B. thetaiotaomicron,* inhibits NF-κB signaling, whereas intestinal *Lactobacillus* prevent the degradation of the NF-κB inhibitor IκB and are potently anti-inflammatory.

Th17 Stimulation

While immunosuppression appears to be a dominant feature of a healthy microbiota, especially the suppression of type 2 responses, this cannot be overdone. Body surfaces still need to be defended.

Activation of the aryl hydrocarbon receptor (AhR) by tryptophan metabolites from some *Lactobacillus* species enhances Th17 differentiation and the release of IL-17. These, in turn, produce IL-22 that protects epithelial membranes by inducing the production of antibacterial peptides. However, AhR also promotes the differentiation of FoxP3$^+$ Treg cells and IL-10-producing Th1 cells. AhR ligands are generated by tryptophan metabolism by certain *Lactobacillus* species. Commensal-derived adenosine triphosphate also supports the differentiation of Th17 cells.

Th17 cells regulate inflammation, maintain the intestinal epithelial barrier, and mount type 17 immune responses (Fig. 7.5). Under the influence of IL-23, they produce the proinflammatory cytokines IL-17A, IL-17F, and IL-22. Like Treg cells, the development of Th17 cells is regulated by signals from the microbiota and cytokines. Thus, Treg cells, when acted on by proinflammatory cytokines, can convert to IL-17 effectors and "break" tolerance. Under these circumstances, the Th17 cells can become IFN-γ producers that functionally resemble Th1 cells. It is likely that many intestinal Th1 cells develop via this pathway. However, a healthy microbiota is required for the production of Th17 cells. Th17 cell development is specifically stimulated by the attachment of segmented filamentous bacteria (SFB) to enterocytes. SFB cause enterocytes to produce serum amyloid A, which acts as a cytokine and stimulates IL-23 production by

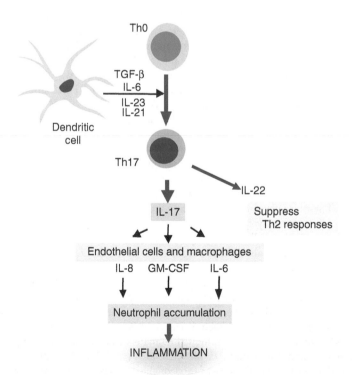

Fig. 7.5 Control of the development of Th17 cells and their subsequent functions.

macrophages leading to IL-22 and IL-17 secretion. These trigger the development of Th17 cells. Lamina propria macrophages and DCs can detect SFB-derived molecules via their TLRs and produce IL-23 and TGF-β, so promoting further Th17 cell differentiation. Th17 cells regulate the abundance of SFB by promoting the production of antibacterial peptides such as β-defensins, lipocalins, and calprotectin by enterocytes.

Systemic Regulatory Effects

Bacterial metabolites and regulatory factors can leak from the intestine to the bloodstream. Therefore, signals from the microbiota are conveyed from the intestine to many other organs. These signals influence the development of T cells and the balance between helper T cell subsets throughout the body. In addition, Treg cells generated by commensal bacteria in the intestine can emigrate to remote tissues and influence the overall T cell balance of the body. For example, the presence of clostridial clusters in the colon increases the numbers of IL-10-producing Treg cells in the spleen and lung, where they play a role in suppressing allergic responses. A major cause of excessive type 2 immune function and consequent increase in atopic disease results from a decline in the activities of these systemic Treg cell populations.

Dysbiosis

The development of the immune system and the growth of the intestinal microbiota occur simultaneously in young animals. Therefore, changes in the microbiota at this time can have long-term consequences on immune system development. Two variants of the "hygiene hypotheses" have been put forward based on the human experience. One suggests that there is a fixed early-in-life "set-point" in infants, with the diversity of the microbiota at that specific age determining the future course of allergic sensitivity. An alternative version suggests that the diversity of the microbiota affects the immune balance; however, this can be recalibrated over time following exposure to childhood infections and environmental microbes. It is unclear which is correct. However, it is clear that if the microbiota becomes imbalanced by a loss of diversity or of certain key species, then the signals regulating the immune responses will change and allergies may result.

MECHANISMS OF DYSBIOSIS

The surfaces of the body represent vulnerability sites to invasion. Therefore, they are under constant scrutiny by immune cells, especially T cells. These surface barriers are not just physical, they also use chemical and biological mechanisms to maintain their integrity. Evolutionary pressures have ensured that the body must strike a balance between protecting itself from invasion while simultaneously maintaining an environment where symbiotic microorganisms can survive and thrive. This mutually beneficial situation must be managed by constant cross-talk and mutual negotiations. In effect, the immune system depends on signals from the microbiota for its appropriate development and function.

Environmental Effects

Newborn animals emerge from the almost-sterile uterus into a world dominated by bacteria. The birth process itself ensures that they encounter and are initially colonized by organisms from the vagina and skin of the mother. Even their first breath will result in the inhalation of large numbers of organisms. Over the subsequent weeks and months, the surfaces of the newborn are colonized by a diverse microbial population. Each of these surfaces acquires its own unique microbiota. The intestinal tract is first colonized by facultative anaerobes such as *Staphylococci* and *Streptococci*, with these gradually replaced by obligate anaerobes such as Clostridia and *Bacteroides*. By the time children reach between two and five years of age, their microbiota starts to resemble that of adults.

Prior to that time, the composition of the microbiota is unstable and readily disrupted by antibiotic use. Some of these colonizing organisms can regulate the developing immune system, which is important since the body depends on these bacteria to establish the correct balance between Th1 and Th2 responses.

The composition and functions of this population are affected by many factors. The most important of these in humans include the route of birth (vaginal or caesarian), their diet, and exposure to other infants and animals.

The development of an allergic phenotype occurs during early life in young animals. Healthy infants harbor intestinal bacteria that protect against food allergies. Germ-free mice experimentally colonized by a healthy human microbiota are protected against allergic responses to cow's milk, whereas mice that receive bacteria from allergic infants are not. Changes in the microbiota prior to two years of age have profound long-term consequences (Fig. 7.6). For example, one study found that dysbiosis in children at three months of age was predictive of asthma and wheeze development at one year. Similarly, children who were lacking certain key organisms in their microbiota had a higher risk of developing food allergies and aeroallergies by two years of age. These children had decreased Treg and increased Th2 cells, suggesting an imbalance had already developed in their T cell populations. Retrospective studies on human infants have demonstrated that early administration of acid-suppressive medications such as H2 receptor blockers,

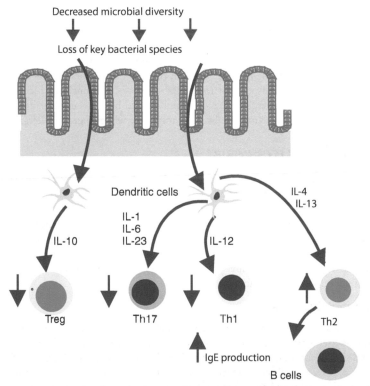

Fig. 7.6 Consequences of a decline in microbial diversity. This decline reduces the immunosuppressive effects of a healthy microbiota. Because of this imbalance, excessive inflammatory and immune responses may develop. The prime targets are the major helper T cell and Treg populations. Most, except Th2 cells, are downregulated.

proton pump inhibitors, or antibiotics during their first six months predisposed them to the developing allergic diseases later in childhood. Presumably this is a result of drug-induced changes in the composition of their intestinal microbiota. Thus, the development of the immune system, its maturation, and its regulation are driven by the microbiota. This dysbiosis does not necessarily involve the absolute loss of individual bacterial species. However, the composition of the microbiota and its diversity may be greatly reduced.

Studies of environmental effects on the microbiota of developing puppies and their owners have found that allergies are most common in urban dogs living in single-person households without other animal contacts. They are least common in rural dogs with an opposite lifestyle. In enclosed urban spaces such as apartments or subways, the human microbiota predominates. Because of this exposure, bacteria commonly found on human skin predominate on the skin of urban dogs also. Human-derived bacteria are also enriched on allergic dogs compared to healthy dogs. Conversely, environmental bacteria predominate on the skin of rural dogs. Thus, both living environment and lifestyle independently shape the skin microbiota and an animal's risks of developing type 2 immune responses.

Similar studies have been conducted on piglets. Major differences have been found in the piglet gut microbiota depending on the environment in which they are raised. These differences also influence the expression of their immune system genes. For example, pigs raised in a very clean environment have decreased microbial diversity and express more genes related to inflammation such as those encoding type 1 interferon, major histocompatibility complex class I, antibacterial peptides, and chemokines. Conversely, outdoor pigs with a much more diverse microbiota expressed more genes linked to T cell function such as T cell antigen receptors and CD8 and the polymeric immunoglobulin receptor.

High-fat and sugar and low fiber diets can produce significant changes in the microbiota that influence T cell function. For example, mice fed a high-fat diet for 12 weeks were sensitized to a food allergen when subsequently challenged. The high-fat-fed mice had higher allergy scores than those on a control diet. The high-fat group also had a decreased microbial diversity, and increased numbers of mast cells in the gut and intestinal permeability. When this microbiota was transferred to germ-free recipient mice, there was no transfer of obesity; however, they too developed an increased susceptibility to food allergies.

Antibiotic Use

Antibiotic treatment is an important cause of dysbiosis, especially if administered to young children at an age where the composition of their microbiota is still evolving. Such treatment can radically alter the composition of their intestinal microbiota, increase the risk of developing infections with organisms such as *Clostridioides difficile*, and permit the overgrowth of other unwanted pathogens. Antibiotics alter the composition of the microbiota, resulting in an increased risk of obesity. (Obese individuals have more Firmicutes and fewer *Bacteroides* than lean ones.) However, much remains to be learned about this very complex subject. The most significant dysbiosis leads to the development of allergies. Even oral antifungal drugs can disrupt the intestinal fungal mycobiota in mice and increase the severity of airway allergic disease. Antibiotic use during pregnancy directly influences the development and composition of the newborn microbiota. By one year of age, up to half of human infants will have been exposed to antibiotics.

Germ-free mice have high serum IgE levels during early life. These can be greatly reduced by bacterial colonization, indicating that the microbiota suppresses IgE production. If low doses of the antibiotic vancomycin are fed to neonatal mice, the diversity of their gut microbiota is reduced, their Treg cell numbers drop, and they suffer from severe allergic lung disease. Antibiotic feeding also increases eosinophil infiltration, IgE levels, and airway hyperresponsiveness. Even adult mice treated with oral antibiotics develop increased IgE levels and blood basophil numbers. They also develop increased airway inflammation following allergen challenge. Preventing this high IgE response in germ-free mice requires colonization by a complex and diverse microbiota, not just a few selected species.

Dysbiosis and Food Allergies

The prevalence of allergies to foods has increased because of intestinal dysbiosis. For example, the microbiota of children with an egg allergy is significantly different from those who are not allergic. Changes in these early microbiota can also predict the resolution of food allergies. For example, the composition of the microbiota in children at 3–6 months of age correlates with the resolution of milk allergy around the age of eight. Clostridia and Firmicutes enrichment is especially important. Germ-free mice or mice treated with antibiotics before weaning developed higher IgE levels against peanut allergens in a food sensitization model; however, this was prevented by reconstitution with a Clostridial mixture. The Clostridia increased Treg cells, IgA, and IL-22 that collectively reduced the uptake of allergens. A high fiber diet had a similar beneficial effect.

There is a correlation between a high-fat diet, obesity, and the development of food allergies in experimental mice. Feeding a high-fat diet to mice results in the dysregulation of intestinal mast cells. While this did not appear to affect mast cells at a steady state, once food allergies were triggered, there was increased accumulation of mast cells in their intestinal walls. In addition, a high-fat diet resulted in a decrease in microbial α-diversity, reflecting changes in the availability of nutrients, especially fatty acids. This dysbiosis conferred increased susceptibility to food allergies independent of obesity. The effect of long-term feeding a high-fat diet persisted even after the diet was changed back to a control diet. Thus, the disruption of the core microbiome may be irreversible. Transfer of this disrupted microbiota to other germ-free mice transfers the predisposition to food allergies.

Skin Microbiota

The skin has its own complex microbiota. Normal skin harbors trillions of microorganisms. In humans, they amount to approximately a million organisms per square millimeter of skin. These are not only found on the surface of keratinocytes, but they also extend deep into sebaceous glands and hair follicles. The diversity of these skin commensals is much less than in the gut because of less friendly environmental conditions. Populations of Proteobacteria and Oxalobacteraceae predominate, but these may differ significantly at different sites because of these environmental differences. Sebaceous sites are colonized by lipophilic organisms such as *Propionibacterium*. Moist sites are mainly occupied by *Staphylococci* and *Corynebacterium* (Fig. 7.7). Fungi, especially *Malassezia* species, may dominate many sites.

Given the sheltering effects of hairs and feathers, it is likely that the skin microbiota in domestic animals is even more complex than in humans, varying greatly between individuals and different skin sites. For example, there is a higher microbial diversity in haired skin compared to mucocutaneous junctions. The highest microbial diversity was found in the canine axilla and on the dorsum of the nose. On average, approximately 300 different bacterial species have been identified on the dorsal canine nose.

The skin microbiota can be divided into a resident population that is relatively stable and consistent—a true commensal population and a population of transient bacteria that may only persist on the skin for hours or days. Both populations contain a mixture of commensals and potential pathogens, yet invasion and disease are relatively uncommon.

The precise composition of the skin microbiota depends on the location (hairy, wooly, or bald skin; back versus skin in the axilla, groin, or ear) and disease presence such as seborrhea or atopic dermatitis (AD). There is also great variation between individuals. Grooming activities have some influence on these microbial populations; however, their significance remains unclear. Provided

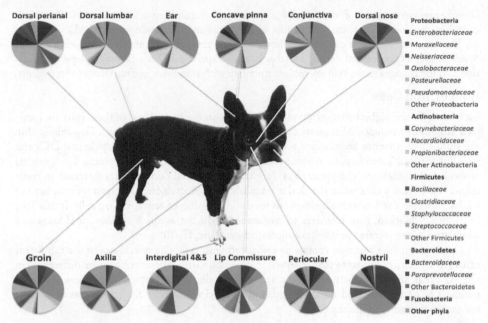

Fig. 7.7 **Composition of the microbiota on canine skin.** (From Rodrigues Hoffmann A, Proctor LM, Surette MG, Suchodolski JS. et al. The skin microbiome in healthy and allergic dogs. *PLoS One* 8;9(1):e83197. doi:10.1371/journal.pone.0083197 eCollection 2014.)

the animal can reach them, atopic lesions will be subject to scratching and licking, and it is inevitable that soil bacteria from the claws and oral bacteria from the tongue will be introduced into these lesions. Therefore, the microbiota in these lesions will differ between accessible and inaccessible sites.

Healthy and allergic cats also show differences in the diversity of their skin microbial populations. There are higher proportions of *Staphylococci* in allergic cats than in non-allergic cats, a finding similar to that in dogs and humans.

The skin microbiota of dog owners is more similar to that of other dog owners than that of non-dog owners, which might explain why living with dogs and sharing some of their microbes may help reduce the risk of developing allergies in children. Dog ownership by children at three months of age is associated with a 90% reduction in the development of food allergies (Owning two dogs is even better.) The situation regarding cats is less clear.

IMMUNE REGULATION

The skin microbiota, like that in the intestine, exerts an immunosuppressive effect on local inflammatory and allergic responses. Like their intestinal counterparts, commensal skin bacteria can produce SCFAs that act as immunoregulatory factors, reduce the skin pH and make the microenvironment less attractive to potential pathogens. Some skin bacteria can induce keratinocytes to secrete antibacterial peptides and complement components that will influence the microbiota composition and enhance immunity to pathogens.

Studies comparing the transcriptome of the skin of germ-free mice with normal mice have found major differences in the genes encoding both innate immunity and antimicrobial proteins. Commensal bacteria act via a pathway involving the IL-1 receptor to drive skin T cell responses.

Commensal colonization of hair follicles is required to recruit Treg cells to the skin. Thus, skin microbial dysbiosis is associated with a loss of Treg cells and the development of AD.

The skin microbiota in canine AD shows reduced diversity and an increased prevalence of *S. aureus* and a concomitant decline in other bacterial species. AD is a chronic, relapsing condition and the changes in the skin microbiota fluctuate with skin flares and responses to treatments.

Role of Treg Cells

Skin contains the highest concentrations of Treg cells in the body. Most of these cells are localized around hair follicles. Microbiota control the balance between effector and Treg cells within the skin. They influence keratinocyte production of IL-1 and its effects on epidermal DCs and so influence local T cell responses. Some skin bacteria can activate antigen-specific T cell subsets across intact epithelium. The presence of Treg cells in neonatal skin mediates tolerance to commensal bacteria at a time when the skin is establishing its microbiota. In human infants, but not adults, skin colonization with *S. epidermidis* results in an influx of activated Treg cells. If this Treg cell influx is blocked, then tolerance to commensals will not occur. *S. epidermidis* is known to stimulate DCs to secrete the immunosuppressive cytokine, IL-10.

Otitis externa is a common complaint associated with AD. The microbiota of the canine ear canal has a diversity similar to that observed in other skin sites. However, there are differences in the ear canal microbiota between atopic and healthy dogs. Thus, atopic dogs show increased numbers of *Staphylococci* and *Ralstonia* spp. and reduced numbers of *Escherichia* species in their ear canals compared to healthy dogs.

Gut-Skin Axis

The risks of developing allergic skin disease are greatly increased if the diversity of the gut microbiota is decreased. The gut and skin have many common features. They are both well vascularized and innervated barrier structures that house a dense commensal population. They interact extensively so that some dermatoses are closely linked to gastrointestinal dysfunction, and the gut microbiota directly influences skin health (Fig. 7.8). This is largely a result of the

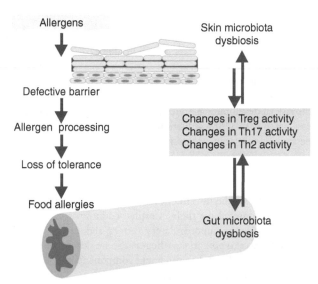

Fig. 7.8 The gut-skin axis. Intestinal or skin dysbiosis can both cause alterations in the T cell balance throughout the body. Reduced skin barrier function can also permit allergen sensitization through the skin. This is one possible mechanism of sensitization to food allergens.

increase in IL-10 production and a decrease in IL-17 production by Treg cells. This is a consequence of microbiota-mediated stimulation of systemic Treg cell numbers and functions. Butyrate-producing bacteria are found in the intestine in higher numbers in healthy infants than in children with severe AD. This is probably linked to the proven immunomodulatory effects of SCFAs.

In humans, the development of AD generally precedes food allergies, and AD-associated cutaneous inflammation is a significant risk factor for the development of food allergies. A defective skin barrier may drive this response simply by allowing allergens to avoid oral tolerance pathways. Thus, exposure to allergens by the skin route together with antigen processing by skin DCs may cause a loss of oral tolerance. Prior sensitization via the skin may permit oral allergies to peanuts, eggs, or wheat to develop. Loss of function mutations in human skin filaggrin can also allow a peanut allergy to develop. (Peanut allergens are stable and can persist in house dust and on skin.) This raises a question regarding animals that feed from a bowl or trough. Their nasal planum may come into significant contact with potential food allergens, especially when feeding. Likewise, the stratified squamous epithelium in the oral cavity could be a site of allergen entry. There is some evidence that migrating T cells may commute between the skin and gut and transfer allergic sensitization.

Respiratory Microbiota

Like all body surfaces exposed to the external environment, the upper respiratory tract, including the nose, throat, and oral cavity, houses a complex microbiota. The oral cavity also has a very diverse and obvious microbiota. (It is no coincidence that the first bacteria were observed by Anton van Leeuwenhoek when he examined the "gunk" between his teeth using the first microscopes.) Many nasal bacteria occur on the skin, whereas others are common environmental bacteria. Newborn mice have a lung microbiota dominated by Firmicutes and Gammaproteobacteria; however, these are gradually replaced by Bacteroidetes as the animals age. This change is associated with a switch from Th2 to Th1 skewing.

Contrary to previous belief, the lower respiratory tract and healthy lungs are not sterile. Healthy lungs harbor a microbial population closely related to but much less dense than that found in the upper respiratory tract. This is derived from the upper respiratory tract via the movement of inhaled air particles. The bronchi contain approximately 2000 bacterial genomes per square centimeter. Lung tissues contain between 10 and 100 bacterial cells per 1000 lung cells. These include both aerobes and anaerobes and like other surfaces; the composition of these populations differ greatly between individuals. The predominant phyla are Firmicutes and *Bacteroidetes* with lower numbers of Proteobacteria, Actinobacteria, and Fusobacteria. These organisms generally live within the mucus layer of the airways and include not only bacteria, but also yeasts, and viruses, especially bacteriophages.

IMMUNE REGULATION

It is unclear just how airway dysbiosis affects allergic disease development. One study in a mouse model of house dust mite-induced lung inflammation has shown that susceptibility was age dependent and associated with an increased load of Bacteroidetes in the lung. Younger mice exposed to dust mite antigens generated a much greater Th2 response than did older mice. The development of this resistance to Th2 in older mice was associated with changes in the airway microbiota, including an overall increase in bacterial numbers and a shift of the predominant organisms from Gammaproteobacteria and Firmicutes to Bacteroidetes. It is also possible to reduce airway allergic sensitization in mice by oral supplementation with beneficial organisms such as *Bifidobacterium* or bacterial metabolites such as SCFAs. Exposure to *E. coli* can suppress the allergic responses to inhaled ovalbumin in mice by activating DCs, inducing a Th1 response that reduces the Th2 response.

As on other surfaces, a balance is normally maintained between immune tolerance and inflammation. The airway microbiota clearly plays a role in resistance to respiratory infections and the development of asthma. Thus, in the absence of the microbiota, the airways are prone to mount an exaggerated Th2 responses. As on other body surfaces, the presence of microbiota stimulates Treg cell activity that suppresses these responses, explaining the protective effects of inhaled microorganisms (as in a farming environment) on the development of allergies in children.

Gut-Lung Axis

Immune responses in the lungs are influenced by the gut microbiota. Cross-talk occurs between the microbiota of the lung and the gut (Fig. 7.9). Allergic lung diseases are commonly linked to gastrointestinal dysbiosis and the intestinal microbiota changes in response to some lung diseases. The intestinal tract has an enormous and diverse microbiota; the lower respiratory tract is much less complex. The Firmicutes and Bacteroidetes predominate in both locations. The two populations develop simultaneously after birth. Many organisms colonize the intestine first and then the lungs. Changes in diet affect the microbiota at both sites. As discussed in Chapter 13, many chronic lung diseases are linked to a loss of microbial diversity in the airways. As in the gut, there is a correlation between a loss of microbial diversity in childhood and developing allergic respiratory disease in later life. This interaction between the gut and lungs is mediated via the production of immunomodulatory SCFAs such as butyrate and propionate within the intestine. As expected, most signaling appears to be one way from the gut to the intestine. However, the influenza virus in the lung may also affect the intestinal microbiota. The intestinal microbiota can also regulate pulmonary adaptive responses. Thus, the presence of segmented filamentous bacteria in the intestine can influence pulmonary resistance to bacteria and fungi.

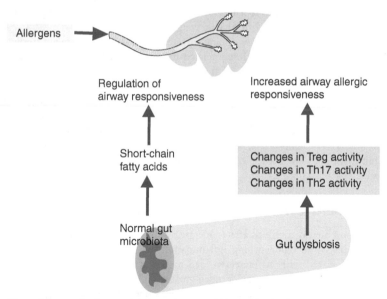

Fig. 7.9 The gut-lung axis. A normal, balanced gut microbiota maintains homeostasis in the airways largely through the release of immunosuppressive short-chain fatty acids. In dysbiosis, this regulation is disrupted and increased airway responsiveness can result. Given the relative sizes of the intestine and airway microbiota, the balance of the conversion is largely from gut to airways.

Helminth Parasites

Allergic reactions, in general, resemble those induced by intestinal helminths or biting insects. Both involve Th2 activation and IgE production. This has led to the suggestion that the immune system in allergic individuals is tricked into reacting to innocuous antigens as if they were parasites. Intestinal helminths, for example, trigger a local allergic reaction that results in "self-cure" in lambs. Reactions to parasites decline once the invader has gone. Therefore, it has been suggested that the development of allergic disease is simply an anti-parasite response "gone wrong." It is unlikely to be as simple as this, but this may be one component of the complex pathogenesis of some allergic diseases.

Helminth parasites can directly suppress the immune system to such an extent that they may inhibit the development of allergic diseases. Thus, children with schistosomiasis are significantly less prone to allergy than unparasitized children. Likewise, large long-term studies indicate that parasitized infants are much less likely to develop asthma. There are many reports of helminth infestations suppressing graft rejection and prolonging allograft survival (Box 7.1). A logical question, therefore, is whether the disappearance of such parasites in developed countries is responsible in part for the rise in allergic diseases.

Studies in experimental animals such as mice have confirmed the immunosuppressive properties of parasitic helminths, while cell transfer experiments have supported the theory that this suppression is largely due to enhanced Treg cell activity. Thus, parasites can directly promote Treg cell activities and IL-10 production, while their removal restores immune functions and immunity to parasites. In addition, many parasite products can suppress IL-12 production and promote Th2 responses. Macrophages in parasitized animals often develop an M2 phenotype that favors tissue repair and wound healing rather than phagocytosis and microbial killing. It is also clear that extent of parasite-induced suppression depends on the size and duration of the infestation and varies among helminth species. Early life parasite infestation is the most effective in preventing the development of allergic disease. The presence of intestinal helminths also affects the composition of the microbiota, which may also have secondary effects on the functions of T cell populations.

BOX 7.1 ■ Worms and Allergies

While the intestinal microbiota primarily consists of bacteria, archaea, and some viruses, it may also contain other organisms, such as parasitic worms. These intestinal worms can influence the development of type 2 immune responses. First, they trigger the body's immune system to mount a defensive response against themselves. Second, their presence may also influence the development of the atopic state. For example, studies have been undertaken to determine whether the presence of the parasitic nematode *Toxocara canis* in the gastrointestinal tract of dogs influenced the development of house dust mite hypersensitivity. One group of young beagles was infected with *T. canis* while a second group was not. Both groups were then sensitized by epicutaneous administration of house dust mite allergens. When the animals were assessed, it was found that the *T. canis*-infected dogs had higher levels of antibodies against mite antigens, as expected. They also had higher levels of total IgE. However, they had lower skin lesion scores and less pruritus. Thus, the worms increased their sensitization to the house dust mite but had a protective effect by inducing a polyclonal IgE response that saturated mast cell FcεRI and prevented cross-linking and degranulation.

Fischer N, Rostaher A, Zwickl L, Deplazes P, Olivry T and Favrot C. A *Toxocara canis* infection influences the immune response to house dust mite allergens in dogs. *Vet Immunol Immunopathol.* 2018;202:11-17.

Suggested Reading

Blander JM, Longman RS, Iliev ID, Sonnenberg GF, Artis D. Regulation of inflammation by microbiota interactions with the host. *Nat Immunol.* 2017;18(8):851-860.

Chermprapai S, Ederveen THA, Broere F, et al. The bacterial and fungal microbiome of the skin of healthy dogs and dogs with atopic dermatitis and the impact of topical antimicrobial therapy, an exploratory study. *Vet Microbiol.* 2019;229:90-99.

Dang AT, Marsland BJ. Microbes, metabolites, and the gut-lung axis. *Mucosal Immunol.* 2019;12(4):843-850.

Ennamorati M, Vasudevan C, Clerkin K, et al. Intestinal microbes influence development of thymic lymphocytes in early life. *Proc Natl Acad Sci U S A.* 2020;117(5):2570-2578.

Hakanen E, Lehtimaki J, Salmela E, et al. Urban environment predisposes dogs and their owners to allergic symptoms. *Sci Rep.* 2018;8(1):1585. doi:10.1038/s41598-018-19953-3.

Kyburz A, Muller A. The gastrointestinal tract microbiota and allergic disease. *Dig Dis.* 2016;34(3):230-243.

Lambrecht BN, Hammad H. The immunology of the allergy epidemic and the hygiene hypothesis. *Nat Immunol.* 2017;18(10):1076-1083.

Lehtimäki J, Sinkko H, Hielm-Björkman A, et al. Skin microbiota and allergic symptoms associate with exposure to environmental microbes. *Proc Natl Acad Sci U S A.* 2018;115(19):4897-4902.

Maizels RM. Regulation of immunity and allergy by helminth parasites. *Allergy.* 2020;75(3):524-534.

Marsella R, Santoro D, Ahrens K. Early exposure to probiotics in a canine model of atopic dermatitis has long-term clinical and immunological effects. *Vet Immunol Immunopathol.* 2012;146(2):185-189.

McCoy KD, Ignacio A, Geuking MB. Microbiota and the type 2 immune responses. *Curr Opin Immunol.* 2018;54:20-27.

Mulder IE, Schmidt B, Stokes CR, et al. Environmentally-acquired bacteria influence microbial diversity and natural innate immune responses at gut surfaces. *BMC Biol.* 2009;7:79. doi:10.1186/1741-7007-7-79.

O'Neill CA, Monteleone G, McLaughlin JT, Paus R. The gut-skin axis in health and disease: a paradigm with therapeutic implications. *BioEssays.* 2016;38(11):1167-1176.

Ohnmacht C, Park JH, Cording S, et al. Mucosal immunology. The microbiota regulates type 2 immunity through RORγt$^+$ T cells. *Science.* 2015;349(6251):989-993.

Older CE, Diesel A, Patterson AP, et al. The feline skin microbiota: the bacteria inhabiting the skin of healthy and allergic cats. *PLoS One.* 2017;12(6):E0178555. doi:10.1371/journal.pone.0178555.

Petersen EBM, Skov L, Yhyssen JP, Jensen P. Role of the gut microbiota in atopic dermatitis: a systemic review. *Acta Derm Venereol.* 2019;99(1):5-11.

Rodrigues Hoffmann A, Proctor LM, Surette MG, Suchodolski JS. The microbiome: the trillions of microorganisms that maintain health and cause disease in humans and companion animals. *Vet Pathol.* 2016;53(1):10-21.

Rooks MG, Garrett WS. Gut microbiota, metabolites and host immunity. *Nat Rev Immunol.* 2016;16(6):341-352.

Allergic Diseases

CHAPTER 8

Anaphylaxis

In 1902, two physiologists, Charles Richet and Paul Portier, went on an oceanographic voyage on a yacht, the "Princesse Alice II," at the invitation of Prince Albert of Monaco, a keen marine biologist. On the voyage, they studied the toxins of the sea anemone, *Actinia*. One project was to make an antitoxin by immunizing dogs. They attempted to immunize a dog called Neptune by first giving him a very low dose of *Actinia* toxin. Twenty-two days later, they boosted Neptune with a second dose of the antigen. Within seconds, Neptune began to gasp for air, collapsed, developed bloody vomiting, and died within 25 minutes. Richet immediately recognized that this was a new phenomenon. To describe this lack of protection, he first used the Greek word aphylaxis; however, anaphylaxis sounded better, and the name stuck. Charles Richet was awarded the Nobel Prize for this discovery in 1913.

Anaphylaxis is defined as a serious, generalized or systemic, allergic or hypersensitivity reaction that can be life-threatening. While anaphylaxis is usually a rapid event—hence the term immediate hypersensitivity—up to 20% of human cases may show biphasic allergic reactions in which the signs of anaphylaxis may recur several hours after the initial reactions have resolved. Some patients may even develop these late-phase reactions without an obvious early phase.

Anaphylaxis is triggered by rapid exposure to an allergen in a highly sensitized animal. In its most extreme form, allergen binds to high-affinity immunoglobulin E (IgE) linked to FcεRI on large numbers of mast cells. Receptor cross-linking results in generalized mast cell degranulation and the release of large amounts of mediators, especially histamine. If the histamine release rate from these mast cell granules exceeds the ability of the body to adjust to the changes in its vascular system, the victim may collapse and die. The clinical signs of anaphylaxis are determined by the specific organ system involved in the response, which differs among the major domestic mammals. In general, most clinical symptoms are the direct result of generalized and intense smooth muscle contraction in the bronchi, gastrointestinal tract, uterus, and bladder. Such contraction is mediated by histamine and other vasoactive molecules suddenly released by large numbers of degranulating mast cells and basophils.

Conventional practice has been to reserve the term anaphylaxis for those reactions mediated by IgE, i.e., immediate-type hypersensitivity. The term anaphylactoid was reserved for non-IgE-mediated reactions. However, in 2003, the World Allergy Organization suggested that the term anaphylactoid be abandoned and that all such episodes be defined as anaphylactic. Currently, anaphylactic reactions are classified into the following:

1. Immunologic IgE-mediated: Typical allergic reactions mediated by IgE responses to allergens such as insect venoms, foods, and drugs.
2. Immunologic non-IgE-mediated: Very similar to IgE-mediated reactions but caused by immune complexes, complement activation, or autoimmunity.
3. Non-immunologic: Reactions caused by physical factors such as cold, heat or exercise, certain drugs, and chemotherapeutic agents that cause mast cells to degranulate.

IgE-Dependent Anaphylaxis

The common cause of IgE-mediated anaphylaxis in humans and domestic animals is the rapid intake of specific allergens, including insect and reptile venoms, some foods, latex allergens, or vaccines, and drugs such as the β-lactam antibiotics.

ALLERGEN UPTAKE

Anaphylaxis is a very rapid process. It can develop when allergens are injected intravenously through a syringe or insect bite. Alternatively, the allergen may be ingested and rapidly absorbed from the stomach or intestine. Once these allergens enter the bloodstream, they are captured by dendritic cells (DCs). Perivascular DCs continually probe nearby blood vessels by extending their processes (dendrites) through blood vessel walls and directly sample any allergens they encounter. Using non-specific mannose-binding receptors, these DCs can readily capture a broad range of circulating allergens. These allergens are not internalized or processed but are incorporated into microvesicles. The microvesicles, ranging from 50 to 1000 nm in size, then bud off from the membrane of the DC2 cells into the perivascular space. Direct cell–cell contact between the DCs and mast cells may also occur, although it is not essential for the triggering of anaphylaxis. When mast cells coated with high-affinity IgE encounter and their receptors are cross-linked by these allergen-loaded vesicles, they respond by rapid degranulation. (Fig. 8.1).

Another reason why anaphylaxis can develop so quickly after the administration of an allergen is that mast cells, as described in Chapter 3, can extend their cytoplasmic processes through blood vessel walls into the vessel lumen. These processes collect any circulating IgE and this IgE can capture any allergen molecules they may encounter. Thus, allergens do not have to leave blood vessels or enter tissues to encounter mast cells.

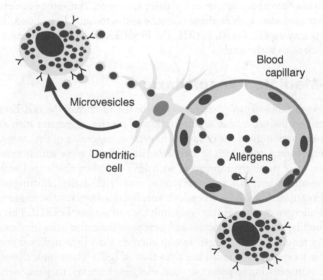

Fig. 8.1 Ways that an antigen can be captured by mast cells. One pathway involves allergen capture by dendritic cells (DCs). The DCs then release antigen-coated microvesicles into the tissues, where they can bind to mast cell-bound IgE. The second way is by direct capture of circulating allergens from the blood-stream by mast cell cytoplasmic processes that insert themselves between vascular endothelial cells directly into the capillary lumen.

IgE RESPONSES

Serum IgE is normally present in the bloodstream at a very low concentration. In humans, this is between 5 and 500 ng/mL in healthy individuals compared to 10 mg/mL for IgG. IgE is found at somewhat higher levels in the blood of allergic individuals (Table 2.1). However, the amount of IgE is much less important than its affinity for the allergen and its degree of glycosylation.

Studies on food allergic patients indicate that high- but not low-affinity IgE is an absolute requirement for mast cell degranulation and anaphylaxis. (As described in Chapter 2, this high-affinity IgE is generated by the somatic mutation of IgG1 driven by follicular helper T cells rather than conventional type 2 helper cells.) Serum IgE assays do not distinguish between low- and high-affinity IgE, which is reflected in the poor correlation between blood IgE levels and the degree to which an animal may be sensitized.

Some patients may develop anaphylaxis when IgE is undetectable. Conversely, allergen-specific IgE can be found in patients who show no signs of allergic disease. For example, the vast majority of humans who possess IgE antibodies to Hymenoptera venoms have no systemic reactions to a sting, perhaps because this is a low-affinity or poorly glycosylated IgE. Thus, the presence of large amounts of IgE alone does not predict clinical reactivity to any specific allergen.

ROLE OF BASOPHILS

Basophils express high levels of FcεRI and the activating IgG receptor FcγRIIA and they likely participate in anaphylaxis. However, it is difficult to determine how significant this is given the dominance of mast cells in the process. Neutrophils may also contribute to the process by releasing myeloperoxidase; however, blood platelets that release platelet-activating factor (PAF) are likely to be of even greater significance. PAF is an incredibly potent mediator (see Fig. 5.2) and its biological activity can be detected at concentrations as low as 10^{-12} M. Anaphylaxis is associated with profound thrombocytopenia and platelet activation. Activated platelets in humans can also release other mediators such as platelet factor 4 and serotonin. In addition, depending on the species, platelets may express FcεRI, FcεRII, and FcγRIIA. Basophils, a source of PAF, may also form close associations with platelets.

Non-IgE-Mediated Anaphylaxis

Under some circumstances, anaphylaxis may occur in the absence of the IgE/FcεR/mast cell axis. This may be caused by inadvertent administration of protein aggregates such as immune complexes, inadvertent activation of the complement system, triggering of the coagulation system, or the direct action of some drugs such as acetylsalicylic acid and some autoimmune diseases.

For example, mice passively immunized with IgG and then challenged with its specific allergen can develop an anaphylaxis-like response that is clinically indistinguishable from the IgE-mediated reaction. This IgG-dependent anaphylaxis involves the triggering of mediator release by IgG-allergen complexes that cross-link the cell surface FcγRIII. This pathway largely involves neutrophils; however, monocytes and basophils have also been implicated. This type of response usually requires a much larger dose of allergen than IgE-mediated reactions. (The affinity of IgG for its receptors is much less than that of IgE.) These high allergen doses are not likely to occur in insect sting responses or food allergies; however, they may occur in some drug reactions (Chapter 14). In addition, activation of this IgG pathway in mice triggers PAF but not histamine release. Occasional cases of anaphylaxis in humans in the absence of IgE have been described, suggesting that IgG-mediated anaphylaxis may occur in people. For example, the IgG-neutrophil-PAF pathway is implicated in anaphylactic responses to some neuromuscular blocking agents.

The activation of the complement system by any of its pathways generates two small peptides, C3a and C5a, that can trigger a severe hypersensitivity response and hence are called anaphyla-toxins. These anaphylatoxins bind to receptors on mast cells, basophils, and other cells. They induce mast cell and basophil degranulation and may directly increase blood vessel permeability and smooth muscle contraction. This pathway may act synergistically with IgE responses in some food allergy cases.

C5a is the most potent to the two anaphylatoxins and can degranulate mast cells and stimulate platelets to release histamine and serotonin. C5a is a powerful attractant for neutrophils and macrophages. It increases vascular permeability, causes lysosomal enzyme release from neutro-phils and thromboxane release from macrophages, and regulates some T cell responses. The other small complement peptide, C3a, can kill bacteria such as *Escherichia coli, Pseudomonas aeruginosa, Enterococcus faecalis*, and *Streptococcus pyogenes*. C3a acts like other antimicrobial peptides by dis-rupting bacterial membranes. When produced in sufficient amounts, C3a and C5a can kill an animal.

Anaphylaxis-like reactions may also be triggered by agents that cause mast cell and basophil degranulation, including physical factors such as temperature extremes or exercise. They can also be triggered by drugs such as radiocontrast agents and some chemotherapeutic drugs. These also include heparan sulfate, aspirin, some non-steroidal anti-inflammatory drugs (NSAIDs), anti-biotics, opiates, and some neuromuscular blocking agents. They may not all work the same way, i.e., heparan sulfate activates the kinin system; NSAIDs may block cyclooxygenase activity and suppress prostaglandin E_2 production but increase levels of cysteinyl leukotrienes. Aspirin can increase FcεR1-mediated basophil activation. Fluoroquinolone antibiotics and neuromuscular blocking agents such as tubocurarine can activate mast cells by binding directly to MRGPRX2, the G-protein coupled receptor for substance P.

If the kinin system is activated, it generates bradykinin, a very potent vasodilator (Chapter 5), but it also activates blood clotting factor XII. This may trigger blood coagulation and consequent consumption of factors V, VIII, and fibrinogen and perhaps result in disseminated intravascular coagulation.

Domestic Mammal Anaphylaxis

Although anaphylaxis is the most dramatic and severe type I hypersensitivity reaction, it is more usual to observe local allergic reactions, the sites of which are referable to the administration route of the allergens. For example, inhaled allergens provoke inflammation in the upper respiratory tract, trachea, and bronchi, resulting in fluid exudation from the nasal mucosa (rhinitis) and tra-cheobronchial constriction (asthma). Aerosolized allergens will also contact the eyes and provoke conjunctivitis, itchiness, and intense lacrimation. Ingested allergens may provoke diarrhea and colic as intestinal smooth muscle contracts violently. If sufficiently severe, the resulting diarrhea may be hemorrhagic (Table 8.1).

DOGS

Severe allergic reactions that are anaphylactic in origin are not widely reported in dogs. Those that have been, include reactions to antimicrobials, vaccines, and insect venoms. The major organ systems affected by canine anaphylaxis are the gastrointestinal tract and the liver (Fig. 8.2). The severity of anaphylaxis is directly related to the pooling of blood in the liver. Histamine, the prime mediator in this species, is released by mast cells in the gastrointestinal tract. This flood of hista-mine into the portal system massively and abruptly increases the blood flow to the liver. However, at the same time, the outflow of blood from the liver is restricted by contraction of the hepatic venous sphincters, located where the hepatic veins enter the inferior vena cava (Fig. 8.3; Box 8.1).

TABLE 8.1 ■ Anaphylaxis in the Domestic Species and Humans

Species	Shock Organs	Symptoms	Pathology	Major Mediators
Horse	Respiratory tract Intestine	Cough Dyspnea Diarrhea	Emphysema Intestinal hemorrhage	Histamine Serotonin
Ruminants	Respiratory tract	Cough Dyspnea Collapse	Lung edema Emphysema Hemorrhage	Serotonin Leukotrienes Kinins Dopamine
Swine	Respiratory tract Intestine	Cyanosis Pruritus	Systemic hypotension	Histamine
Dog	Hepatic veins	Collapse Dyspnea Diarrhea Vomiting	Hepatic engorgement Visceral hemorrhage	Histamine Leukotrienes Prostaglandins
Cat	Respiratory tract Intestine	Dyspnea Vomiting Diarrhea Pruritus	Lung edema Intestinal edema	Histamine Leukotrienes
Human	Respiratory tract	Dyspnea Urticaria	Lung edema Emphysema	Histamine Leukotrienes
Chicken	Respiratory tract	Dyspnea Convulsions	Lung edema	Histamine Serotonin Leukotrienes

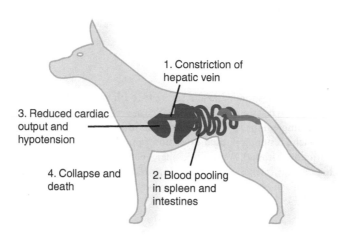

Fig. 8.2 Pathogenesis of anaphylaxis in a dog.

Hepatic portal vein vascular resistance can increase over 200% within 12 s during an anaphylactic episode. As a result, there is a massive drop in the venous return to the heart; therefore, cardiac output also drops abruptly, resulting in a compensatory tachycardia. The rise in intrahepatic vein pressure results in a massive influx of fluid to the liver, which is followed by liver enlargement and edema of the gallbladder wall.

BOX 8.1 ■ Hepatic Venous Sphincters

Venous sphincters are rings of smooth muscle cells associated with endothelial cells and mast cells adjacent to the vascular endothelium inside the elastic lamina. These sphincters are capable of spontaneous contraction and regulate blood flow. They also respond to vasoactive agents. Comparative studies have shown that dogs are unique in that they possess sphincters on the hepatic vein within 3 cm of its junction with the vena cava. Sublobular blood vessels within the hepatic parenchyma also possess these smooth muscle sphincters. The sphincters protrude into the vessel lumen either as circular or spiral bundles. Mediators such as histamine or endothelin 1 can cause them to contract and increase portal vein pressure. Corrosion casts of the hepatic blood vessels show a series of these sphincters arranged along the hepatic vein (see Fig. 8.3). Under normal conditions, the resistance caused by these sphincters is insignificant. However, administration of histamine or the histamine-release agent 48/80 results in their contraction. The greatest constriction occurs in the small branches (~100–400 μm dia) of sublobular veins.

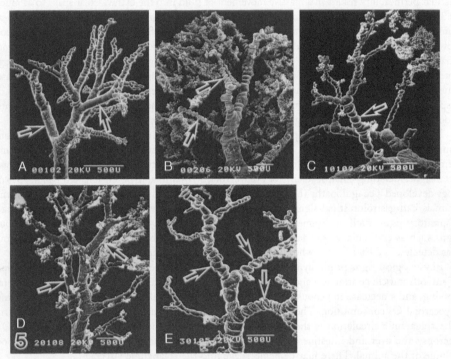

Fig. 8.3 Latex cast of hepatic blood vessels from a dog showing the presence of numerous constrictions, denoting the location of venous sphincters. Vascular casts of sublobular veins. The constriction of these sphincters results in clinical anaphylaxis in this species. (From Yamamoto K. Ultrastructural study of the venous sphincter in the sublobular vein of the canine liver. *Microvasc Res*, 1998;55(3):219. With Permission).

The resulting increased thickness and distinctive striation pattern of the gallbladder wall (>3 mm) are readily detected by ultrasound. This "gallbladder halo sign" is a useful confirmatory diagnostic test for anaphylaxis. Likewise, liver damage results in a significant rise in alanine transaminase, which may remain elevated for more than 24 h. Another diagnostic aid is a significant drop in body temperature. Hypotension is a prominent feature of dogs in anaphylaxis. In a recent study, the overall mortality in dogs with severe anaphylaxis was 14.9% (10/67 cases).

Clinical signs of dogs undergoing anaphylaxis include initial excitement followed by vomiting, bloody defecation, and urination. There may be a complete cessation of respiration for the first one or two minutes following the challenge. As the reaction progresses, dogs collapse with weakness and depressed respiration, become comatose, convulse, and die in less than an hour. Cutaneous signs may be slow to develop or absent in canine anaphylaxis. When they do occur, they include generalized erythema due to systemic vasodilation, urticaria, pruritus, and facial edema. However, only about half of affected dogs show this erythema and it can be very subtle and difficult to see.

Respiratory signs include dyspnea resulting from bronchoconstriction, pharyngeal edema, excessive mucus production, bronchospasm, and coughing. The depressed respiratory function is due to the release of histamine and leukotrienes within the lungs and a subsequent increase in airway resistance. The drop in cardiac output can account for a decline of 80% in the pulmonary blood flow. This decreased pulmonary circulation and redistribution of blood account for the fall in pO_2. However, the prime clinical feature is severe and prolonged hypotension. The histamine-induced increase in vascular permeability results in a massive movement of fluid into the extravascular space to as much as 35% of the total blood volume of the animal. Neurological signs may include weakness and seizures. However, with the drop in cardiac output, compensatory reflexes effectively redistribute blood flow to the brain, the adrenals, and the diaphragm. Therefore, these organs can maintain a normal flow. Non-specific gastrointestinal signs include vomiting and diarrhea. Antemortem hemorrhagic enteritis may be a consequence of the portal hypertension and associated mast cell heparin release. The rapid dramatic drop in cardiac output and mean arterial pressure account for the cessation of respiration and the deaths that occur within a few minutes. If an animal survives these initial events, blood flow to other organs will begin to return to normal after approximately 30 min.

Recent studies on canine anaphylaxis have found that serum phosphorus and prothrombin time were significantly higher in non-surviving dogs. Non-survivors also had lower body temperatures (histamine causes heat loss due to peripheral vasodilation). All dogs showed cardiovascular signs, including collapse, tachy- or bradycardia, arrhythmia, hypotension, and pallor. 85% of dogs developed a coagulopathy (high prothrombin and partial thromboplastin times); 94% of the animals had gastrointestinal signs, including abdominal pain, vomiting, and diarrhea; 67% had respiratory signs, such as dyspnea, wheezing, coughing, and cyanosis; and 27% had cutaneous signs such as erythema, angioedema, urticaria, and pruritus. The presence of gallbladder edema was detected in 84% of cases, whereas peritoneal effusions occurred in 65% of cases.

Physiological signs primarily result from occlusion of the hepatic vein due to a combination of smooth muscle contraction and hepatic swelling, resulting in portal hypertension and visceral pooling, and a decrease in venous return, cardiac output, arterial pH, mean arterial pressure, and myocardial O_2 consumption. The reduced cardiac output is caused by a drop in venous return. The splanchnic circulation is the largest blood reservoir in the body and very compliant. On necropsy, the liver and intestine are massively engorged, holding up to 60% of the total blood volume of the animal. There may be hemorrhage into the splanchnic viscera.

Identified mediators include histamine, prostaglandins, and leukotrienes. Histamine is the most important of these and some of its activity is driven via H3 receptors. Therefore, the classical H1 antihistamines are of limited clinical benefit. Anaphylactic reactions may resolve spontaneously within hours depending on the severity of the reaction and the ability of the animal to mount compensatory processes. Thus, the dog will produce epinephrine in its distress as well as angiotensin II and endothelins. (Endothelins are potent vasoconstrictor peptides that normally maintain vascular tone.)

CATS

In cats, the major organs affected by anaphylactic shock are the lungs and respiratory tract. Following an intravenous challenge with a parasite allergen such as from heartworms or other helminth parasites, cats undergoing anaphylaxis show vigorous scratching around the face and head as histamine is released into the skin, permeability increases, and facial swelling results. This is followed by sustained respiratory distress with severe dyspnea, tachypnea, and wheezing because of upper and lower airway edema, resulting in increased lung resistance. Cats may also develop systemic hypotension, salivation, vomiting, incoordination, hemorrhagic diarrhea, bradycardia, hypothermia, collapse, and death. The reported mortality is approximately 13%. Depending on the severity of the shock and the survival time of the animal, cats may exhibit retching, defecation and flatulence, urination, and bleeding from the nose or anus. Necropsy reveals bronchoconstriction, emphysema, pulmonary hemorrhage, and edema of the glottis. The major mediators in the cat are histamine and leukotrienes.

Because of extreme dyspnea, cat blood shows decreased O_2 saturation. In cats that die, there may be a sudden onset of apnea, suggesting a loss of input from the respiratory center in the brainstem because of acute hypotension. The most consistent hematological change is an increase in hematocrit values because of hemoconcentration secondary to increased vascular permeability and a loss of intravascular fluid.

HORSES

The major shock organs of horses are the lungs and intestine. During anaphylaxis, bronchial and bronchiolar constriction leads to coughing, dyspnea, and eventually apnea. On necropsy, severe pulmonary emphysema and peribronchiolar edema are commonly seen. In addition to the lung lesions, edematous hemorrhagic enterocolitis may cause severe diarrhea.

Experimental anaphylaxis in ponies sensitized by inoculation of whole bovine serum has a characteristic pattern. Within 2 min of beginning allergen infusion, there is a fall in carotid artery pressure accompanied by a rise in pulmonary blood pressure and a brief fall in vena cava pressure. By 3 min, the vena cava pressure increases transiently coinciding with a period of apnea. After about 8–10 min, the venous pressure returns to normal. Carotid pressure returns to normal by 15 min and pulmonary artery pressure normalizes after 20–25 min.

In other experimental anaphylaxis studies in ponies, the initial apnea was followed by 2–3 min of rapid breathing. There was another period of apnea lasting 3–4 min and after a short period of shallow rapid breathing, respiration returned to normal by 12 min. During the shock phase, there was marked hemoconcentration. The total leukocyte count decreased within 5–10 min but returned to normal by 30–40 min. This decrease involved neutrophils and monocytes, whereas the lymphocyte numbers remained unchanged. Simultaneously, there was a severe thrombocytopenia with the platelet count dropping to about 25% of normal. Mast cells demonstrated some dispersal of granules into the surrounding tissues. The lungs were congested and edematous. There was significant emphysema and bronchiolar edema. Two to four minutes after allergen infusion started, there was a 5- to 6-fold increase in plasma histamine, and it remained elevated for at least 20 min. Simultaneously, there was an increase in whole blood kinin activity that peaked at 5 min but returned to normal by 10–12 min. Plasma concentrations of serotonin were reduced significantly within 30–60 s of infusion. They remained below normal for at least 20 min.

CATTLE

Cattle may develop acute allergic reactions ranging in severity from pruritic urticaria to acute anaphylaxis with pulmonary edema and sudden death; however, this is a rare event. Anaphylaxis usually develops within 10–20 min of allergen administration but may take significantly longer. In cattle, the major target organs are the lungs, specifically the pulmonary vasculature (Figure 8.4). Anaphylaxis is characterized by the rapid onset of profound systemic hypotension and pulmonary hypertension, with the latter resulting from constriction of the pulmonary vein,

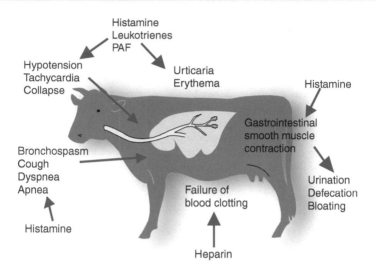

Fig. 8.4 Pathogenesis of bovine anaphylaxis. The proximal cause of death in most species results from extreme constriction of the bronchial smooth muscle and subsequent asphyxiation. However, in cattle, pulmonary hypertension results in death from pulmonary edema.

leading to pulmonary edema. The smooth muscle of the bladder and intestine contract, causing urination, defecation, and bloating. Initial signs include severe dyspnea with open mouth breathing, anxiety, salivation, urticaria, and lacrimation. Edema of the face, eyelids, lips, perineum, and udder may develop. Animals may extend their tongue and walk backward in an effort to take deeper breaths. Bloody foam may appear at the nose and mouth, followed by staggering, collapse, recumbency, and death.

Experimental calves were sensitized by repeated injections of horse serum. 14–21 days later, they were anesthetized and challenged with the same allergen. Their systemic arterial pressure fell rapidly after infusion, followed by a transient rise and further hypotension before it returned to normal. Pulmonary arterial pressure rose about the same time as the fall in systemic pressure. This dropped, rose again, and then dropped slowly to normal. Increased vena cava pressure was delayed for about 20 seconds at a time that coincided with a period of apnea. Initial bradycardia lasted for about 3 min before being followed by tachycardia. Repeated allergen administration 30–60 minutes later induced a milder anaphylactic response. It was not possible to evoke a third response. There was a 10-fold increase in plasma histamine concentration within the first minute after allergen injection.

The main mediators of anaphylaxis in cattle are histamine, serotonin, kinins, and leukotrienes. Dopamine enhances histamine and leukotriene release from the lung, thus exerting a form of positive feedback. Because of the anticoagulant properties of heparin from mast cell granules, blood from affected animals may not coagulate. In contrast to the other species, in cattle, β-stimulants such as isoproterenol potentiate histamine release from leukocytes, whereas α-stimulants such as norepinephrine inhibit histamine release. In addition, epinephrine potentiates histamine release in the bovine. The significance of these anomalous effects is unclear.

The only effective treatments for experimental anaphylactic shock in calves were sodium meclofenamate or a combination of disodium cromoglycate and diethylcarbamazine, suggesting that the prime mediators were histamine, serotonin, and most importantly leukotrienes (slow reacting substance-A). (Sodium meclofenamate is an NSAID that acts as a cyclooxygenase inhibitor and inhibits leukotrienes, disodium chromoglycate inhibits mast cell degranulation, and diethylcarbamazine inhibits arachidonic acid metabolism.) Normally, histamine relaxes tracheal muscles. However, when a calf undergoes anaphylactic shock, it triggers muscle contraction. Relaxation is mediated via H2 receptors, whereas contraction is mediated via H1R. Thus, there is a switch in histamine receptor usage during bovine anaphylaxis.

SHEEP

In sheep anaphylaxis, pulmonary signs predominate because of constriction of the bronchi and pulmonary vessels. Smooth muscle contraction also occurs in the bladder and intestine with predictable results.

Experimental anaphylaxis in sheep sensitized against ovalbumin and then given an intravenous dose of the allergen resulted in a clinical response similar to that observed in other species. Within 15–30 s, the injection triggered dyspnea, nose licking, defecation, and urination. The sheep stood still but attempted to stay upright by spreading their legs. Within 2 to 5 min, they sat on their haunches. Some went into lateral recumbency. Breathing became labored and the animals coughed violently. Sheep began to recover within 10–15 min after the injection; however, the handling of animals exacerbated the symptoms of severe dyspnea and frothing from the nose. By 40–60 min, the animals had returned to normal. These clinical signs were accompanied by a fall in systemic blood pressure and a rise in pressure in the pulmonary artery accompanied by hypertension in the vena cava and hepatic vein. There was a marked rise in tracheobronchial resistance. There were no significant lesions observed at necropsy, although renal cortical necrosis was associated with prolonged hypotension. Based on the use of selective pharmacological inhibitors such as sodium meclofenamate, the major mediators involved were bradykinin and leukotrienes. Antihistamines and serotonin inhibitors had no protective effect.

PIGS

In pigs, anaphylaxis is largely caused by systemic and pulmonary hypertension, leading to dyspnea and death. In some pigs, the intestine is involved, whereas in others no gross intestinal lesions are observed. The most significant mediator identified in this species is histamine.

Experimental anesthetized pigs previously sensitized to ovalbumin received an intravenous infusion of ovalbumin into the ear vein. Thirty seconds after the start of the infusion, their blood pressure dropped rapidly. This corresponded to a significant increase in pulmonary arterial pressure that lasted for 3–4 min. Dyspnea or apnea developed between 30 s and 4 min after the infusion started. All the pigs died from cardiovascular shock within 5–12 min. There were no gross or histopathological lesions seen on necropsy. Plasma histamine rose sharply within a minute of the infusion to 140% of normal levels. Total leukocyte counts dropped significantly within 2 min and the animals developed thrombocytopenia. Clinical signs included respiratory distress, apnea, uncoordinated movement, convulsions, and collapse. Cutaneous congestion occurred around the eyes, nose, and ears. In less acute cases, animals developed retching, vomiting, defecation, and nasal and facial pruritus. Histamine is probably the major mediator; however, the delayed onset of dyspnea may have been due to slower-acting mediators, such as leukotrienes or bradykinin.

HUMANS

The most common triggers of anaphylaxis in humans include foods such as peanuts, tree nuts, fish and shellfish, milk and eggs; latex; some drugs including penicillin and aspirin; and insect stings from bees, wasps, hornets, and fire ants. Death has been estimated to occur in approximately 17% of human anaphylactic cases. The commonest causes of anaphylaxis in children and young adults are food allergies. The most common causes of anaphylaxis in older individuals are drugs and insect stings. Mild cases are associated with flushing, urticaria, and angioedema. In moderate cases, dizziness, dyspnea, and nausea occur, while severe disease is characterized by bronchospasm, cyanosis, loss of consciousness, incontinence, acute myocardial infarction, respiratory arrest, and death. The triggering allergen is often undetermined; so that up to 50% of these cases may be classified as idiopathic.

Biphasic Anaphylaxis

It has been traditionally recommended that in anaphylaxis cases in humans, the patient should be monitored for 4–6 h after the initial event in case of possible recurrence. However, in up to 20% of affected humans, a second reaction may occur up to 72 h after the initial event, with a mean time delay of approximately 8 h. The pathogenesis of this delayed response is unclear, although it is recognized that it is IgE mediated. At one time it was believed to result from inadequate treatment of the initial event. Another possible cause was a delayed absorption of food allergens from the gut. However, neither explanation can account for all cases. Studies in mouse models have suggested that these delayed responses are due to the late release of PAF. Suggestions that corticosteroid administration can decrease the incidence of these biphasic reactions are controversial.

Late-Phase Reactions in Animals

Relatively few anaphylaxis studies have been performed in domestic species and it is unclear whether they too mount a biphasic response. Evidence suggests that they may develop delayed cutaneous reactions. Thus, when skin testing dogs suffering from allergic dermatitis, an inflammatory reaction may develop 6–24 h after allergen injection. There is an influx of neutrophils, eosinophils, and basophils into the skin, which is eventually followed by infiltrating Th2 and later Th1 cells (Fig. 8.5). Approximately a third of sensitized dogs develop this skin lesion by 6 h. The histology of this lesion closely resembles that of spontaneous atopic dermatitis. These delayed reactions may result from differential mast cell degranulation. Thus, a delayed wave of mediator release from mast cells, especially leukotrienes and newly synthesized cytokines, may account for the reaction.

Anaphylaxis Biomarkers

Many attempts have been made to devise a blood test for humans that would accurately reflect the anaphylactic process and exclude other possible causes of acute collapse. For example, can

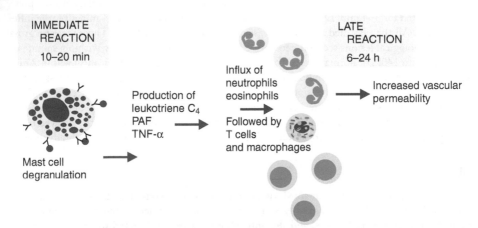

Fig. 8.5 Pathogenesis of the late-phase response in anaphylaxis.

mast cell products be detected in the bloodstream? None have been uniformly successful, either because of poor specificity and sensitivity or because of a lack of immediate availability. Total tryptase activity assay is most widely used in humans. However, its usefulness varies with the route of allergen exposure. For example, tryptase assay results correlate poorly with the severity of food allergies. Plasma histamine measurement is another such assay; however, this peaks within 5–10 min of onset and declines to baseline after 1 h. Therefore, it is often impractical. In dogs suffering from anaphylaxis, hepatocytes may be severely damaged, which can be measured by assaying alanine transaminase, an enzyme found in the hepatocyte cytosol. It is a sensitive indicator of liver damage with a half-life in plasma of 60 h. During canine anaphylaxis, alanine transaminase rises to peak at 24–48 h but may take as long as 3 weeks to return to normal. As stated previously, ultrasonography of the canine gallbladder wall shows thickening due to edema with characteristic striations.

TREATMENT OF ACUTE ANAPHYLAXIS

Anaphylaxis is a life-threatening medical emergency. Deterioration can occur very rapidly, and time is of the essence. Prompt recognition and aggressive management must be initiated before performing diagnostics. Clinical onset may occur within a minute of exposure to an allergen. Epinephrine (adrenaline chloride) administered intramuscularly is the first-line therapy for anaphylaxis and should be given immediately (Fig. 8.6). It counteracts the pathophysiologic changes in anaphylaxis by acting through α_1-adrenergic receptors to induce vasoconstriction and reduce airway edema, and acts through β_1-adrenoceptors to stimulate the heart rate and contractility. Epinephrine also acts through β_2-adrenoceptors to dilate the airways by relaxing the smooth muscle, thus relieving obstruction and blocking the further release of mediators from the mast cells. It causes a rise in blood pressure, improved oxygenation, and increased blood glucose levels.

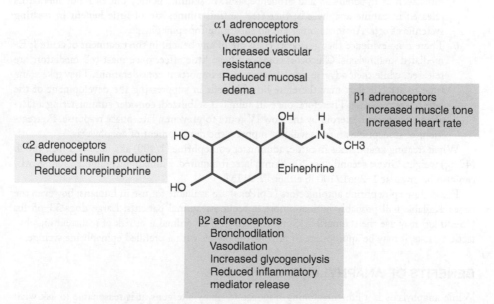

Fig. 8.6 Structure and pharmacology of epinephrine. It acts through four different adrenoceptors to induce its effects. Most of these effects counteract those of the mediators released in anaphylaxis.

(Epinephrine also has a biphasic effect where low doses may result in vasodilatation and increased mediator release.)

Initiate treatment immediately. If an animal is undergoing acute anaphylaxis, take the following steps:

1. Stop administering the allergen.
2. In the case of dogs and cats, administer epinephrine 1:1000 at a dose of 0.01 mg/kg intramuscularly (IM). (Maximum dose is 0.3 mg in animals under 40 kg and 0.5 mg in larger dogs). This may be repeated every 5–15 min if necessary, because epinephrine has a very short duration of action. If very severe and shock has developed, place an intravenous (IV) catheter and administer 0.1 mg/kg of 1:10,000 epinephrine by slow IV infusion while monitoring blood pressure and perfusion. Alternative routes of epinephrine administration include intracardiac or intratracheal. Avoid subcutaneous administration because epinephrine is a potent vasoconstrictor and its absorption is delayed.

   In the case of foals, administer epinephrine 1:1000 at 0.01–0.02 mg/kg (0.5–1 mL for a 50 kg foal). It is given slowly IV or IM. In adult horses, administer epinephrine at 0.01 mg/kg (3–8 mL for a 450 kg horse) slowly IV. If the condition is mild, this dose may be doubled and administered IM. Repeat every 10–20 min as necessary.
3. Secure the airway, intubate if necessary, and administer high-flow oxygen to any animals showing respiratory symptoms.
4. Provide isotonic shock crystalloid fluids (normal saline or lactated Ringer's solution) IV to help restore adequate blood pressure in hypotensive animals. The volume required depends on the animal's response but may be as high as 90 mL/kg for dogs and 60 mL/kg for cats.
5. Administer an H1-antihistamine such as diphenhydramine every 8–12 h if necessary. It may be given PO or IM at a dose of 1–4 mg/kg in dogs and 0.5–2 mg/kg in cats. Antihistamines may be effective in less severe anaphylaxis, especially in ameliorating skin and nasal symptoms. They are ineffective in treating the cardiovascular and respiratory symptoms such as hypotension and bronchospasm. Histamine is only one of many mediators released in canine anaphylaxis; therefore, antihistamines are of little benefit in treating systemic effects. Antihistamines are no substitute for epinephrine.
6. There is no evidence that glucocorticoids are of any benefit in the treatment of acute IgE-mediated anaphylaxis. Glucocorticoids can have little effect once mast cell mediators are released, while their adverse side-effects remain important considerations. They take some time to act but they may therefore be of benefit in suppressing the development of the late-phase response. Therefore, once an animal is stabilized, consider administering a fast-acting glucocorticosteroid by the slow IV route to prevent a late-phase response. Pretreatment of susceptible animals will not suppress the development of anaphylaxis.

When treating anaphylaxis in cattle, administer epinephrine (1/100) at a dose of 1 mL/100 lb (45 kg) weight. Give a second dose 10–20 min later if required. Flunixin meglumine (50 mg/mL) can also be given at 1–2 mL/100 lb either IV or IM.

Fixed-dose epinephrine autoinjectors (EpiPens) are available for use in humans; however, the doses available will probably be inappropriate for most animal patients. Large dogs 33–65 lbs (15–30 kg) may use the standard 0.15 mg EpiPen Jr. If an animal is at risk of recurrent anaphylactic attacks, it may be appropriate to provide the owner with a prefilled epinephrine syringe.

BENEFITS OF ANAPHYLAXIS

While anaphylaxis is a life-threatening response to many allergens, it is reasonable to ask what good it does and why has it evolved. Components of animal venoms often result in allergic sensitization and may provoke anaphylaxis. However, experimental studies in mice have shown that the development of a type 2 immune response to honeybee venom improves mouse survival. This response to bee venom phospholipase A_2 reduces the mouse's temperature decline in response to the venom. This effect depends on IgE and its high-affinity receptor FcεRI. Mast cells plus IgE and FcεRI can protect against snake venoms. The release of large amounts of mast cell proteases, especially carboxypeptidase A and chymase, in response to envenomation, result in the rapid proteolytic destruction of venom proteins. Thus, the response will be beneficial if the victim also survives the anaphylaxis.

Suggested Readings

Alexander F, Eyre P, Head KW, Sanford J. Effects of anaphylaxis and chemical histamine liberators in sheep. *J Comp Pathol.* 1970;80(1):19-30.

Caldwell DJ, Petras KE, Mattison BL, Wells RJ, Heffelman VL. Spontaneous hemoperitoneum and anaphylactic shock associated with Hymenoptera envenomation in a dog. *J Vet Emerg Crit Care (San Antonio).* 2018;28(5):476-482.

Choi HW, Suwanpradid J, Kim IH, et al. Perivascular dendritic cells elicit anaphylaxis by relaying allergens to mast cells via microvesicles. *Science.* 2018;362(6415):656-667.

Eyre P, Lewis AJ. Acute systemic anaphylaxis in the horse. *Br J Pharmacol.* 1973;48(3):426-437.

Eyre P, Lewis AJ, Wells PW. Acute systemic anaphylaxis in the calf. *Br J Pharmacol.* 1973;47(3):504-516.

Finkelman FD, Khodoun MV, Strait R. Human IgE-independent systemic anaphylaxis. *J Allergy Clin Immunol.* 2016;137(6):1674-1680.

Hume-Smith KM, Groth AD, Rishniw M, LA Walter-Grimm, SJ Plunkett, DJ Maggs. Anaphylactic events observed within 4 h of ocular application of an antibiotic-containing ophthalmic preparation: 61 cats (1993-2010). *J Feline Med Surg.* 2011;13(10):744-751.

Kapin MA, Ferguson JL. Hemodynamic and regional circulatory alterations in dog during anaphylactic challenge. *Am J Physiol.* 1985;249(2 Pt 2):H430-H437.

Lemanske RF Jr, Kaliner MA. Late phase allergic reactions. *Int J Dermatol.* 1983;22(7):401-409. doi:10.1111/j.1365-4362.1983.tb02158.x.

Lihua L, Yoshikawa S, Ohta T, et al. Large particulate allergens can elicit mast-cell mediated anaphylaxis without exit from blood vessels as efficiently as do small soluble allergens. *Biochem Biophys Res Commun.* 2015;467(1):70-75.

Litster A, Atwell R. Physiological and haematological findings and clinical observations in a model of acute systemic anaphylaxis in Dirofilaria immitis-sensitized cats. *Aust Vet J.* 2006;84(5):151-157.

Quantz JE, Miles MS, Reed AL, White GA. Elevation of alanine transaminase and gallbladder wall abnormalities as biomarkers of anaphylaxis in canine hypersensitivity patients. *J Vet Emerg Crit Care (San Antonio).* 2009;19(6):536-544.

Reber LL, Hernandez JD, Galli SJ. The pathophysiology of anaphylaxis. *J Allergy Clin Immunol.* 2017;140(2):335-348.

Shmuel DL, Cortes Y. Anaphylaxis in dogs and cats. *J Vet Emerg Crit Care (San Antonio).* 2013;23(4): 377-394.

Smith MR, Wurlod VA, Ralph AG, Daniels ER, Mitchell M. Mortality rate and prognostic factors for dogs with severe anaphylaxis: 67 cases (2016-2018). *J Am Vet Med Assoc.* 2020;256(10):1137-1144.

Wells PW, Pass DA, Eyre P. Acute systemic anaphylaxis in the pig. *Res Vet Sci.* 1974;16(3):347-350.

Yamamoto K. Ultrastructural study on the venous sphincter in the sublobular vein of the canine liver. *Microvasc Res.* 1998;35(3):215-222.

CHAPTER 9

Atopic Dermatitis

The word atopy is derived from the Greek "*atopia*" meaning a strange disease, and it was first used in 1923 by Arthur Coca and Robert Cook. They defined atopy as the hereditary predisposition to develop allergies to environmental allergens. They included asthma, food allergy, eczema, and hay fever, among the atopic diseases. Eczema is a term used for atopic dermatitis (AD) in humans. AD refers to several similar genetically-predisposed inflammatory and pruritic allergic skin diseases with characteristic clinical features. Such skin diseases are often associated with the production of immunoglobulin E (IgE) antibodies to environmental allergens. AD is complex and multifactorial. It is characterized by the development of chronically inflamed and itchy skin lesions. It is very common in humans, and as many as 20% of children and 10%–15% of adults may be affected. Its apparent prevalence in dogs is determined by the nature of the veterinary practice, geographical region, and diagnostic criteria. Estimates range from 20%–50% of dogs presenting as dermatology patients to 3%–15% in broad-based general practice. AD is also recognized in cats, horses, and goats.

AD is not simply an IgE-mediated skin disease driven by exposure to environmental or food allergens in genetically predisposed animals. It also involves immune dysregulation, skin barrier defects, and microbial dysbiosis. It is often complicated by secondary Staphylococcal or Malassezia yeast infections. It is best considered as a syndrome with multiple endotypes. In acute cases it is primarily driven by excessive cutaneous Th2 responses with contributions from ILC2 cells. In chronic cases and infected lesions, Th17, and Th1 cells, are also active participants.

Introduction

Atopic dermatitis (AD) is a term that encompasses several chronic skin diseases typically presenting with inflammatory lesions and intense pruritus. The syndrome is frustrating to treat because it is influenced by many different environmental factors. At its simplest, it may be considered to be a local skin hypersensitivity response to environmental allergens. However, it is made vastly more complex and difficult to treat because of interactions with other factors that determine its progression and outcome.

For many years, it was widely believed that AD in dogs was a disease triggered by inhaled environmental allergens. It was thus called "allergic inhalant dermatitis." However, after reconsideration and analysis, it is now generally understood that most initiating allergens enter the body through the epidermis. Recent advances in our knowledge of the biology of this disease, such as the role of skin barrier defects and the distribution and histology of its lesions, make a transepidermal allergen transfer much more plausible. Experimental models of the disease involving the cutaneous application of allergens also support the transepidermal route of sensitization.

It is now generally accepted that the pathogenesis of most forms of AD begins with a skin barrier defect manifested by dry, itchy skin and associated with changes in the cutaneous microbiota (Fig. 9.1). Environmental allergens and bacteria breaching the skin barrier trigger the expression of proinflammatory cytokines, including thymic stromal lymphopoietin (TSLP) and interleukin 33 (IL-33), and as a result, activate type 2 helper (Th2) cells, basophils, and mast cells. This local type 2 immune response generates IL-31, a key mediator of itch. These responses eventually result in the development of dermatitis, which is initially erythematous and edematous

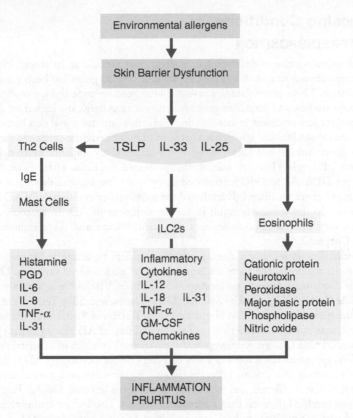

Fig. 9.1 Overview of the pathogenesis of atopic dermatitis. This represents the most widely accepted outside:inside hypothesis where the disease is triggered by extrinsic environmental allergens and skin barrier defects.

BOX 9.1 ■ Urticaria vs Angioedema

When mast cells degranulate, their contents such as histamine or bradykinin cause a local increase in vascular permeability. The movement of fluid into the skin intercellular tissues results in local swelling. In human skin, a clear difference can be readily seen between urticaria with pruritic wheals and normal skin. There is usually a relatively well-defined margin to the lesions and surrounding epidermal erythema. This may also be seen in species such as dogs (see Fig. 12.9). However urticarial lesions are much more difficult to discern in cats, with their highly elastic skin and lack of defined margins. Angioedema, in contrast, is swelling that occurs deeper within the skin. It is much more diffuse and difficult to see in furred animals. Urticaria and angioedema often occur together.

---

and are described as an urticarial type (*Urtica dioica* is the name of the "stinging nettle," a plant that has hollow stinging hairs that inject histamine into the skin when touched). Urticarial lesions are extremely pruritic; consequently, scratching may mask the true nature of the lesion. The inflammatory cell infiltrate in these urticarial lesions is typical of type 2 allergic inflammation. The lesions are infiltrated with B cells, macrophages, and mast cells, while IL-4, IL-13, and TSLP expression is higher than non-lesional skin (Box 9.1).

Predisposing Conditions

GENETIC PREDISPOSITION

Humans and animals prone to developing an allergic state are said to be atopic. However, the genetics of atopy are not simple. A complex network of over 30 genes has been associated with the human disease. These genetic studies have included genome-wide linkage studies, genome-wide association studies, and candidate gene associations. In general, the important genetic factors influence three key processes: innate immunity, adaptive immunity, and skin barrier function.

Initial studies looked for the associations between immune response genes and atopic lesions in dogs. No direct linkage was found between the major histocompatibility complex (DLA) haplotype and IgE levels. However, animals that possessed the major histocompatibility complex haplotypes DLA-A3 and -R15 developed atopy more frequently. Likewise, there was no apparent linkage between median IgE levels and the subsequent development of AD in puppies. High IgE levels do not inevitably result in the development of AD. In practice, serum IgE levels provide very limited information regarding sensitization and disease susceptibility, as discussed in Chapter 2.

While heritability varies, atopic disease prevalence differs significantly between breeds, although this varies regionally and there is a large amount of within-breed variation. Thus, the list of susceptible dog breeds depends on location. For example, Vizslas are commonly affected in Hungary, while Cavalier King Charles Spaniels, Great Danes, and Silky Terriers are commonly affected in Australia. A study on West Highland White Terriers in Switzerland provided an AD heritability estimate of 0.31. Another study of the heritability of AD among British guide dogs (mainly Labradors and Golden Retrievers and their crosses) resulted in a heritability value of 0.47. Therefore, approximately a third to a half of a dog's risk of developing AD is derived from its genotype. This study also indicated that the risks are higher when both parents are atopic, less when only one parent is affected, and much lower if neither is affected. Golden Retrievers have higher total and specific IgE levels than Labrador Retrievers. Two loci on canine chromosome 5 are associated with serum IgE levels in storage-mite sensitized Labradors. AD is, in practice, most common in West Highland White Terriers, Labrador and Golden Retrievers, German Shepherd dogs, Cocker Spaniels, Boxers, Bulldogs, and Shar-Peis. However, these reflect their breed popularity. There is no sex predilection. Chocolate-colored Labrador Retrievers are at greater risk than yellow or black dogs.

Both susceptibility and protective gene loci have been identified in dogs as a result of genome-wide linkage and association studies. Careful clinical evaluation has recognized several disease phenotypes that differ in such features as the age of onset, presence of hot spots, gastrointestinal disorders, flexural dermatitis, and the distribution of skin lesions. Some breeds may develop lesions in specific areas. Thus, French Bulldogs often develop lesions in the axillae, eyelids, and flexural surfaces. German Shepherd dogs, in contrast, develop lesions on the elbows, hind limbs, and thorax.

Candidate genes associated with atopy include those encoding the skin protein filaggrin (*FLG*), genes that affect T cell function and IgE production, and the TSLP receptor gene. Loss of function mutations in the filaggrin gene are well recognized in humans with AD and may also occur in dogs. (Filaggrin deficiency occurs in 10% of Northern Europeans and accounts for 20%–30% of AD cases in humans.) However, studies on the heritability of AD in West Highland White Terriers have shown that the filaggrin gene is not involved in this breed. Conversely, this mutation is involved in AD in Golden Retrievers. (That is not to say that West Highland Whites do not have barrier defects, simply that they are not due to mutations in the filaggrin gene.) Prospective studies on the development of atopic dermatitis in a cohort of West Highland White terriers have shown a reduction in circulating Treg cell numbers at 3 months and 1 year of age in animals destined to develop atopic dermatitis. Healthy animals had 4.5% Treg cells, while atopic puppies had 3.1% Treg cells at 3 months of age. By 1 year, healthy puppies still had 4% Treg cells, while atopic puppies had 2.9%. Some variants of the gene for the TSLP receptor are also associated with canine AD. As discussed in Chapter 5, TSLP is one of the master cytokines released by damaged keratinocytes. It contributes to the Th2 response and the itch sensation. Changes in its receptor affinity may increase or decrease its activity. Other genes that may be linked to the pathogenesis of AD include those encoding a tyrosine kinase involved in regulating the activation of B and T cells. In another study that examined a population of German Shepherd dogs, an association was found with the gene encoding plakophilin-2 (*PKP2*), a protein involved in epidermal cell–cell adhesion through corneodesmosomes and skin barrier formation. In conclusion, canine AD is a disease syndrome in which multiple genes play a role in association with environmental factors.

ENVIRONMENTAL FACTORS

For the past 100 years or so, biological and chemical environmental factors have increasingly acted to disrupt the physical integrity of the skin epithelial barrier, triggering the production of the three major epithelial cytokines and increasing barrier permeability. Environmental factors such as proteases in allergens, detergents, tobacco smoke, ozone, diesel exhaust fumes, nanoparticles, and microplastics contribute to barrier dysfunction (Box 9.2).

BOX 9.2 ■ Pollution, Smoking, and Allergies

The aryl hydrocarbon receptor (AhR) was originally identified by toxicologists investigating how environmental pollutants such as the aromatic hydrocarbons affected the body. AhR is a transcription factor activated by small molecules from the diet, microbiota, and environment, and controls cellular responses to aromatic hydrocarbons such as dioxanes and bisphenols. AhR plays an important role in regulating immune responses and the intestinal barrier. Thus, it is expressed at high levels in antigen-presenting cells, intraepithelial lymphocytes, Th17, and regulatory T (Treg) cells. Ligand binding to the AhR stimulates IL-23 production and a Th17 cell response. Defective AhR signaling results in increased intestinal permeability, severe intestinal inflammation, and the development of allergies. AhR-knockout mice mount enhanced Th2 responses and produce high IgE and IgG1 levels.

Air pollutants such as diesel exhaust particles on skin cells can bind to AhR. This receptor then translocates to the epithelial cell nucleus and upregulates the genes encoding IL-33 and TSLP, both of which trigger pruritus. Additionally, the AhR upregulates a protein called artemin in keratinocytes. Artemin acts to promote sprouting of peripheral nerve fibers into the epidermis and upregulates expression of the capsaicin and wasabi receptors. (Both of these detect chemical irritants.) Collectively, these changes induce extreme skin sensitivity. This can explain how some allergic individuals develop "allodynia," where mild skin stimulation triggers intense pruritis or pain.

Other ligands of AhR include the mediators serotonin and dopamine, products from the yeast *Malassezia*, and from intestinal bacteria such as *Lactobacillus* and some foods. All have been associated with AD development in pets. It is no coincidence that dogs in households where cigarettes are smoked are significantly more likely to develop AD than those living in non-smoking homes. This is probably related to AhR activation and damage of the stratum corneum via the generation of reactive oxygen species.

Hidaka T, et al. The aryl hydrocarbon receptor AhR links atopic dermatitis and air pollution via induction of the neurotrophic factor artemin. *Nat. Immunol.* 2017; 18:64-73.

Ka D, et al. Association between passive smoking and atopic dermatitis in dogs. *Food Chem. Toxicol.* 2014;66:329-333.

Scott SA., et al. Microbial tryptophan metabolites regulate gut barrier function via the aryl hydrocarbon receptor. *Proc Natl Acad Sci USA.* 2020; doi:10.1073/pnas.2000047117

Studies on the environmental and social factors predisposing to the development of AD in retrievers suggest that they include being reared in an urban environment, being male, being neutered, receiving flea control, and being permitted on upholstered furniture. Conversely, protective factors included living with other dogs (but not cats) and walking in rural areas, including woodlands, fields, and beaches. Collectively, these suggest that decreased air quality in cities may be a significant risk factor, which was supported by the fact that smoking by owners predisposes to AD development. As stated in Chapter 7, the urban microbiota may also be a predisposing factor.

SKIN BARRIER

The skin consists of the epidermis, the dermis, and the subcutis that collectively form a strong, multicellular, tight, defensive barrier. The outermost layer of the epidermis, the stratum corneum, consists of layers of dead cells—flattened, anucleate corneocytes that have undergone a form of cell death called "corneoptosis." These corneocytes lack a plasma membrane, which has been replaced by a structure called the cornified envelope. This envelope consists of a layer of an insoluble protein called loricrin that is highly cross-linked by transglutaminases, linked to keratin filaments, and surrounded by a ceramide-rich lipid envelope. The cornified envelope serves as a scaffold to which the lipids attach. Therefore, these corneocytes are effectively coated with a layer of lipids (Fig. 9.2). This structure has been likened to a brick wall where the corneocytes act as bricks and the lipid envelope serves as the mortar. The keratinocytes together with the highly hydrophobic lipids in the stratum corneum form a physical barrier that serves to keep water in and invaders out. In addition, the keratin within these cells is bundled together by a protein called filaggrin to form a dense protein–lipid matrix. Dog epithelium may contain much less lipid than human skin, perhaps because of the additional protection afforded by hair.

Normal Skin

Lipids. Extracellular lipids account for almost 10% of the mass of the stratum corneum. The layers of lipids surrounding keratinocytes consist of about 50% ceramides, 25% cholesterol and its esters, and 15% free fatty acids. These lipids are derived from specialized secretory organelles called epidermal lamellar bodies and synthesized by keratinocytes in the upper stratum spinosum and stratum granulosum. Ceramides are waxy lipids composed of fatty acids attached to sphingosine. There are many possible combinations of fatty acids and sphingosines, making at least 12 different ceramides. The lamellar bodies deliver the lipids and enzymes that are needed to

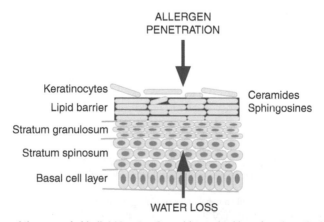

Fig. 9.2 **Location of the normal skin lipid barrier.** Ceramides and sphingosines form the basis of the intercellular "cement" that connects keratinocytes and prevent water loss and allergen penetration.

generate the ceramides and free fatty acids required for the development of mature lamellar membranes. Simultaneously, the lamellar bodies generate proteases that degrade corneodesmosomes, permitting the corneocytes to separate, loosen, and eventually be shed from the skin surface. Provided the skin lipid barrier is intact, it will minimize water evaporation and block ingress of environmental allergens.

Proteins. One of the most important proteins in the cornified envelope is filaggrin. Filaggrin is a histidine-rich, filament-associated protein involved in cross-linking keratin fibers within the envelope so that they become densely packed, and is a major component of the skin barrier. Filaggrin is first synthesized as a large polyprotein tetramer containing four filaggrin monomers called profilaggrin (Fig. 9.3). Profilaggrin is stored in keratohyalin granules in the stratum granulosum. As these cells differentiate into corneocytes at the boundary between the stratum granulosum and the stratum corneum, the profilaggrin is broken down into filaggrin monomers. These monomers then aggregate keratin filaments into keratin fibrils. Eventually, however, filaggrin is further broken down by skin proteases into its amino acids. These are then deaminated into urocyanic acid and pyrrolidone carboxylic acid. These acids draw water osmotically into corneocytes and generate an "acid barrier" with significant antimicrobial properties. For example, they inhibit the growth of *Staphylococcus aureus*. The acid pH is required for the proper synthesis of ceramides, activation of skin proteases, and in the desquamation process.

In addition to filaggrin, several other tightly cross-linked, insoluble proteins are key components of the corneocyte barrier. These include envoplakin, periplakin, and involucrin. Defects in the genes encoding any of these can also impair skin barrier function. Antimicrobial peptides, including defensins and cathelicidins, are also delivered to the intercellular sites by secretion from the contents of lamellar bodies.

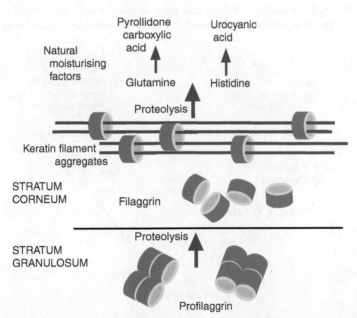

Fig. 9.3 Function of filaggrin. Profilaggrin in the stratum granulosum is broken down to filaggrin monomers. These monomers bundle keratin filaments within the stratum corneum to form a physical barrier. Further proteolytic degradation of filaggrin generates natural moisturizing factors such as pyrollidone, carboxylic acid, and urocyanic acid.

As described previously, a genome-wide survey suggested that there was a significant risk focus for canine AD on canine chromosome 27. *PKP2* was identified as the top candidate gene in German Shepherd dogs. Plakophilin-2 (PKP2) is a key component of desmosomes, the structures that bind epithelial cells together. It is present in skin and cardiac muscle, and is important in cell signaling and gene transcription. This finding resulted in a hunt to determine whether *PKP2* was present in the skin of atopic dogs. Skin biopsies revealed that it was present in keratinocytes, dendritic cells (DCs), and skin T cells. However, there was no apparent difference in its expression between AD lesions and normal skin control samples.

Skin Barrier Defects

It is widely believed that rather than being a consequence of AD, skin barrier defects may be its major predisposing cause. Defects in either the skin barrier protein filaggrin or in skin lipids such as the ceramides and sphingosine-1-phosphate permit water loss and the penetration of allergens and microbes, and increase the interactions between the skin immune system and environmental irritants.

One way to measure the integrity of the skin lipid barrier is to determine transepidermal water loss (TEWL). Evidence shows that the destruction or removal of the canine stratum corneum will increase TEWL. While difficult to measure in dogs and often difficult to replicate, evidence shows that destruction or removal of the canine stratum corneum will increase TEWL. TEWL is also increased in the skin of atopic beagles compared to control dogs. This is especially evident in skin locations prone to AD and is greater in younger than older animals. TEWL is increased in both lesional and non-lesional skin in natural cases of AD.

Lipid Defects. In many canine AD cases, the initial lesion appears to be a defect in the epithelial lipid barrier, leading to a decrease in its thickness (Fig. 9.4). Decreased ceramide levels or short-chain fatty acids in the skin have been associated with increased TEWL in humans. IL-4 and IL-13 interfere with the activities of fatty acid elongases in the skin. A ceramide defect occurs in human AD and it is both a primary causal defect and a secondary consequence of AD. In

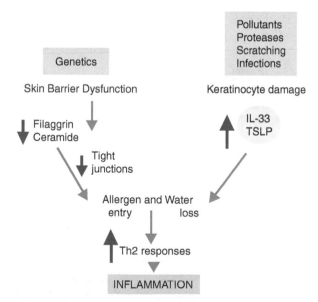

Fig. 9.4 Some of the consequences of skin barrier dysfunction and its relationship to allergic inflammation. Its causes can be environmental or genetic.

experimental canine AD, a decrease in ceramides is linked to epithelial inflammation. The proportion of ceramides is also reduced in lesional and non-lesional skin in AD dogs. Thus, experimental studies are consistent with a primary ceramide deficiency in dogs. There are wide variations in the free ceramide content in the skin of healthy dogs. Therefore, there may be large amounts of free glucosylceramides present in the skin of atopic dogs but not in the skin of normal dogs.

Sphingosine-1-phosphate is another important component of the skin lipid barrier. It is both a structural lipid and a signaling molecule because it modulates allergen capture by Langerhans cells. The mean level of sphingosine-1-phosphate is lower in lesional atopic skin than in healthy canine skin.

In atopic skin, the lipid lamellae in the barrier may be thinner and fragmented or discontinuous, whereas the spaces between the corneal cells may be wider. Electron microscope studies suggest that the continuity and thickness of the intercellular lamellae are decreased in non-lesional atopic dog skin compared to normal dog skin. Another feature of atopic skin is the presence of bands of variable density in the lipid layers, which may reflect fluctuating levels of ceramide associated with acute inflammatory episodes. In both humans and dogs, these ultrastructural changes are accompanied by a loss of epidermal ceramides.

Protein Defects. In humans, mutations in the filaggrin gene are important risk factors for AD development. A subset of AD dogs also have reduced filaggrin expression because of the loss of its C-terminal end. Single nucleotide polymorphisms within the canine filaggrin gene have been associated with some forms of canine AD. These loss of function mutations may be important in some breeds. However, these mutations are not consistently present and similar defects may occur in healthy animals. Thus, the importance of filaggrin in canine AD remains unclear. It is possible that filaggrin defects only account for a subset of canine AD cases or that filaggrin defects are secondary to other causes of AD.

Skin is also rich in proteases. These skin proteases include calpain-1, caspase-14, furin, and matriptase. Studies on the skin of atopic dogs have indicated elevated levels of calpain-1, caspase-14, and matriptase. These changes are also apparent in non-lesional skin from atopic dogs. A loss of filaggrin production by keratinocytes is accompanied (in mice) by the upregulation of IL-1 production, which is activated by proteases and contributes significantly to AD inflammation.

The cells of the epithelia are bound together by intercellular protein complexes called tight junctions. Other adherence structures include adherens junctions, which are located under the tight junctions and form a second barrier to invasion. The tight junctions seal the apical borders of the cell layer and block the free passage of allergens, pollutants, and microbes into the body. Desmosomes generally bind epithelial cells to basement membranes and connect epithelial cells. The skin of atopic dogs may develop defects in the expression of the tight junction proteins, such as claudin-1, occludin, and zonula occludens-1. These tight junctions normally bind cells in the stratum granulosum tightly to reinforce the physical barrier. If the tight junctions break down, then cells fall apart and allergens can more easily penetrate the skin. Hair follicles may be especially susceptible to tight junction defects.

Allergic Inflammation

Th2-mediated inflammation can worsen any barrier defects or induce such defects. This may permit skin DCs to capture and present environmental allergens to Th2 cells and promote the inflammatory state. Scratching also damages the integrity of the skin lipid barrier and stimulates the release of TSLP that further promotes Th2 cell functions.

House dust mite allergens such as Der f 1 have significant protease activity and once in contact with the skin, may damage the skin barrier. They can reduce the expression of adhesion and tight junction proteins in the stratum corneum such as corneodesmosin and claudin-1. Likewise, proteases of the kallikrein family are responsible for the desquamation of keratinocytes. They too may become dysregulated in AD, promote acanthosis, and induce TSLP production. Epithelial proteases such as kallikreins and cathepsins may also directly trigger neuronal pathways to induce itch.

ENVIRONMENTAL ALLERGIES

The sum of the external factors that an individual animal is exposed to throughout their lifetime (the exposome) includes non-specific factors that affect dog populations; specific factors such as humidity, diet, behavior, pollution, and allergens; and host factors such as the animal's skin microbiota and host-cell interactions. Given its location, the skin is the organ that directly interacts with the exposome and where environmental influences would be expected to have the greatest influence.

The most important route of allergic skin sensitization is percutaneous. There may be hyperplasia of the Langerhans cells in lesional skin, which suggests that the Langerhans cells respond to allergens that have penetrated the skin barrier. γ/δ T cells are also present in lesional skin. These are specialized T cells, many producing IL-17, that serve to protect epithelial barriers and support the concept of an ongoing type 2 response to environmental allergens within the skin lesions. The syndrome associated with sensitization to known environmental allergens is known as "extrinsic AD."

Environmental Allergens

Extrinsic AD is associated with exposure to environmental allergens such as molds and pollens and as a result, many cases are seasonal. Surveys suggest that approximately 30% of affected dogs show seasonal responses (range 15%–62%). Non-seasonal extrinsic AD may be associated with allergies to house dust mites (*Dermatophagoides farinae* and *D. pteronyssinus*), animal danders, and the yeast *Malassezia pachydermatis*. Diverse environmental allergens implicated in the pathogenesis of AD include biological particles generated by many different plants, molds, other mammals, and arthropods (Fig. 9.5).

Pollens. Many atopic dogs are sensitized against pollen-derived allergens. This sensitization is usually directed against plants that rely on the wind to spread their pollen long distances. To increase their fertilization chances, these plants have evolved small, light, aerodynamic pollen

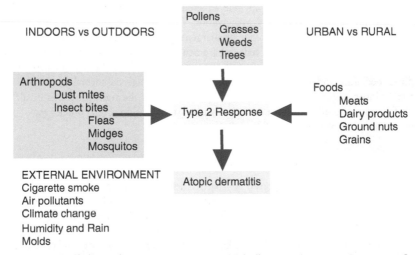

Fig. 9.5 Summary of the major types of environmental allergens that can trigger type 2 allergic responses in the skin.

grains that allow them to be transported hundreds of miles. Most pollens and mold spores are approximately 20–60 μm in diameter and lodge in the eyes and nasal passages. Smaller airborne particles around 10μm in diameter can be inhaled and penetrate the lower respiratory tract. Pollen grains initially contain a single fertilized cell that eventually develops into a male gametophyte. Their allergens are usually glycoproteins found within the pollen protoplast that are released when the pollen lands on a moist surface and rehydrates. The allergens escape via small apertures in the pollen coat and can cover the entire pollen surface. In addition to their glycoproteins, pollens may also release lipids that can bind to toll-like receptors, and promote type 2 immune responses. These lipids include saturated and unsaturated fatty acids, glycophospholipids, and lipopolysaccharides from the microbiota on the pollen surface. Therefore, simple aqueous pollen extracts may not contain all the biologically active substances released by pollen grains and may underestimate their allergenicity when used for skin testing or immunotherapy. Many grass and tree pollens contain active cysteine and serine proteases that can disrupt the epithelial barrier by degrading the proteins in tight junctions.

There is a very high frequency of cross-reactions between different species of grass pollens. Pollen counts are affected by temperature, humidity, and wind speed. Warmer temperatures promote pollination. As measured over the past 20 years, across the United States, higher temperatures have already begun to result in higher pollen counts and lengthened allergy seasons. Pollen seasons have increased on average by 0.9 days per year. Simultaneously, the proportion of dogs sensitized to grass pollens has increased from 14.4% in 1999–2002 to 27.7% in 2007–2010. Pollen counts in the United States may be accessed at www.pollen.com. Canadian pollen counts are available at https://www.aaaai.org/global/nab-pollen-counts/canada.

Tree pollens range from 20 to 60 μM in diameter. The major allergenic pollens originate from box elder (*Acer negundo*), cedar, and oak trees. As with other plants, their prevalence varies regionally; however, cross-reactivity between species is uncommon. Tree pollination usually occurs in spring (between December and April) and tends to be brief. Tree pollen allergies are most significant in industrialized societies in temperate climate zones. However, they are becoming a greater problem in subtropical climates.

Wind-pollenated grasses such as Bermuda grass, Johnson grass, ryegrass, and Kentucky bluegrass release large amounts of pollen during spring and summer (May through July), the growing season. Seasonal patterns are more obvious in northern regions. Maximum pollen levels occur in the afternoons on hot, dry, windy days. Grass pollen ranks second to ragweed as the leading aeroallergen in humans in the United States.

Wind-borne weed pollens are generally produced by non-colorful, annual flowers that do not attract insects. Weed pollination generally occurs from late summer through October. In the United States, the pollen from the common ragweed (*Ambrosia* spp.) is the most important cause of allergies. It predominates in the central plains and agricultural areas in the eastern United States. A single plant can release a million pollen grains daily that can be detected up to 400 miles away. It is highly seasonal with peak pollen counts occurring during the third week of September (National Asthma Week). Other important pollen sources include sagebrush (*Artemesia*), English plantain (*Plantago*), yellow dock (*Rumex*), lamb's quarters (*Chenopodium*), and pigweed (*Amaranthus*). These, of course, differ between countries. For example, in Australia, red clover pollen is the most prevalent allergen based on intradermal skin testing of dogs.

Molds. Mold spores are also common aeroallergens. The fungi that form hyphae may be specialized to produce reproductive spores that are dispersed by wind, water, or insects. Some molds sporulate under low humidity conditions, whereas others prefer high humidity to achieve maximal dispersal. Mold allergies are subject to acute exacerbations because of temporary high concentrations of these spores. Examples include exposure to freshly mown grass or working in poorly ventilated barns. Some sources of important mold allergens include *Alternaria, Fusarium,*

Cladosporum, *Aspergillus*, and *Penicillium*. The reported sensitization level to fungal allergens is highly variable, reflecting animal housing, geographical differences, and a lack of standardization.

Arthropods. Another major source of airborne allergens is those derived from common but microscopic environmental mites, especially dust and storage mites. The most important of these mites are *Dermatophagoides fariniae*, *D. Pteronyssinus*, *Acarus sero*, and *Tyrophagus putrescantiae*. Epidermal allergens such as hairs and skin squames from other mammal species, including humans and feather dust from selected bird species, may also cause sensitization. Trends suggest that house dust mites and shed epidermal allergens are important in both North America and Europe, whereas pollen and mold allergens may be more important in North America, and pollens and mites are common in Australia.

SECONDARY INFECTIONS

Keratinocyte production of antimicrobial peptides is affected by the presence of AD. Human studies have suggested that these are downregulated, whereas a canine study suggested the opposite. It is clear, however, that dogs with AD suffer from frequent secondary infections. Recurrent staphylococcal skin and ear infections are common in AD dogs. Atopic lesions are predisposed to infections by *S. pseudintermedius* and the yeast *Malassezia pachydermatis*. Both these organisms can act on keratinocytes to cause damage and promote the release of the three master cytokines (TSLP, IL-33, and IL-25) that cause inflammation and pruritus. They also provide a source of conventional allergens to further promote Th2 responses, IgE production, and mast cell degranulation. The mast cell proteases may then attack and degrade the skin barrier. Thus, these secondary microbial infections may initiate AD development and then perpetuate it. These secondary infections are discussed in detail in Chapter 10.

Pathogenesis

EXTRINSIC AD

Extrinsic AD originates from a combination of genetic predisposition, Treg defects, and disruption of the skin epidermal barrier. Therefore, environmental allergens may penetrate the skin and be captured and processed by allergen-processing DCs and Langerhans cells. In response to DC activation and damage, keratinocytes then release the three epidermal cytokines, TSLP, IL-25, and IL-33. Keratinocytes are also a major source of proinflammatory cytokines, which expand the numbers and activities of skin-resident ILC2s. These stimuli collectively promote an intense, local Th2 response. Th2 cells secrete cytokines such as IL-4, IL-5, IL-13, and IL-31, and trigger IgE production. The most important of these is IL-13, which binds to mast cells so that when exposed to allergens, they release their mediators and trigger intense inflammation.

Below the surface of normal skin, there is a large resident population of regulatory T (Treg) cells in the dermis, accounting for almost half the total $CD4^+$ cell population in the skin. (This is in contrast to the situation in lymphoid organs such as the spleen or lymph nodes where only 5%–10% of the $CD4^+$ cells are Treg cells.) Normally, Treg cells reside in the skin, where they exert immunosuppressive and anti-inflammatory effects through the production of IL-10. As in other sites, this Treg cell population is influenced by products originating in the skin microbiota, such as short-chain fatty acids, vitamin A, and ultraviolet radiation. A cast of supporting cell types, including immature DCs and keratinocytes, act together to maintain the skin immune system in a quiescent state. When this changes in response to allergen exposure and the factors described above, these Treg cells may change their phenotype and differentiate into Th2 cells with a consequent IgE response and into Th17 and Th1 cells generating more inflammation.

Allergic Sensitization

In the majority of cases, dogs with AD show evidence of an IgE response to aeroallergens based on either intradermal skin testing or serologic assays. This is especially true of animals sensitized to house dust mites and pollens. However, neither total nor allergen-specific IgE levels correlate with lesional severity in dogs. IgE is bound to the surface of Langerhans cells in the epidermis of atopic dogs, contributing to the capture and processing of allergens. It is also found on dermal mast cells. Total IgE is elevated in the blood of atopic humans; however, this is less consistent in dogs. (IgE levels in normal dogs [24–410 µg/mL] are approximately 100 times higher than in humans [see Table 2.1]). Therefore, there is no correlation between total IgE in serum and disease status in normal and atopic dogs. (However, see the discussion on IgE affinity and functional heterogeneity in Chapter 2.) Normal IgE levels differ between breeds and depend greatly on flea infestation and intestinal parasite status. Neutering decreases IgE levels in Labradors and Golden Retrievers. Much of the normal IgE in serum consists of low-affinity antibodies directed against abundant environmental allergens.

In contrast to total IgE, allergen-specific IgE levels often correlate well with disease presence and severity. This forms the rational basis for treating these animals by specific immunotherapy. Several studies have also found elevated IgE levels in healthy, non-atopic dogs.

Allergens are trapped by Langerhans cells and presented to γ/δ T cells. γ/δ T cells play a critical role in the pathogenesis of AD, with type 2 responses and cytokines predominating during the acute phase over the first 24 h and mixed type 1 and 2 responses in the later, chronic disease (48–96 h). Lesions from patients with both intrinsic and extrinsic forms of AD are infiltrated with T cells and DCs. However, Th17-derived cytokines are elevated only in those with intrinsic AD. Conversely, lesions from patients with extrinsic AD have higher levels of the Th2 cytokines IL-4, IL-13, and IL-5. The suppressive cytokine TGF-β is under expressed in both types of AD. In chronic skin lesions, there is overexpression of IL-4 and some Th1 cytokines, including IL-2, IFNγ, and TNF-α, implying the development of a mixed response. Leukotrienes may also be elevated in many cases of AD and may contribute to the pruritus. Dogs with AD may have elevated levels of IL-17 as well as IL-31.

Allergen-specific IgG is sometimes present in the serum of experimentally or naturally sensitized AD dogs. However, these IgG antibodies may simply reflect allergen exposure rather than allergic sensitization. Early studies attributed atopic disease to an IgG subclass termed IgGd. However, IgG nomenclature has changed and the precise identity of IgGd is unclear. Despite much speculation, there is currently no evidence that IgG antibodies play a significant role in the pathogenesis of canine AD.

The development of a type 2 immune response in AD is probably secondary to the influx of environmental or food allergens because of epithelial barrier dysfunction. In other words, the primary defect is in the skin permeability barrier and is followed by the influx of allergens and a subsequent type 2 response (The outside-inside hypothesis). An alternative explanation is that there is a process associated with the atopic state in which the type 2 response in the skin results in secondary barrier defects, the inside-outside theory. Of course, both theories could be correct and simply reflect two different disease endotypes. Once AD develops, by whatever route, the skin response becomes a self-perpetuating cycle of inflammation, itch, and skin damage.

Cytokines. Keratinocytes respond to injury, environmental allergens, and toxins and invading bacteria by producing a mixture of antibacterial peptides, cytokines, and chemokines (Fig. 9.6). One of the cytokines they produce is TSLP. TSLP is upregulated in inflamed skin, especially when associated with epidermal barrier dysfunction or physical damage. This TSLP is produced by keratinocytes and mast cells in response to antimicrobial peptides such as β-defensins and cathelicidins. TSLP acts on Th2 cells to promote IL-4, IL-5, and IL-13 production, which then promote IgE production.

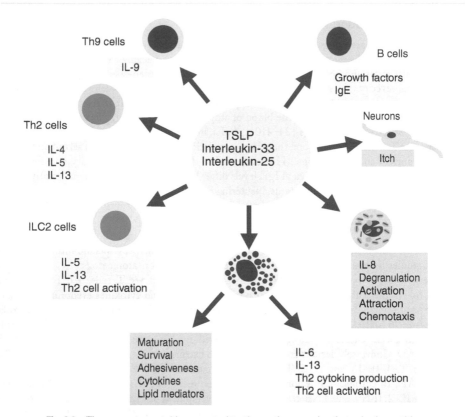

Fig. 9.6 Three master cytokines central to the pathogenesis of atopic dermatitis.

While AD has generally been considered a type 2 response dominated by Th2 cells and their cytokines, other Th cell subsets are also clearly involved in the process. Thus, Th17 cells may also participate and promote neutrophil-dominated pathology. Their normal role is to protect against bacterial invasion at epithelial surfaces.

Some dermal DCs produce IL-25, enhancing the production of Th2 cytokines (especially from ILC2 cells) and downregulating filaggrin synthesis. IL-33 also downregulates skin filaggrin. Th22 cells secrete IL-22 that promotes and regulates skin inflammation, especially epithelial cell proliferation and the production of antimicrobial peptides. IL-22 can be detected in chronic skin lesions and its genes are upregulated in acute AD lesions. However, dysregulation of the IL-17/IL-17RA axis plays a key role in some inflammatory skin diseases. IL-17-deficient mice develop severe skin inflammation due to the activities of Th2-derived IL-5. Thus, IL-17 exercises a protective effect. IL-21 is a Th1 cytokine that is involved in skin inflammation, including enhanced proliferation of keratinocytes, lymphocytes, and NK cells. It promotes the development of Th17 cells. Both IL-21 and its receptor are upregulated in human atopic skin lesions.

Transcriptomics

It is now possible to extract RNA from tissue samples and sequence them. This provides a snapshot of which genes are turned on in that tissue at the time of sampling. Olivry and his colleagues examined the transcriptome of acute AD lesions induced in dogs by extracts of the house dust mite *D. farinae*, a very common and important allergen. In these acute lesions, there was significant upregulation of the genes encoding proteins involved in type 2 immune responses. These included

IL-4, IL-5, IL-9, IL-13, IL-22, IL-31, and IL-33. Chemokine genes that were activated included CCL5 and CCL17. Other proinflammatory genes activated included those for IL-6, IL-18, lymphotoxin-β, as well as cathepsin S, mast cell chymase, tryptase, mastin, neuromedin-B, nerve growth factor, and several enzymes involved in leukotriene synthesis. Transcriptome profiles of the blood lymphocytes in dogs with AD showed increases in $CD8^+$ T cells and Treg cells. Likewise, there was increased expression of TNF-α and decreased IL-10 and TGF-β expression. The increase in Treg cells together with a decline in IL-10 and TGF-β suggests that Treg cell function is somehow impaired.

In summary therefore, these AD lesions showed evidence of activation of both innate and adaptive immune pathways and pruritogenic, cytokine-mediated pathways. With the activation of so many pathways, no single drug is likely to "cure" the condition.

INTRINSIC AD

There are well-documented reports of dogs suffering from a clinical disease indistinguishable from AD, but these dogs have neither elevated total IgE nor allergen-specific skin reactivity. This has been called "atopic-like" dermatitis in dogs and a similar disease, intrinsic AD, is seen in humans. There are several possible mechanisms of this. In humans, intrinsic AD occurs in older individuals. There is no apparent genetic predisposition and their skin barrier function is normal. These cases may be attributed to some internal causation resulting in the development of allergic inflammation in the skin. Allergic inflammation can be triggered in the absence of IgE and antigens by non-specific activation of ILC2 cells and the release of the three master cytokines, IL-33, TSLP, and IL-25, from damaged keratinocytes. Intrinsic AD lesions contain relatively low IL-4, IL-5, and IL-13 levels.

Clinical Disease

The average onset age of canine AD is between 3 months and 3 years. Atopic dogs commonly present with pruritus prior to the development of obvious skin lesions. Examination at this time may simply reveal diffuse erythema. Dogs subsequently develop the allergic triad: face rubbing, axillary pruritus, and foot licking. AD lesions have a characteristic distribution in the dog (Fig. 9.7). They occur most commonly around the mouth and eyes, the ears, on the front feet, the ventral abdomen, and in the inguinal and axillary regions, although they may be found anywhere on the body (Fig. 9.8). These lesions are secondary to the intense pruritus and vary from acute erythema and focal urticaria to chronic changes, including crusting, scaling, hyperpigmentation, lichenification, and pyoderma. Some animals may also develop simultaneous rhinitis, otitis externa, blepharitis, or conjunctivitis. Secondary bacterial or yeast infections complicate the disease. Depending on the inducing allergen, the disease may or may not be seasonal and relapsing. Once it starts, it gets progressively and inexorably more severe unless treated.

HISTOPATHOLOGY

Histopathology demonstrates the presence of a chronic hyperplastic spongiotic perivascular dermatitis (Fig. 9.9). There is hyperkeratosis, melanosis, and leukocyte exocytosis. The lesion is infiltrated with mononuclear cells that appear to consist primarily of T cells.

Within the skin, the number of DCs varies. DC2s are present in high numbers in the dermis, and there are fewer DCs in the subcutis and adipose tissue. Given that the offending allergen(s) cross the cutaneous barrier, allergen-presenting DCs, especially Langerhans cells, likely play a key role in initiating these responses. Epidermal Langerhans cell numbers and macrophages are increased in AD lesions in dogs. In human AD patients, T cell infiltration predominates. These appear to be primarily Th2 cells. Similarly, the predominant T cells in the blood of human cases

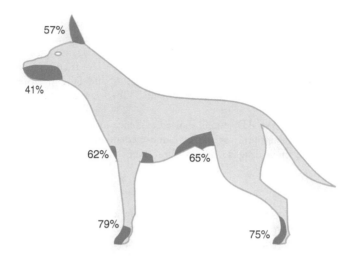

Fig. 9.7 Distribution of atopic dermatitis (AD) lesions in affected dogs. (Data from Wilhem S, Kovalik M, Favrot C. Breed-associated phenotypes in canine atopic dermatitis. *Vet Dermatol* 2010; doi: 10.1111/j.1365-3164.2010.00925.x)

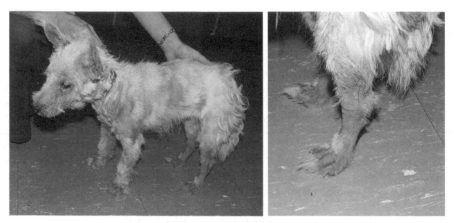

Fig. 9.8 A dog with chronic atopic dermatitis. Note the erythema, lichenification, and alopecia affecting the skin of the face, feet, and flexural areas. (From Pucheu-Haston C. Atopic dermatitis in the domestic dog. *Clin Dermatol.* 2015;34:299–303.)

tend to be Th2 cells. T cells predominate in canine AD skin and include both α/β and γ/δ cells. The α/β T cells predominate in the dermis, whereas γ/δ T cells are greatly increased in the epidermis as befits a cell population tasked with epithelial defense. B cells are not a major cell population in atopic skin lesions.

Mast cell density varies between different sites. Their highest density occurs in the pinnae, and high numbers are also found in the facial skin and perineum. Their lowest density occurs in the footpads and nasal planum. There is also a dense population of mast cells in the interdigital skin. It is unclear whether mast cell numbers are increased in AD skin lesions, especially when these

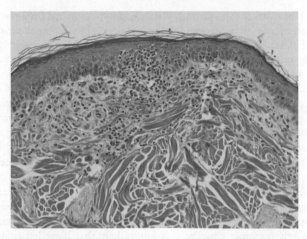

Fig. 9.9 Histopathology of a canine atopic dermatitis lesion. Note the relatively mild inflammatory response and lymphocytic infiltration. (Courtesy of Dr. Dominique Weiner.)

site-specific variations are considered. Basophils are present in mouse models of AD, where they associate with ILC2 cells.

Eosinophils are rare in normal healthy skin, and their numbers increase minimally in AD lesions. Many of these eosinophils have degranulated and they do not appear to be major participants in the skin reactions. Their significance may depend on the specific allergens involved. Likewise, neutrophils are not major participants in the AD process provided secondary bacterial invasion has not developed. Their numbers increase significantly in response to secondary staphylococcal invasion.

DIAGNOSIS

AD is a progressive, life-long disease and intervention is necessary to control it and improve the animal's quality of life. Constant scratching makes both pets and owners uncomfortable. It can be controlled but rarely cured.

There is no single diagnostic test or clinical feature that definitively indicates a diagnosis of AD. Thus, the diagnosis relies largely on identifying several criteria that are recognized as being associated with the disease. The more such criteria are recognized, the greater the specificity and sensitivity of the diagnosis, i.e., the greater the chances of a correct diagnosis. Once a combination of such criteria is recognized, it then becomes essential to eliminate other differential diagnoses. For example, it is obviously important to rule out other causes of itch such as flea allergy dermatitis, demodicosis, scabies, adverse food reactions, and *Malassezia* dermatitis.

Other ectoparasites, in addition to fleas, should be excluded by the use of skin scrapings from lesional skin. It is also essential to rule out *Demodex gatoi* in cats and Culicoides hypersensitivity in horses.

Food allergies should be considered if the dog has a non-seasonal allergy with itching. Gastrointestinal signs may or may not be present. Carefully managed food trials are required for the diagnosis of food allergies (Chapter 11).

Allergy Testing

Following the identification of canine IgE and the detection of its presence in the skin of atopic dogs, intradermal skin testing with dilute allergen solutions became a standard procedure. However, the division of AD into intrinsic and extrinsic disease endotypes resulted from the observation that there was no consistent correlation between IgE levels as determined by intradermal skin test results and the severity of clinical AD in dogs. Many AD cases do not have detectable IgE antibodies to environmental allergens as determined by skin testing. In one study, 26% of dogs with AD had no detectable IgE as measured by a skin test response. Serological assays that measure IgE antibodies to the offending allergens rarely correlate well with disease severity or intradermal skin tests. Blood IgE levels may drop to undetectable levels, whereas levels in the skin and skin reactivity remain high. Intradermal testing of pruritic dogs shows that many are sensitive to house dust mites, various pollens, and epidermal allergens, and some seasonal allergens. However, skin testing of clinically normal dogs also elicits positive reactions to these same allergens. Allergen-specific IgE may also be detected in dogs that have no clinical signs of AD, whereas IgE levels cannot discriminate among normal dogs, dogs with parasites, or dogs with AD.

Additionally, about a quarter of canine cases are unreactive to intradermal allergen inoculation and lack any allergen-specific IgE as determined by serology. These are classified as intrinsic AD cases. Some of these IgE-negative cases may represent early stage disease when the animal has yet to develop an IgE response; however, it is more likely that these individuals represent an intrinsic endotype that employs alternative pathways to induce inflammatory responses as sometimes occurs in anaphylaxis.

Scoring Systems

Much to their credit, veterinary dermatologists have long sought to establish a quantitative basis to describe the severity of AD. Only in this objective way can treatments be rationally assessed. Subjective estimations of disease severity are subject to recall error and bias, i.e., what constitutes mild, moderate, or severe is a matter of opinion.

The first such scoring system was called the Canine Atopic Dermatitis Extent and Severity Index (CADESI). This has gone through several versions because of thorough reassessment and analysis. The first well-validated version of these indices (CADESI-03) was designed for use in clinical trials and to measure the efficacy of treatments. However, it was complex and time consuming, requiring 248 evaluations of erythema, lichenification, excoriation, and self-induced alopecia at 62 specified skin sites on a scale of 0 to 5. The maximum point score added up to 1240. Because of its complexity, other simpler schemes have been developed for use in clinical practice. For example, an alternative scoring system is called the Canine Atopic Dermatitis Lesion Index. This system quantifies lesions at five sites: head and pinnae, forefeet, hind feet, ventral thorax and axillae, and ventral abdomen and the inguinal region. Each site is graded on a 0 to 5 scale for erythema, excoriation, and erosion, and on a 0 to 5 scale for alopecia, lichenification, and hyperpigmentation. Thus, the maximum possible score is 50. The time needed to complete it is about a sixth of that needed for CADESI-03; however, its results strongly correlate with the CADESI-03 score.

A revised and simplified version of the CADESI scale (CADESI-04) was designed to record the severity of 3 lesions, erythema, lichenification and alopecia/excoriation, at 20 body sites on a 4-point scale with a maximum score of 180. It has also been validated and shown to be reliable.

In 2010, Claude Favrot proposed the following diagnostic criteria for canine AD:
1. Initial pruritus without lesions beginning in dogs between 6 months and 3 years. The reported mean age of onset varies from 1.7 to 2.7 years. Some reports suggest that food-allergic dogs can develop their disease when less than 1 or over 6 years of age.
2. Dogs living mostly indoors.
3. Corticosteroid-sensitive pruritus at least initially.
4. Chronic or recurrent yeast infections.
5. Lesions affecting the front feet and pinnae.

6. Ear margins are usually unaffected.
7. Dorsolumbar regions are unaffected (these are more characteristic of flea allergy, and ventral involvement may be associated with house dust mite allergy).

If five of the above criteria are positive, the diagnostic sensitivity is 85% and the specificity is 80%. If six are positive, the sensitivity drops to 58% and the specificity rises to 88%.

Other features to consider include determination of whether the dermatitis is chronic or chronic-relapsing. There may be a family history of atopy. The animal may belong to a susceptible breed. The disease may be occurring in a region where AD is common. However, dogs suffering from other conditions such as food allergies or scabies will also satisfy these criteria. Non-cutaneous lesions may be associated with AD. For example, conjunctivitis has been reported in 21%–30% of dogs with AD. Rhinitis is less common (<10%) and highly variable. Otitis externa is a common feature of AD, with more than 80% of affected dogs having ear problems. It has been claimed that 75% of chronic otitis externa cases are associated with atopic disease. Another study suggested that 43% of chronic otitis externa are due to allergies. Food-allergic dogs are also prone to develop otitis externa. Pyoderma may be present in 68% of cases.

Clinical signs can be seasonal or non-seasonal, or non-seasonal with seasonal exacerbation, depending on the allergens involved. Approximately 80% of affected dogs are symptomatic in the spring, summer, and fall. The remaining 20% show signs in the winter. Presumably, in the summer, outdoor living and pollen counts are high, whereas in the winter, pollen counts are much lower.

TREATMENT

Treatment of canine AD is best considered a two-stage process. The first stage is to treat the patient to reduce inflammation and achieve disease remission. The second stage is to prevent recurrences. AD can be treated and controlled but rarely cured. In treating an AD dog, a life-long management plan should be drawn up and adhered to.

Constant scratching is stressful for both dogs and their owners. The first task in working up a pruritic dermatitis case is to ascertain the cause by excluding food and flea allergies. The International Committee on Allergic Diseases of Animals has provided guidelines for the treatment of canine AD. It is due to be updated every 5 years.

Restore the Skin Barrier Function

Repairing the skin barrier function is critically important in treating this disease. Current attempts to restore the epidermal barrier function have centered on the oral or topical use of lipids and ensuring that an animal's nutrition is optimal. Topical therapy with emollients and applying moisturizers in humans results in a reduction in disease severity, enhances the effectiveness of other treatments, and reduces the number of flares.

Oral therapy includes providing important nutrients such as essential fatty acids, pantothenate, choline, histidine, and inositol. Oral treatment with essential fatty acids may increase the lipid content of the stratum corneum and improve barrier function, although there is little objective evidence to support their clinical efficacy. There is also little evidence to suggest that AD results from a deficiency of these vitamins or fatty acids.

Topical lipid emulsions may also be applied to provide substitutes for the missing skin ceramides and repair the barrier. The use of topical formulations containing the major barrier lipids, ceramides, cholesterol, and fatty acids, is justified, but these have rarely been critically evaluated. Topical treatment with synthetic pseudoceramides and plant extracts containing glycyrrhetinic acid have shown encouraging results (Chapter 17).

Control Secondary Infections

Many cases of AD are exacerbated by secondary fungal and bacterial infections. Infection often plays a key role in an itchy animal. Thus, appropriate antifungal or antibacterial therapy is essential. Likewise, mite infestations must be ruled out.

Anti-Inflammatory/Immunosuppressive Therapy

Acute disease treatment with the goal of clinical remission involves elimination of the cause, controlling pruritus with frequent baths using mild shampoos, and reducing inflammation with glucocorticoid sprays or oclacitinib. Reducing skin inflammation and its associated itch generally requires the use of broad-spectrum anti-inflammatories such as oral corticosteroids that are rapidly effective. Topical corticosteroids may also be used to treat acutely inflamed or lichenified lesions. Thus, therapy should seek to reduce the type 2 inflammatory responses and the other inflammatory endotypes while leaving other defensive pathways intact. Spray formulations of glucocorticoids such as triamcinolone or hydrocortisone aceponate may be effective in controlling focal pruritus, but care must be taken to avoid skin atrophy. Topical corticosteroids are used to treat acute exacerbations. Until recently, the only effective medications were glucocorticoids. However, their long-term use is associated with diverse adverse effects (Chapter 17). The use of oclacitinib (Apoquel-Zoetis), a rapid-acting inhibitor of IL-31 signaling through Janus kinase receptors, can be used to control pruritus in association with glucocorticoid therapy (Chapter 17).

Once reactive treatment has brought the acute disease under control, then topical glucocorticoid sprays may be used to prevent disease flares. More recently, an alternative has presented itself with the calcineurin inhibitor cyclosporine. This blocks the transcription of many proinflammatory genes. It primarily inhibits the production and release of IL-2, but its secondary effects include IL-4 suppression and IFN-γ production. It is generally given orally for 4–6 weeks before a positive response is seen. Then, the dose may be reduced to a maintenance level. Another calcineurin inhibitor, tacrolimus, is applied topically; however, it is expensive, but it can be used to control focal pruritus if skin atrophy is developing. Antihistamines are of limited usefulness.

For chronic AD cases, preventative strategy includes avoiding factors that may cause flares, supporting skin and coat health by bathing, and fatty acid intake. Allergen-specific immunotherapy and proactive intermittent topical glucocorticoids are the only treatments likely to delay or prevent the flares.

Targeted Immunotherapy

AD treatment in humans is being revolutionized by the use of targeted immunotherapy with new drugs and monoclonal antibodies. A monoclonal antibody, dupilumab, has been approved for use in humans. This targets the common chain of the IL-4/IL-13 receptor and is very effective as an AD treatment. Monoclonal antibodies such as Cytopoint-Zoetis that block signaling by IL-31 are also very effective in canine AD treatment because the inhibition of IL-31 signaling stops itch.

Allergen-specific immunotherapy is currently the only long-term solution to the problem of AD. However, its success rate is variable, and it may produce temporary remissions rather than a permanent unresponsiveness. This is discussed in detail in Chapter 16. The possibility of removing the offending allergens from the animal's environment should also be discussed with the animal owner. This is often difficult or impossible to achieve; however, it is a potential, inexpensive, long-term solution that should, at least be considered.

Feline Atopic Skin Syndrome

Most skin diseases in cats resemble those in dogs, while feline atopic skin syndrome (FASS) does not. In most respects, FASS has similar pathogenesis and complications as the canine disease. Allergic skin disease in cats is less common than in dogs and may present very differently. There appears to be a familial predisposition in some cases, and some breeds such as Abyssinian cats may also be predisposed.

FASS is believed to be a result of sensitization to environmental allergens; however, its symptoms overlap with feline food allergy and flea allergy dermatitis. Before diagnosing FASS, flea, mange mite, lice, fungal, and bacterial infections, and food allergies must first be ruled out. Generally, cats will present with one of four common skin reactions. These include intense pruritus on the face, pinnae, and neck with associated, possibly severe, scratch lesions and self-induced alopecia caused by excessive grooming and licking. Other non-cutaneous signs may include otitis externa, conjunctivitis, rhinitis, and sinusitis associated with sneezing or coughing. None of the above features are pathognomonic and there is currently no conclusive evidence that it is mediated by IgE.

Most allergies in cats result in the development WS of components of the eosinophilic granuloma complex. These include milary dermatitis, eosinophilic plaques, eosinophilic granulomas, or indolent ulcers described in Chapter 4 (Fig. 9.10). The presence of eosinophilia is also a feature of most of these cats.

Malassezia overgrowth is not uncommon; therefore, once detected, cats should receive systemic antifungal medication. Mild cases may receive fatty acid supplementation and antihistamines. Severe or refractory cases may receive glucocorticoids (1–2 mg/kg prednisolone once daily) and then taper the dose while maintaining control. Alternatively, a cyclosporine microemulsion may be applied topically. Oclacitinib has not been extensively studied in cats. The monoclonal antibody against IL-31, lokivetmab, must not be used in cats because it is caninized and will induce antibodies against the foreign dog protein in the treated cats.

AD is not simply an IgE-mediated skin disease driven by exposure to environmental or food allergens in genetically-predisposed animals. It also involves immune dysregulation, skin barrier defects, and microbial dysbiosis. It is often complicated by secondary staphylococcal or

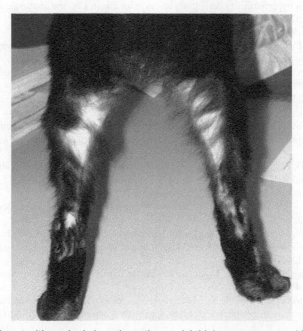

Fig. 9.10 An atopic cat with marked alopecia on the caudal thigh, a common pruritic site in this species. (From Trimmer AM, Griffin, CE, Rosenkrantz WS. Feline immunotherapy. *Clin Tech Small Anim Pract* 2006; 21:157-161.)

Malassezia yeast infections. It is best considered a syndrome with multiple endotypes. In acute cases, it is primarily driven by excessive cutaneous Th2 responses with contributions from ILC2 cells. In chronic cases and infected lesions, Th17 and Th1 cells are also active participants.

Suggested Readings

Agler CS, Friedenberg S, Olivry T, Meurs KM, Olby NJ. Genome-wide association analysis in West Highland White Terriers with atopic dermatitis. *Vet Immunol Immunopathol*. 2019;209:1-6. doi:10.1016/j.vetimm.2019.01.004.

Ardesjo-Lundgren B, Tengvall K, Bergvall K, et al. Comparison of cellular location and expression of plakophilin-2 in epidermal cells from nonlesional atopic skin and healthy skin in German Shepherd dogs. *Vet Dermatol*. 2017;28(4):377-e88.

Asahina R, Maeda S. A review of the roles of keratinocyte-derived cytokines and chemokines in the pathogenesis of atopic dermatitis in humans and dogs. *Vet Dermatol*. 2017;28(1):16-e5.

Barnard N. A clinician's guide to making a diagnosis of atopic dermatitis in dogs. *Pract*. 2020;42(4):188-196. doi:10.1136/inp.m1440.

Bizikova P, Pucheu-Haston CM, Eisenschenk MN, Marsella R, Nuttall T, Santoro M. Review: role of genetics and the environment in the pathogenesis of canine atopic dermatitis. *Vet Dermatol*. 2015;26(2):95-e26.

Bizikova P, Santoro D, Marsella R, Nuttall T, Eisenschenk MN, Pucheau-Haston CM. Review: clinical and histological manifestations of canine atopic dermatitis. *Vet Dermatol*. 2015;26(2):79-e24.

Brement T, Laly MJ, Combarros D, Guillemaille D, Bourdeau PJ, Bruet V. Reliability of different sets of criteria in diagnosing canine dermatitis applied to a population of 250 dogs seen in a veterinary teaching hospital. *Vet Dermatol*. 2019;30(3):188-e59.

Brown SJ, McLean WH. One remarkable molecule: filaggrin. *J Invest Dermatol*. 2012;132(3 Pt 2):751-762.

Diesel A. Cutaneous hypersensitivity dermatoses in the feline client: a review of allergic skin disease in cats. *Vet Sci*. 2017;4(4):25-35.

Elias PM. Skin Barrier function. *Curr Allergy Asthma Rep*. 2008;8(4):299-305.

Fanton N, Santoro D, Cornegliani L, Marsella R. Increased filaggrin-metabolizing enzyme activity in atopic skin: a pilot study using a canine model of atopic dermatitis. *Vet Dermatol*. 2017;28(5):479-e111.

Gedon NK, Mueller RS. Atopic dermatitis in cats and dogs: a difficult disease for animals and owners. *Clin Transl Allergy*. 2018;8:41-52.

Halliwell R, Banovic F, Mueller RS, Olivry T. Immunopathogenesis of the feline atopic syndrome. *Vet Dermatol*. 2021;32(1):13-e4.

Harvey ND, Shaw SC, Craigon PJ, Blott SC, England GCW. Environmental risk factors for canine atopic dermatitis: a retrospective, large-scale, study in Labrador and golden retrievers. *Vet Dermatol*. 2019;30(5):396-e119.

Hensel P, Santoro D, Favrot C, Hill P, Griffin C. Canine atopic dermatitis: detailed guidelines for diagnosis and allergen identification. *BMC Vet Res*. 2015;11:196. doi:10.1186/s12917-015-0515-5.

Imai Y. Interleukin-33 in atopic dermatitis. *J Dermatol Sci*. 2019;96(1):2-7.

Kashiwagi M, Hosoi J, Lai JF, et al. Direct control of regulatory T cells by keratinocytes. *Nat Immunol*. 2017:18-334-343.

Lauber B, Molitor V, Meury S, et al. Total IgE and allergen-specific IgE and IgG antibody levels in sera of atopic dermatitis affected and non-affected Labrador and golden retrievers. *Vet Immunol Immunopathol*. 2012;149(1-2):112-118.

Leung DYM, Berdyshev E, Goleva E. Cutaneous barrier dysfunction in allergic diseases. *J Allergy Clin Immunol*. 2020;145(6):1485-1497.

Majewska A, Gajewska M, Dembele K, Maciejewski H, Prostek A, Jank M. Lymphocytic, cytokine and transcriptomic profiles in peripheral blood of dogs with atopic dermatitis. *BMC Vet Res*. 2016;12(1):2174-2188.

Marsella R, Sousa CA, Gonzales AJ, Fadok VA. Current understanding of the pathophysiologic mechanisms of canine atopic dermatitis. *J Am Vet Med Assoc*. 2012;241(2):194-207.

Mueller RS, Janda J, Jensen-Jarolim E, Rhyner C, Marti E. Allergens in veterinary medicine. *Allergy.* 2016;71(1):27-35.

Nuttall TJ, Marsalla R, Rosenbaum MR, Gonzales AJ, Fadok VA. Update on pathogenesis, diagnosis and treatment of atopic dermatitis in dogs. *J Am Vet Med Assoc.* 2019;254(11):1291-1300.

Olivry T, Banovic F. Treatment of canine atopic dermatitis; time to revise our strategy? *Vet Dermatol.* 2019;30(2):87-90.

Olivry T, Bensignor E, Favrot C, et al. Development of a core outcome set for therapeutic clinical trials enrolling dogs with atopic dermatitis (COSCAD'18). *BMC Vet Res.* 2018;14(1):238-246.

Olivry T, Saridomichelakis M, Nuttall T, et al. Validation of the canine atopic dermatitis extent and severity index (CADESI)-4, a simplified severity scale for assessing skin lesions of atopic dermatitis in dogs. *Vet Dermatol.* 2014;25(2):77-e25.

Pucheu-Haston CM, Bizikova P, Eisenschenk MN, Santoros D, Nuttall T, Marsella R. Review: the role of antibodies, autoantigens and food allergens in canine atopic dermatitis. *Vet Dermatol.* 2015;26(2):115-e30.

Pucheu-Haston CM, Santoroi D, Bizikova P, Eisenschenk MN, Marsella R, Nuttall T. Review: innate immunity, lipid metabolism and nutrition in canine atopic dermatitis. *Vet Dermatol.* 2015;26(2):104-e28.

Rostaher A, Dolf G, Fischer NM, et al. Atopic dermatitis in a cohort of West Highland White terriers in Switzerland. Part II: estimates of early life factors and heritability. *Vet Dermatol.* 2020;31(4):276-e66. doi:10.1111/vde.12843.

Santoro D, Marsella R, Pucheu-Haston CM, Eisenschenk MN, Nuttall T, Bizikova P. Review: pathogenesis of canine atopic dermatitis: skin barrier and host-micro-organism interaction. *Vet Dermatol.* 2015;26(2):84-e25.

Sozener ZC, Cevhertas L, Nadeau K, Akdis M, Akdis CA. Environmental factors in epithelial barrier dysfunction. *J Allergy Clin Immunol.* 2020;145(6):1517-1528.

CHAPTER 10

Malassezia and Staphylococci

Body surfaces are, of course, not sterile. Dense and complex populations of commensal bacteria and fungi are found on all surfaces. Healthy skin is inhabited by a well-balanced mixture of bacteria and fungi. These organisms interact with the immune system systemically and at the local level. Should the commensal microbiota or the environment change, for example, when allergic or inflammatory skin disease develops, some organisms exploit the situation by invading the affected areas and causing disease exacerbation. However, it is often difficult to determine whether the overgrowth of a microorganism in an allergic skin lesion is a cause or the result of the disease. This dilemma is readily seen in canine atopic dermatitis (AD) cases infected with the yeast *Malassezia pachydermatis* or the bacterium *Staphylococcus pseudintermedius*. In dogs with AD, approximately one-third suffer concurrent yeast infections and two-thirds have secondary bacterial infections.

Failure of the skin permeability barrier predisposes to secondary infections, while pathogen colonization aggravates the permeability defect. The antimicrobial barrier is also defective in AD cases. Both defensins and cathelicidins are downregulated because of defective lamellar body functions. Reduced levels of free fatty acids and sphingosine reduce antimicrobial activity in the skin and as a result, secondary infections are common.

Malassezia

Fungi are common members of the natural skin microbiota (the mycobiota). As commensals, they interact with the immune system of their host and play an important role in regulating host immune responses. They are a major predisposing factor in some forms of dermatitis; however, other factors such as host immunity, epithelial barrier dysfunction, and environmental factors also play a role.

BIOLOGY OF MALASSEZIA

Among the most common commensal skin fungi are the lipophilic yeasts of the genus *Malassezia*. (These were named after Louis-Charles Malassez, a French anatomist.) In humans, *Malassezia* yeasts account for more than 90% of all commensal skin fungi. Their preferred habitat is the stratum corneum of the skin of wild and domestic carnivores and humans. (They are rare in rodents.)

Malassezia are oval, bottle-shaped, or peanut-shaped yeasts. They have a thick, multilayered cell wall and bud from one pole. This cell wall is rich in chitin and chitosans and, as discussed later, these molecules may stimulate keratinocyte functions and type 2 helper (Th2)- and Th17-mediated immune responses. The *Malassezia* cell wall also contains β-(1,3)-glucans and β-(1,6)-glucans. These two polymers cross-link to form a very stable complex. This structure is very different from the cell walls of other fungal species because these glucan polymers can act as ligands for pattern recognition receptors such as dectin-1 and as a result will trigger both innate and adaptive immune responses.

Malassezia are classified as Basidiomycetous fungi. Within the Basidiomycetes, only *Malassezia* and *Cryptococcus* are significant pathogens. A total of 18 *Malassezia* species have been recognized and at least 14 of these have been found on the skin of mammals. *Malassezia* yeasts have a relatively small genome (approximately half the size of other yeasts). Uniquely, all of them lack a fatty acid synthase gene. They cannot synthesize long-chain fatty acids and are totally dependent on a source of exogenous lipids for their growth. They are, in effect, specialized skin commensals. In humans, *M. restricta* and *M. globosa* are the most abundant species. However, in dogs, the mycobiota is much more diverse and *Malassezia* species are relatively less abundant. *M. pachydermatis* is the most frequently identified species on dog and cat skin. (Its species name, meaning "thick skin," is derived from the fact that it was first isolated from an Asian rhinoceros with severe dermatitis.) Other species have been identified rarely, such as *M. nana* in the ear canal and *M. slooffiae* in the claw fold. Their distribution is uneven, favoring some sites over others. They colonize the skin of neonates within the first few days of life. *Malassezia* are commonly isolated from the anal sacs, vagina, rectum, and perioral/lip region of healthy dogs. They are also found in the interdigital area, haired skin of the lower lip, chin, and external ear canal. The organisms are readily moved between sites by licking and grooming behavior. (Speciation is unclear and gene sequencing suggests that there may be multiple sequence types of *Malassezia* present on normal skin.) However, in one report, it was found that the *Malassezia* population on normal healthy dog skin was genetically very diverse, whereas the population on the skin of atopic dogs was almost monogenic. Thus, a genetically distinct *Malassezia* sequence, type Id, was recovered from 91% of AD dogs. This isolate produced more phospholipase A2 and was active at a higher pH than other isolates.

Malassezia yeasts thrive on the skin environment. They are highly lipophilic and prefer seborrheic skin sites. Because they lack the gene for fatty acid synthetase, *Malassezia* express an expanded set of diverse lipid hydrolyzing enzymes, such as lipases, phospholipases, and sphingomyelinases that enable them to metabolize fatty acids from animal skin. Therefore, they utilize sebum triglycerides and fatty acids as energy sources. These *Malassezia* enzymes can effectively disrupt the epidermal lipid barrier.

Presence on Skin

M. pachydermatis readily colonizes the skin of healthy dogs because it can adhere strongly to corneocytes. It binds via mannosyl carbohydrate residues on the cell surface. While normally commensals, *Malassezia* yeasts can also cause opportunistic infections should the local skin immune environment or microclimate change. Therefore, they can be isolated from diverse skin diseases ranging from dandruff to AD, otitis externa, seborrheic dermatitis, and folliculitis.

If *Malassezia* is as common as it is believed, it may be found on almost all dogs, whether atopic or not, and colonization rates may be misleading. However, atopic dogs may differ from normal dogs in the distribution of the yeast and its population density. Another difference may result from the overgrowth of less common genotypes of *Malassezia* within AD lesions.

Pathogenesis

The increased moisture and lipid availability in seborrheic skin lesions encourage fungal growth. As a result, *Malassezia* skin and ear infections are common in canine AD. The exudate from these lesions is a better nutrient source for the yeasts than healthy normal skin. *Malassezia* also bind strongly to apoptotic keratinocytes, while the release of lipases and phospholipases by the yeast disrupts the skin integrity and keratinocyte adhesion by degrading the lipid barrier. *Malassezia* biofilms may also be generated, which can contribute to its pathogenicity (Fig. 10.1). *Malassezia* may contribute to skin barrier dysfunction through the production of free fatty acids from sebum triglycerides.

Immediate Responses. *Malassezia* yeasts growing on the stratum corneum produce diverse antigens that can act as allergens. Keratinocytes can recognize these *Malassezia* products via their

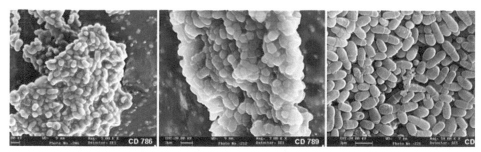

Fig. 10.1 Scanning electron microscopy showing biofilm structures of *Malassezia pachydermatis* strains from dogs with skin lesions. The biofilm is organized in a multilayer form with variable amounts of extracellular matrix. (From Figueredo LA, Cafarchia C, Desantis, Otranto, D. Biofilm formation of *Malassezia pachydermatis* from dogs. *Vet Microbiol*. 2012;160:126–131.)

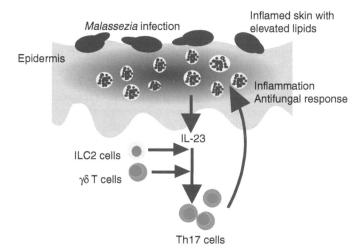

Fig. 10.2 Pathogenesis of *Malassezia* hypersensitivity in atopic skin disease. This is primarily a type 17 response.

toll-like receptors and their aryl hydrocarbon receptors. As a result, keratinocytes upregulate the production of the immunosuppressive cytokines interleukin 10 (IL-10) and tumor necrosis factor-β. *Malassezia* cell wall carbohydrates can also penetrate the skin and be captured by dendritic cells (DC). They may then act as antigens and stimulate adaptive immune responses. These can include local type 2 immune responses and protective type 1 responses. Many of the constituent proteins of the yeast can act as allergens and thus trigger antibody production and hypersensitivity responses (Fig. 10.2).

Like the other the microbiota members of the skin microbiota, *Malassezia* yeasts interact with the immune system of the host in many ways. When triggering inflammation, they can induce IL-1β, IL-6, IL-8, and tumor necrosis factor-α production from keratinocytes. They may also promote the release of the three master cytokines, IL-25, IL-33, and thymic stromal lymphopoietin (TSLP).

Colonization with *Malassezia* in atopic skin may be associated with high levels of specific immunoglobulin E (IgE), positive intradermal and patch tests, and induction of lymphocyte proliferation in humans. One major antigen, Mala f 1, induces histamine release from human basophils. *Malassezia*-specific IgE antibodies, positive intradermal tests, and stimulation of blood lymphocytes have all been attributed to *Malassezia* infection in dogs. Several distinct antigens have been characterized, including proteins of 45, 52, 56, and 63 kDa. Thus, *Malassezia* can trigger a type 2 immune response with subsequent IgE production and act as a conventional environmental allergen in canine skin. While dogs with AD and *Malassezia* dermatitis show greater skin test reactions than normal dogs, given the ubiquitous presence of *Malassezia* in the normal mycobiota, some positive reactions would be anticipated in healthy animals.

Local treatment with corticosteroids or cyclosporine permits *Malassezia* overgrowth, presumably as a result of suppression of local immune defenses.

Malassezia infections occur with greater than expected frequency in some dog breeds, including Basset Hounds, Dachshunds, English Setters, Cocker Spaniels, Shih-Tzus, Boxers, and West Highland White and Australian Silky Terriers. The presence of deep skin folds is considered a risk factor. However, not every dog with *Malassezia* dermatitis is atopic and not every atopic dog will develop *Malassezia* dermatitis. Overgrowth is not related to either sex or age.

Th17 Responses. To defend itself against fungal invasion, the body commonly employs type 17 immune responses. *Malassezia* are highly effective in triggering these responses in the skin. Mice that are deficient in either IL-17 or its triggering cytokine, IL-23, suffer from uncontrolled *Malassezia* growth. When *Malassezia* invades atopic skin lesions, it triggers an influx of neutrophils and monocytes associated with selective activation of the IL-17 pathway and an increase in their recruiting cytokines, IL-17A and IL-23. These cytokines are mainly produced by γ/δ T cells. These are innate defensive T cells found on body surfaces that respond rapidly to invasion, much faster than conventional α/β T cells. Thus, the initial immune response to *Malassezia* is mediated by Th17 cells, although later it may switch to a mixed Th17–Th2 response.

Clinical Features

Malassezia lesions may be localized or generalized. The most prominent features of skin lesions secondarily infected with *Malassezia* are a marked erythema associated with the production of a "greasy" exudate accompanied by pruritus of variable severity. Affected animals may also develop alopecia and waxy, greasy, or scaly seborrhea that is yellow or gray in color. Paronychia with a browning of the nail bed, possibly associated with obsessive paw chewing and licking, may also be a feature. Some dogs may develop a severe folliculitis. The primary lesions may be inconspicuous and simply show erythema. However, because of the pruritis and scratching, some dogs develop excoriation, perhaps with secondary bacterial invasion, malodor, alopecia, seborrheic plaques, and eventually, chronic lichenification and pigmentation (Fig. 10.3).

Secondary *Malassezia* infections may also cause otitis externa associated with erythema and itchiness and severe facial and muzzle pruritus. The otitis externa may generate a moist waxy yellow or brownish discharge.

"Hot Spots"

Otherwise called pyotraumatic dermatitis or summer sores, hot spots are superficial skin lesions that originate from self-inflicted trauma to the skin (Fig. 10.4). The most important cause is excessive scratching and licking due to chronic itch. The inflamed and damaged tissues can ooze fluid and are then secondarily invaded by *Malassezia* or *Staphylococcus*. Because of the *Malassezia* overgrowth, the itch worsens, the lesion enlarges, and the animal is acutely uncomfortable. During the initial stages of the disease, the affected site becomes red and inflamed and starts to itch. Superficial necrosis and ulceration may follow. Pus or other exudate may ooze from the damaged skin and dry to form a crust. A local, well defined, area of a wet, sticky coat develops. Local hair loss occurs, and the site may be very painful. While the initial lesion may be small, the affected area can enlarge rapidly within hours. Triggers of hot spots may include ectoparasite bites, allergic reactions such as AD, the presence of foreign bodies, otitis externa, or scratch damage. They

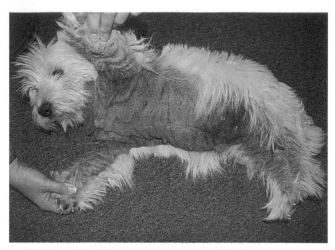

Fig. 10.3 *Malassezia.* Severe alopecia, lichenification, and hyperpigmentation on the entire ventrum of a West Highland White Terrier. The yeast infection was secondary to the allergic dermatitis. (From: Medleau L, Hnilica KA. *Small animal dermatology,* 2nd ed. Saunders; 2006.)

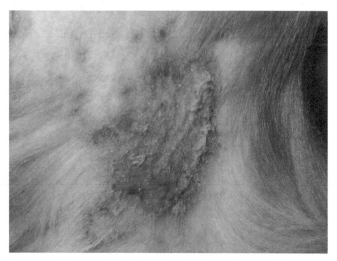

Fig. 10.4 Pyotraumatic dermatitis. These lesions are triggered by locally intense itch. Subsequent scratching can result in secondary *Malassezia* or staphylococcal infections. (Courtesy Dr. Robert Kennis.)

are also associated with hot, humid weather; a heavy, dirty, matted hair coat; and poor grooming. Hot spots should be shaved and then regularly cleaned so that they can dry. Animals should be properly groomed. Culture or cytology should be used to determine the nature of the secondary infection and should be treated as a priority. Medicated shampoos may help in cleaning the affected area. Elizabethan collars may be required to minimize scratching or licking.

Histopathology

Histopathological examination of *Malassezia*-infected lesions generally shows parakeratotic hyperkeratosis, epidermal hyperplasia, and diffuse intercellular edema (spongiosis) with both lymphocytic infiltration and mast cell accumulation (Fig. 10.5A). Mast cells may align themselves along blood vessels in the subepidermis. The lymphocytes are primarily T cells and plasma cells. *Malassezia* yeasts are not always visible in the stratum corneum. The presence of plasma cells in the lesions is consistent with an antibody response, and anti-*Malassezia* IgG antibodies are readily detectable in serum.

Diagnosis

Malassezia yeasts are readily observed in ear or skin scrapings, nail bed debris, acetate tape strip preparations, or skin impression smears, where they bind to clumps of desquamated skin cells. The slide should be heat fixed and stained with modified Wright-Giemsa stain (Diff-Quik), methylene blue, or Gram stain, and examined under oil immersion. *Malassezia* are round or oval, ("footprint-shaped") dark-staining bodies 3–8 μm in diameter (Fig. 10.5(B)). Thus, their presence and numbers are readily assessed by direct microscopic examination. However, there are no definitive guidelines as to what constitutes overgrowth, and high numbers may be found on some clinically normal skin. Culturing on modified Dixon's medium at 32–34°C aerobically (with 5%–10% CO_2) for up to 7 days provides some qualitative data. However, the final diagnosis should rely on both the presence of the yeast and clinical presentation. The precise numbers of the organisms are of less significance than the presence and intensity of pruritus and the severity of the obvious lesions.

Treatment

In mild cases of *Malassezia* dermatitis, topical therapy with antifungal products may suffice. Most isolates of *M. pachydermatis* are susceptible to the azoles; however, the possibility of emerging resistance must always be considered. For severe or generalized disease, or if the animal is suffering from intense, recurrent pruritus, oral antifungal therapy is required. Ketoconazole, fluconazole, and itraconazole are active against *Malassezia*. They inhibit the ergosterol synthesis required for its plasma membrane synthesis. Ketoconazole administered 5–10 mg/kg daily PO for 4 weeks is the usual course of treatment. Other effective treatments include 2% miconazole or oral itraconazole (5 mg/kg). Other issues should also be addressed, including antipruritic and seborrheic therapy. Medicated shampoos such as those containing miconazole and chlorhexidine will make the dog more comfortable, block fungal and bacterial growth, and hasten recovery. It is also essential to identify the underlying cause of the disease. The daily application of skin wipes

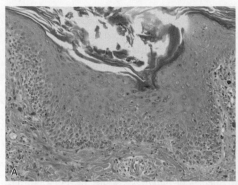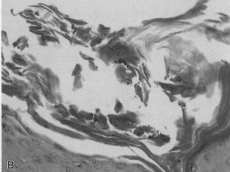

Fig. 10.5 Histopathology of canine *Malassezia* dermatitis showing (A) parakeratotic hyperkeratosis, epidermal hyperplasia, and diffuse intercellular edema (spongiosis) with both lymphocytic infiltration and mast cell accumulation. (B) A higher power view showing the presence of numerous *Malassezia* yeasts. (Courtesy Dr. Dominique Wiener.)

containing chlorhexidine, climbazole, and Tris-EDTA can substantially reduce the *Malassezia* population on treated dog skin. These may be useful adjuncts to topical therapy, especially in areas such as the lips, paws, perianal areas, and skin folds. Allergen-specific immunotherapy is a safe and effective treatment for *Malassezia* hypersensitivity based on reducing the severity of pruritus and the need for drug therapy.

Feline Malassezia Dermatitis

Malassezia dermatitis is much less frequent in cats than in dogs. The most common species involved is *M. pachydermatis* but other species have also been detected on cat skin. They appear to be more prominent in the ear canals of allergic and diseased cats than in healthy cats. Otitis externa is the commonest clinical presentation. The clinical signs include a greasy seborrheic dermatitis, erythema, hypotrichosis, perhaps with paronychia, and greasy brown discoloration. The face is most commonly affected and is often restricted to the chin, where it causes chin acne. Pruritus is less common. Secondary *Malassezia* infection in cats has been associated with retroviral-mediated immunosuppression. Devon Rex and Sphynx breeds appear to be predisposed to these infections. Proven treatments include oral itraconizole at 5–10 mg/kg daily for a 7-day on/7-day off treatment cycle.

Malassezia can infect humans, so its zoonotic potential must always be considered and appropriate hygienic precautions are taken.

Staphylococci

As described in Chapter 7, commensal bacteria will, under stable conditions, prosper and persist on the skin. Simultaneously, their products influence cutaneous homeostasis and local immunity. Should environmental conditions change, some bacteria may take advantage of new opportunities and invade the host. One such change occurs in AD, where the inflammatory environment provides opportunities for *Staphylococci* to exploit the situation to their advantage. Therefore, both dogs and humans with AD may suffer from simultaneous and recurrent staphylococcal skin infections. These bacteria readily invade atopic skin, and their toxins will enhance the resulting inflammatory response. They do this by stimulating both Th2- and Th17-mediated responses and activating lymphocytes via the release of staphylococcal superantigens.

STAPHYLOCOCCAL SKIN INFECTIONS

Normal Skin

Healthy skin is normally quite dry with a low pH and constant desquamation of the upper layer of keratinocytes. It also contains plenty of antibacterial defensins. Nevertheless, up to 90% of healthy humans have *S. aureus* living on their skin while a similar percentage of dogs carry *S. pseudintermedius*. Therefore, superficial infections with these organisms are not uncommon.

Atopic Skin

Staphylococcus thrives in AD lesions. In one human study, 70% of atopic skin samples contained *S. aureus* compared to only 40% of non-lesional samples. In some children, *S. aureus* colonization precedes the development of atopic eczema. Therefore, *S. aureus* is frequently isolated from the skin of AD patients, especially during disease flares. The degree of *S. aureus* colonization is directly correlated with the severity of the atopic lesions.

AD lesions provide a suitable habitat for both species of *Staphylococci* species. For example, the lesional skin pH climbs into the alkaline range because of decreased sweating and reduced production of filaggrin-derived free fatty acids. Mutations in the *flg* gene result in decreased levels of the filaggrin breakdown products urocanic acid and pyrrolidone carboxylic acid. The Th2 cytokines, IL-4 and IL-13, reduce filaggrin expression still further. The increase in IL-4 levels results in the accumulation of fibronectin. *Staphylococci* produce fibronectin-binding proteins that enable them to adhere to the fibronectin and cytokeratin and fibrinogen on the surface of keratinocytes. Once firmly attached, the staphylococcal proteins and enzymes can penetrate the impaired epithelial barrier and stimulate host immune responses and inflammation.

Staphylococcal Toxins

The complex mixture of soluble factors released by Staphylococci contribute directly to the inflammatory and allergic responses in infected skin. For example, staphylococcal delta toxin induces mast cell degranulation and increases IgE levels. Staphylococcal modulins and protein-A trigger cytokine release from keratinocytes. Staphylococcal superantigens preferentially bind to T cell antigen receptors, provoking an unusually strong and prolonged inflammatory response. These superantigens bypass the regular T cell activating pathways to promote IL4 and IL-13 release, leading to barrier dysfunction. They can also stimulate the production of anti-staphylococcal IgE.

Staphylococcal phenol-soluble modulins (PSMs) are a family of peptides that disrupt cell membranes and kill many different cell types. PSMs cause keratinocyte damage and the release of IL-1 and IL-36. PSMs also combine with induced keratinocyte proteases to damage the skin barrier. *Staphylococci* can produce ceramidases and proteases that further disrupt the epithelial barrier. Clumping factor B promotes bacterial adhesion to atopic corneocytes in AD skin by binding the bacterium to corneocyte cytokeratin 10.

Staphylococcal serine proteases are especially effective in promoting IgE responses because of their cleavage and IL-33 activation. *S. aureus* is also unique in that it can induce the rapid release of constitutive IL-33 from human keratinocytes and selectively promote type 2 responses. Epicutaneous *S. aureus* exposure drives T cell-derived IL-36- dependent skin inflammation. IL-36 directly induces T cell production of IL-17A, which is needed for inflammation. These molecules signal through their respective receptors via the adaptor protein MyD88 to induce IL-17A-producing γ/δ T cells and ILC3 cells. Thus, as with *Malassezia*, soluble staphylococcal molecules can trigger Th2 or Th17 responses, or both.

CANINE STAPHYLOCOCCAL INFECTIONS

Staphylococcus pseudintermedius

The predominant *Staphylococcus* species found on dog skin and mucous membranes is *S. pseudintermedius*. Canidae such as dogs and foxes are its natural hosts. Cats are not, although it is occasionally isolated from feline pyoderma cases. *S. pseudintermedius* is found on the skin, hair follicles, mouth, anus, and nasal passages of many healthy dogs. It is transmitted vertically from mothers to their puppies at birth. Some of these infections may be transient, while others can persist indefinitely. As with *S. aureus* in humans, this colonization alone does not directly cause disease. Nevertheless, *S. pseudintermedius* is the predominant cause of canine pyoderma. Primary staphylococcal skin and ear infections occur in dogs, even in the absence of AD. They cause inflammation and pruritus of variable severity. It is also frequently isolated from wounds and canine urinary tract infections.

Atopic Disease

Dogs with AD are more susceptible to colonization and infection with *S. pseudintermedius* than healthy animals. When these infections involve AD lesions, they result in a marked increase in disease severity and animal discomfort. Some veterinary dermatologists believe that some canine AD cases are due entirely to a recurrent staphylococcal pyoderma and antibiotic treatment alone will result in a cure. However, there is little published evidence to support this concept.

Because lesional skin in atopic dogs is predisposed to S. *pseudintermedius* colonization, up to 91% of dogs with AD may have lesions colonized by coagulase-positive staphylococci compared to only 40% of healthy dogs. This increased colonization is due in part to the decreased production of antibacterial peptides and increased adherence because of the presence of Th2 cytokines. Staphylococcal proliferation is also stimulated by decreased competition from other commensals and a locally higher skin pH.

Studies on bacterial diversity at canine skin sites sensitized by topical administration of house dust mite extracts showed changes in the relative abundance of many bacterial species as AD lesions developed. One of the most significant was an increase in the abundance of *S. pseudintermedius* at the challenged site compared to the contralateral control. *S. pseudintermedius* adheres to corneocytes from both inflamed and non-inflamed atopic dog skin to a much greater extent than to corneocytes from normal dogs. This might reflect increased expression of fibronectin induced by the actions of IL-4 on nearby fibroblasts.

These staphylococcal infections may be persistent, and infected dogs eventually develop anti-staphylococcal IgG antibodies. Second, these infected animals mount either a Th2- or Th17-mediated immune response, or a combination of the two, against the invading staphylococci. Third, some *Staphylococcus* strains may release exotoxins that act as superantigens and further promote skin inflammation.

Pathogenesis

Staphylococcal hypersensitivity is a pruritic pustular dermatitis of dogs. Skin testing with staphylococcal antigens suggests that hypersensitivity types I, III, and IV may all be involved. Histological findings of a neutrophilic dermal vasculitis suggest that the type III reaction may predominate. Pruritus-induced self-trauma, other skin environmental changes, and anti-inflammatory therapy may facilitate staphylococcal colonization. The bacteria concentrate in the cornified layers of the epidermis because of increased adherence between the bacteria and keratinocytes. The numbers of *S. pseudintermedius* and their adherence decline as AD improves.

S. pseudintermedius produces a diverse mixture of toxins and other mediators (Fig. 10.6). Thus, approximately a quarter of *S. pseudintermedius* isolates produce superantigens such as staphylococcal enterotoxins A and C. These bind to MHC molecules on DCs, mast cells, and T cells.

Canine keratinocytes express toll-like receptors and protease-activated receptors. When activated by bacterial pathogen-associated molecular patterns or the proteases of house dust mites, they activate the genes associated with innate and adaptive immune responses. Staphylococci also induce the production of TSLP by canine corneocytes. TSLP then acts on DCs to cause them to differentiate into DC2 cells that in turn promote Th2 responses.

Th2/IgE Responses

Staphylococcal proteins can cross the disrupted stratum corneum in AD lesions and trigger immune responses in humans and dogs. This does not require bacterial tissue invasion, simply penetration by soluble factors. Anti-staphylococcal IgG is elevated in both atopic and non-atopic dogs with staphylococcal pyoderma. The IgG antibody titer is higher, as expected, in dogs with the most severe pyoderma.

Staphylococci produce superantigens that can induce inflammation as a result of polyclonal B and T cell activation; however, they are also significant conventional antigens. These superantigens skew the dog's immune response in favor of a type 2 response (Fig. 10.7). Thus, the IgE response to these superantigens determine the severity of AD. Dogs suffering from AD have significantly higher levels of anti-staphylococcal IgE than do non-atopic, non-infected dogs. These IgE levels are also higher in atopic dogs than in dogs with staphylococcal infections resulting from other causes (Box 10.1).

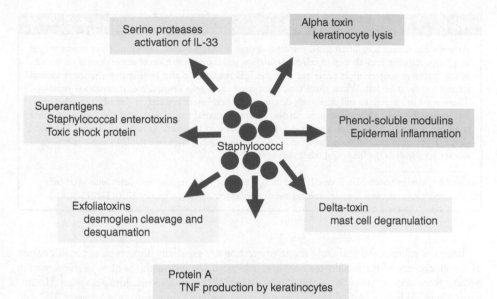

Fig. 10.6 Some of the many staphylococcal products affecting atopic skin disease.

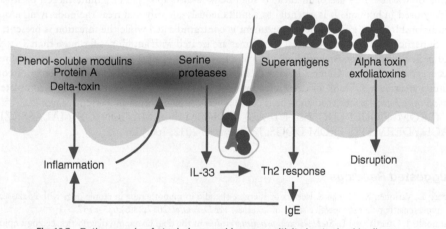

Fig. 10.7 Pathogenesis of staphylococcal hypersensitivity in atopic skin disease.

Diagnosis and Treatment

Given the complex pathogenesis of these lesions, it is essential to identify and treat the underlying cause of the skin lesions and pruritus in addition to treating the bacterial infection. Unlike humans, where *S. aureus* is routinely detected by nasal swabs, canine carriers of *S. pseudintermedius* are best detected by swabbing the perineum and oral mucosa. (A combination of both sites detects about 90% of healthy carriers.) Atopic dogs have a much higher carriage rate than healthy dogs. These differences are most apparent in the ear and conjunctival sac. As many as 75% of atopic dogs may require antibiotic treatment for staphylococcal dermatitis.

BOX 10.1 ■ Mast Cells Are Not All Bad

Animals can mount a significant IgE response against *S. aureus* toxins. Therefore, these toxins trigger an allergic response leading to mast cell degranulation and the exacerbation of atopic dermatitis. So why is this pathway conserved? It turns out that the IgE response is also beneficial—it protects against staphylococcal infection. When these toxin-sensitized mast cells degranulate, they release proteases. These mast cell proteases will effectively destroy snake and insect venoms, as described in Chapter 3. Recently, it has been shown that they can also destroy bacterial toxins, such as the staphylococcal hemolysins and leucocidins. They also limit tissue pathology and bacterial growth and spread. This local skin IgE response has also been shown in mice to protect against systemic staphylococcal infections at distant sites such as the lungs and other skin sites.

(Starkl P, Watzenboeck ML, Popov LM, et al. IgE effector mechanisms, in concert with mast cells, contribute to acquired host defense against *Staphylococcus aureus. Immunity* 2020; 53:793-804)

Bacterial cultures and antibiotic sensitivity testing are especially important, not least because of the emergence of methicillin-resistant staphylococci. Up to two-thirds of *S. pseudintermedius* isolates from dogs may now be methicillin resistant. Many are also multidrug resistant. (In humans, there has been a 24-fold increase in staphylococcal multidrug resistance between 2011 and 2014.)

While waiting for culture and sensitivity results, animals may be treated with chlorhexidine baths or washes. The use of medicated shampoos is also appropriate. Dilute bleach baths are widely used in humans. It is essential to simultaneously identify and treat the underlying atopic condition.However, glucocorticoid treatment is contraindicated while the infection is present.

Superficial primary streptococcal pyodermas are treated with antibiotics for more than 3 weeks and preferably 4 weeks. An antibiotic known to be effective against *S. pseudintermedius* is required. Recovery may be slow. Clinical lesions should have resolved at least 1–2 weeks prior to discontinuing treatment. Chronic or deep infections may require up to 12 weeks to resolve completely. Based on efficacy, safety, cost, and client compliance, cephalosporins are currently favored.

(FROM FIGUEREDO LA ET AL. BIOFILM FORMATION OF MALASSEZIA PACHYDERMATIS FROM DOGS. *Vet Microbiol* 2012; 160:126-131.)

Suggested Readings

Aberg L, Varjonen K, Ahman S. Results of allergen-specific immunotherapy in atopic dogs with Malassezia hypersensitivity: a retrospective study of 16 cases. *Vet Dermatol.* 2017;28(6):633-e157.

Bannoehr J, Guardabassi L. *Staphylococcus pseudintermedius* in the dog: taxonomy, diagnostics, ecology, epidemiology and pathogenicity. *Vet Dermatol.* 2012;23(4):253-e52.

Bond R, Morris DO, Guillot J, et al. Biology, diagnosis and treatment for Malassezia dermatitis in dogs and cats. Clinical consensus guidelines of the World Association for Veterinary Dermatology. *Vet Dermatol.* 2020;31(1):27-e4.

Chermprapai S, Ederveen TH, Broere F, et al. The bacterial and fungal microbiome of the skin of healthy dogs and dogs with atopic dermatitis and the impact of topical antimicrobial therapy, an exploratory study. *Vet Microbiol.* 2019;229:90-99.

Fazakerley J, Nuttall T, Sales D, et al. Staphylococcal colonization of mucosal and lesional skin sites in atopic and healthy dogs. *Vet Dermatol.* 2009;20(3):179-184. doi:10.1111/j.1365-3164.2009.00745.x.

Fazakerley J, Williams N, Carter S, McEwan N, Nuttall T. Heterogeneity of *Staphylococcus pseudintermedius* isolates from atopic and healthy dogs. *Vet Dermatol.* 2010;21(6):578-585. doi:10.1111/j.1365-3164.2010.00894.x.

Guillot J, Bond R. *Malassezia pachydermatis* [a review]. *Med Mycol.* 1999;37(5):295-306.

Ishimaru H, Okamoto N, Fujimura M, et al. IgE sensitivity to Malassezia pachydermatis and mite allergens in dogs with atopic dermatitis. *Vet Immunol Immunopathol.* 2020;226:110070, doi:10.1016/j. vetimm.2020.110070.

Khantavee N, Chanthick C, Sookrung N, Prapasarakul N. Antibody levels to *Malassezia pachydermatis* and *Staphylococcus pseudintermedius* in atopic dogs and their relationship with lesion scores. *Vet Dermatol.* 2020;31(2):111-115. doi:10.1111/vde.12802.

Kim J, Kim BE, Ahn K, Leung DY. Interactions between atopic dermatitis and *Staphylococcus aureus* infection: clinical implications. *Allergy Asthma Immunol Res.* 2019;11(5):593-603.

Krysko O, Teufelberger A, Van Nevel S, Krysko DV, Bachert C. Protease/antiprotease network in allergy: the role of *Staphylococcus aureus* protease-like proteins. *Allergy.* 2019;74(11):2077-2086.

Layne EA, DeBoer DJ. Serum Malassezia-specific IgE in dogs with recurrent Malassezia otitis externa without concurrent skin disease. *Vet Immunol Immunopathol.* 2016;176:1-4.

McEwan NA, Mellor D, Kalna G. Adherence by *Staphylococcus intermedius* to canine corneocytes: a preliminary study comparing noninflamed and inflamed atopic canine skin. *Vet Dermatol.* 2006;17(2):151-154. doi:10.1111/j.1365-3164.2006.00503.x.

Morales CA, Schultz KT, DeBoer D. Antistaphylococcal antibodies in dogs with recurrent staphylococcal pyoderma. *Vet Immunol Immunopathol.* 1994;42(2):137-147.

Rangel SM, Paller AS. Bacterial colonization, overgrowth, and superinfection in atopic dermatitis. *Clin Dermatol.* 2018;35(5):641-647.

Rodrigues Hoffmann A. The cutaneous ecosystem: the roles of the skin microbiome in health and its association with inflammatory skin conditions in humans and animals. *Vet Dermatol.* 2017;28(1):60-e15.

Santoro D, Archer L, Kelley K. A defective release of host defense peptides is present in canine atopic skin. *Comp Immunol Microbiol Infect Dis.* 2019;65:65-69.

Santoro D, Marsella R, Pucheu-Hastomn CM, Eisenschenk MN, Nuttall T, Bizikova P. Review: pathogenesis of canine atopic dermatitis: skin barrier and host-micro-organism interaction. *Vet Dermatol.* 2015;26(2):84-e25.

Wikramanayake TC, Borda LJ, Miteva M, Paus R. Seborrheic dermatitis – looking beyond Malassezia. *Exp Dermatol.* 2019;28(9):991-1001.

Yamakazi Y, Nakamura Y, Nunez G. Role of the microbiota in skin immunity and atopic dermatitis. *Allergol Int.* 2017;66(4):539-544.

CHAPTER 11

Allergies in the Gastrointestinal Tract

The most important allergic diseases affecting the gastrointestinal tract are those directed against antigenic food components. Food allergies include immunoglobulin E (IgE)-mediated responses expressed as food-induced anaphylaxis, immediate gastrointestinal hypersensitivities, acute urticarial attacks, or oral allergy syndromes. They also include non-IgE-mediated food allergies and eosinophilic gastrointestinal disorders. They do not include food intolerances or food poisoning.

Food allergies result from a loss of oral tolerance to food proteins. As a result, exposure to very small quantities of these proteins may trigger mast cell-mediated digestive upsets, urticaria, or dyspnea that can range in severity from mild to lethal. Food allergies must be differentiated from food intolerances in that intolerance is not immune-mediated. For example, lactose intolerance results from lactose malabsorption and a deficiency of the enzyme lactase.

The prevalence of food allergies in humans is increasing. Between 1997 and 2007, the reported prevalence of food allergies in children under 18 in the United States increased from 3.9% to 5% by 2011 and to 8% in 2016. At least 30% of these children have multiple food allergies. Similar numbers have been reported in the UK and Australia, and the number continues to rise. The proportion of patients admitted to the hospital for food allergic responses in the United States increased from 13.2% in 2005 to 18.2% in 2014. Peanut allergies accounted for most of the increase, followed by tree nut allergies. There is a suggestion that the allergy epidemic has occurred in two waves. The first wave was dominated by allergic rhinitis and asthma and began in the 1950s. The second wave has involved food and skin allergies primarily and began in the 1990s.

The Fate of Foods

FOOD TOLERANCE

Normal animals are tolerant to the protein antigens in foods and are immunologically unresponsive to ingested proteins. Dietary proteins are generally not antigenic for two reasons. First, the ingested proteins are degraded by the gut proteases to small, non-immunogenic peptides. Second, any dietary proteins absorbed intact normally generate a strong intestinal regulatory T (Treg) cell response (Fig. 11.1). Treg cells are abundant in the intestinal mucosa, where they mediate tolerance to food antigens and much of the microbiota. Treg cells suppress type 2 helper (Th2) cells, decrease B cell IgE production, suppress effector T cell emigration into tissues, induce interleukin 10 (IL-10) production by dendritic cells (DCs), and inhibit the activation of mast cells, eosinophils, and basophils. A specialized subpopulation of intestinal DCs promotes this Treg cell population, triggering oral tolerance.

Antigenic food components that enter the gut lumen may leak into the body by passing between cells (paracytosis) or through cells (transcytosis). Specialized antigen-capturing cells in the intestine, called microfold cells, bind these food proteins and deliver them to DCs. Other food proteins may penetrate the gut barrier by transcytosis through goblet cells. Intestinal DCs can extend their dendrites between the epithelial cells and capture proteins within the gut lumen. Once these proteins are captured, they are carried by the DCs to the draining mesenteric lymph

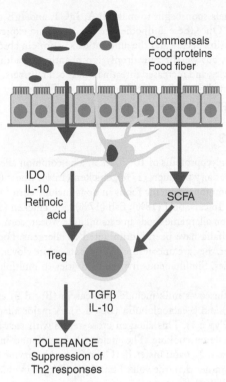

Fig. 11.1 Mechanisms of oral tolerance, which is mediated by the activities of Treg cells within the intestinal wall and maintained by signals derived from the normal microbiota as well as microbial metabolites such as short-chain fatty acids. *IDO,* indoleamine dioxygenase; TGF-b = transforming growth factor-beta.

nodes or Peyer's patches. The DCs produce molecules such as TGF-β and retinoic acid that instruct the responding T cells to differentiate into Treg cells. The Treg cells from the mesenteric lymph nodes of orally tolerant animals secrete the suppressive cytokines TGF-β and IL-10.

A second mechanism by which oral tolerance is induced is through the production of "tolerosomes." These are exosomes shed by enterocytes. They carry MHC class II molecules on their surface and bind peptides sampled from the gut lumen. Purified tolerosomes fed to animals induce tolerance. It is suggested that the presentation of food antigens by tolerosomes selectively induces Treg cell formation.

Approximately 2% of ingested food protein is absorbed as peptide fragments large enough to be recognized by the immune system, although a much smaller fraction of these molecules (<0.002%) is absorbed intact. This protein can reach the portal circulation; however, very little passes the liver and enters the systemic circulation. The Kupffer cells of the liver capture any passing blood-borne food antigens. Antibodies produced in the submucosa may also bind to any adsorbed protein to form immune-complexes that are selectively removed as they pass through the liver.

The Role of IgA

IgA responses are not normally generated against food antigens. However, if weaned calves or pigs are fed a defined high-protein diet such as soy-based milk replacer, although it is initially well absorbed, the animals soon begin to make IgA, IgG1, and IgE antibodies against the soy protein (β-conglycinin). Once these antibodies are produced and expressed on enterocyte surface receptors, immune exclusion occurs and the amount of soy protein absorbed rapidly drops. (Feed intake remains constant, but weight gain drops significantly.) In addition, the animals develop diarrhea, skin test positivity, and increased intestinal mast cell numbers. Thus, antibodies can bind and exclude some potential food allergens from the body. The extent to which normal animals make IgA against food proteins remains unclear.

FOOD ALLERGENS

Most food allergens are glycoproteins of 10–70 kDa. The common allergens in dogs are proteins derived from beef (34%), dairy products (17%), chicken (15%), wheat (13%), soy (6%), and lamb or mutton (5%). Less common allergenic foods in dogs include corn (4%), eggs (4%), pork (2%), rice, and fish (2% each). In cats, beef (18%), fish (17%), and chicken (5%) are important sources of allergens. Less common allergenic foods in cats include wheat, corn, dairy products, and lamb. In pigs, fish meal and alfalfa have been incriminated as allergens. Food allergies have been reported in horses; however, they are uncommon. Wild oats, white clover, and alfalfa are recognized as allergens in this species. Simultaneous hypersensitivities to multiple unrelated food allergens are not uncommon.

The major allergens in cow's milk include αS1-casein (Bos d 8) and whey proteins such as α-lactalbumin (Bos d 4) and β-lactoglobulin (Bos d 5). A major allergen from fish is the carp allergen, parvalbumin (Cyp c 1). This allergen cross-reacts with parvalbumin from many other fish species and it is stable on cooking. The major allergens found in eggs include ovomucoid (Gal d 1), ovalbumin (Gal d 2), ovotransferrin (Gal d 3), and lysozyme (Gal d 4), all of which are present in the egg white rather than the yolk. The major allergen in chicken meat is Gal d 7. This is a heat-stable myosin light chain.

It is important to note that cross-reactivity may occur between related food allergens. For example, cross-reactions have been reported in dogs between beef and lamb and, to a lesser extent, cow's milk. Analysis of serum from dogs that are allergic to both beef and cow's milk shows that the major allergens in these cases are bovine IgG heavy chains and bovine serum albumin. A second major allergen found in both lamb and beef extracts is phosphoglucomutase. Fetal bovine serum is often used for tissue culture purposes in virus vaccines. It is possible that the use of such a vaccine could sensitize an animal against dietary bovine serum albumin. The consumption of foods such as peanuts, milk, eggs, fish, or wheat in early life is associated with a reduced incidence of food allergies. This has been demonstrated in human trials for peanut allergies, but the results for egg allergies are much less clear.

BREAKING TOLERANCE

While oral ingestion of an antigen in food normally induces tolerance, allergic sensitization to food allergens is not uncommon. This sensitization can develop not only against allergens administered orally but also by allergens absorbed through the airways or skin. Animal models suggest that early epidermal barrier disruption caused by genetic defects or local inflammation is associated with the loss of oral tolerance and the development of food allergies. Thus, sensitization to food allergens can occur through the gastrointestinal tract, oral cavity, skin, or respiratory tract.

When oral tolerance breaks down, Treg cells are effectively replaced by Th2 and ILC2 cells, causing type 2 immune responses to develop. Class switching results in IgE production and the development of food allergies (Fig. 11.2). Some infections, primarily those mediated by enteric viruses, may also trigger a Treg to Th1 cell switch and break oral tolerance.

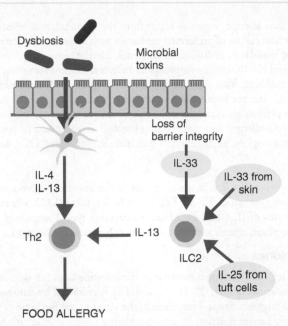

Fig. 11.2   Mechanisms of loss of oral tolerance and the subsequent development of food allergies resulting from dysbiosis. As a result, a Th2 immune response is mounted.

Food allergens are first captured by DCs sampling their environment, including the gut lumen. In the presence of the three epithelial cytokines, IL-25, IL-33, and TSLP, these DCs differentiate into DC2 cells and produce IL-4 and IL-13. These cause the Treg cells to differentiate into Th2 cells. IL-33 is especially effective in dysregulating Treg cell production. The Th2 cells, in turn, release a mixture of cytokines that trigger B cell IgE production. IgE production specific to food proteins is key to the development of food allergies. Long-lived IgE$^+$ plasma cells are responsible for maintaining peanut allergies and memory B cells in the gastrointestinal tract. Intestinal lymphoid tissues are a major source of IgE in these cases.

In many cases of food allergies, the antibodies may be directed against conformational epitopes rather than sequential epitopes. Therefore, when proteins are cooked and the protein denatures, the peptide chains unfold and their conformational epitopes are destroyed. Conversely, sequential epitopes are heat resistant and not destroyed by cooking. Some food allergens such as lipid transfer proteins that are important in fruit, nuts, and cereals may be highly resistant to heat denaturation and cooking. Therefore, allergenicity can increase in cooked or canned foods, and proteins from canned foods appear to be more immunogenic than unprocessed proteins.

IgE Responses

IgE-dependent reactions are elicited very shortly after food exposure in sensitized animals. They result in severe or lethal reactions occurring between a few minutes and 2 hours after ingestion. The reactions may affect the skin in the form of hives or pruritus, the respiratory tract in the form of dyspnea or coughing, or the gastrointestinal tract in the form of vomiting or diarrhea. In very severe cases, anaphylaxis will result. In humans, IgE-mediated allergies to cow's milk, egg, wheat, and soy tend to be outgrown. Allergies to peanuts, tree nuts, and shellfish tend to persist until adulthood.

IgE-dependent food allergic responses result from the degranulation of basophils and mast cells. After the immediate release of preformed mediators such as histamine, there is a second wave of newly synthesized mediators, including leukotrienes, platelet-activating factor, and cytokines such as IL-4, IL-5, and IL-13. Initial symptoms include oral tingling, pruritus, swelling, nausea, abdominal pain, and vomiting. Skin signs can include flushing, angioedema, pruritus, and urticaria. Systemic responses may include hypotension or hypothermia, and anaphylaxis in extreme cases.

The role of neutrophils in food allergies is unclear. In mice, exposure to food allergens can activate neutrophils via IgG-allergen complexes acting through Fc receptors. In peanut allergic individuals, in addition to basophils, other activated cells include monocytes, DCs, and neutrophils.

ILC2 Cells

As described in Chapter 2, ILC2 cells are abundant in the intestinal submucosa. When stimulated by the three master cytokines, IL-33, TSLP, and IL-25, these ILC2 cells respond by rapidly producing large amounts of IL-5 and IL-13 and so promote type 2 responses, mast cell activation, goblet cell hyperplasia, mucus secretion, and smooth muscle contraction.

The Master Cytokines

The switch from a Treg cell to a type 2 response in the intestine as in the skin is mediated by the three epithelial master cytokines, IL-33, IL-25, and TSLP, produced by damaged intestinal epithelial cells. Thus, the triggers of type 2 responses in the intestine are the same as those in the skin.

IL-33 reduces skin barrier function by downregulating filaggrin in keratinocytes. It also increases mucosal permeability in the gut and promotes Th2 skewing of the intestinal immune response. IL-33 does not directly cause the expansion of tuft cells. It activates ILC2 cells that are driven to produce IL-13, which then in turn drives epithelial cell differentiation into tuft cells. IL-25 production is also upregulated in the intestine of animals with food allergies. IL-25 and Th2 cells together enhance ILC2-derived IL-13 production and further promote Th2 responses.

IL-33 can act directly on mucosal mast cells and enterochromaffin cells to trigger the release of mediators such as serotonin from both cell types. The serotonin stimulates gut motility and intestinal secretions. Thus, IL-33 alone is sufficient to promote intestinal allergy. Cross-talk between IL-33 released from injured skin keratinocytes and IL-25 produced by intestinal tuft cells can promote the accumulation of intestinal ILC2 cells in mice. IL-25 produced in response to intestinal parasites also acts on tuft cells to stimulate their release of leukotrienes that also activate ILC2 cells.

Role of IL-9

IL-9 plays an important role in the induction of food allergies and is the most highly upregulated gene in memory T cells from peanut allergic individuals. It is similarly upregulated in egg-allergic individuals. IL-9 acts as a growth factor for mast cells. A population of mucosal mast cells (MMC) that produce unusually large amounts of IL-9 and IL-13 in response to stimulation by IL-33 has been identified in mice. These MMC9 cells also produce large amounts of proteases in response to allergen and IgE receptor cross-linking. They are induced by Th2 cells and promote the development of mature mast cells in the intestine. MMC9 cells may play a significant role in food allergic individuals.

ROLE OF THE MICROBIOTA

The major increase in food allergies occurring over the past 25 years have been influenced by environmental factors, including increases in caesarian births, exposure to pets or living on farms, having older siblings, and early exposure to daycare. All except the first are protective. These factors are all affected by the microbial environment and composition of the intestinal microbiota. There is growing evidence that microbial dysbiosis precedes the onset of food allergies and determines its course. Children with food allergies have distinctly different gut microbiota compared to those without food allergies. This appears to be especially important during early infancy, when it is associated with changes in the microbiota associated with weaning. Weaning is a critical time when persistent oral tolerance is usually established. It has been calculated that every reduction in microbial diversity by a quarter in young children increases their chances of developing a food allergy by 55%. Mouse models have clearly demonstrated that changes in the microbiota can affect susceptibility to food allergies. For example, germ-free mice readily generate high IgE responses and exaggerated allergic responses. Conversely, it is necessary to colonize them with a complete microbiota from normal animals to suppress this IgE response. Likewise, transfer of the fecal microbiota from milk-allergic infants to germ-free mice renders the mice milk allergic. Feeding milk or β-lactoglobulin to these mice increases their IgE levels and the development of diarrhea and anal inflammation. Conversely, fecal bacteria from healthy infants protect germ-free mice from experimental milk allergies.

Microbial colonization reduces IgE production and promotes IgA production by regulating the production of Treg cells in the mucosa (Chapter 7). The colonization of germ-free mice with certain clostridial strains induces IL-22 production, which protects the integrity of the intestinal epithelial barrier and reduces its permeability to dietary proteins. The microbiota also interact with dietary components to suppress food allergies. Most importantly, dietary fiber is metabolized to short-chain fatty acids such as butyrate, propionate, and acetate, which act on the immune system to enhance Treg cells and suppress Th2 responses. Tryptophan metabolites derived from gut bacterial metabolism also act via the aryl hydrocarbon receptor to maintain epithelial integrity and protect against increased intestinal permeability.

SKIN DISEASE AND FOOD ALLERGIES

Another link between atopic skin disease and food allergies occurs because of scratching. Thus, epithelial damage in mice caused by scratching promotes the development of food allergies because mechanical skin injury promotes intestinal mast cell expansion. This expansion occurs in response to the release of IL-33 from keratinocytes and IL-25 from intestinal tuft cells. These two cytokines together activate ILC2 cells. The activated ILC2 cells in turn generate IL-4 and IL-13, which trigger the increase in duodenal mast cell numbers.

Cutaneous Sensitization

In humans, it has long been appreciated that eczema is a major risk factor for the development of food allergies. Atopic dermatitis predisposes to food allergies in infants and there is a growing body of evidence that the site of this food sensitization is the skin. For example, the use of infant diaper creams that contain peanut or almond oil is associated with the development of peanut or almond allergies. Similarly, the use of soap containing wheat proteins predisposes to developing a wheat allergy. Skin exposure to air-borne peanut dust is also a major source of allergic sensitization. Percutaneous sensitization is associated with the development of allergic diseases on other surfaces, such as the lungs and bronchi (Chapter 13).

Cutaneous antigen exposure sensitizes to both immediate and delayed allergies. Both depend on the activation of T cells within the draining lymph nodes of sensitized skin. This is probably caused by the migration of antigen-bearing DCs from the skin to the lymph nodes. The process is regulated by the activities of skin-resident Treg cells. If these Treg cells are suppressed, as occurs in AD, then percutaneous sensitization becomes more effective.

Skin Barrier Defects

There is a clear association between skin barrier defects and the development of food allergies. This is due to increased allergen penetration through the skin barrier and thus effectively

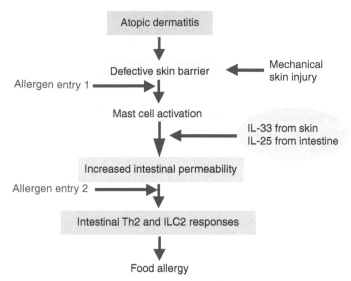

Fig. 11.3   The Dual exposure hypothesis suggests that skin barrier defects permit allergens to enter the body through the skin and bypass the Treg cells in the intestine.

bypassing both skin and oral tolerance pathways. Peanut allergens applied to inflamed skin result in sensitization, whereas early consumption of peanuts will protect against allergies and induce tolerance. Loss of function mutations within the filaggrin gene (*flg*) have been associated with increased risks of developing food allergies. Filaggrin is not expressed in the gastrointestinal tract beyond the oral mucosa. Thus, sensitization against allergens such as peanuts and milk likely results from epidermal barrier defects. Studies on young children with atopic dermatitis due to food allergies suggest that this is a unique dermatitis endotype associated with an immature skin barrier.

Food allergens may be delivered to experimental animals such as mice either by feeding or applying them topically. Under normal conditions, mice develop tolerance to allergens delivered orally. Staphylococcal enterotoxin B can act as an oral adjuvant and promote intestinal immune responses. However, this could be a factor in oral sensitization because *Staphylococci* colonize the skin of patients with AD. The "dual exposure hypothesis" postulates that exposure to allergens through eczematous skin promotes sensitization, whereas early oral exposure promotes tolerance (Fig. 11.3).

Genetic Factors

While family history is associated with the development of allergies, much of this may simply reflect growing up in the same environment as parents and siblings. Studies have demonstrated a high genetic component for peanut allergy susceptibility but not for milk or egg allergies. The only other genetic link identified to date is for filaggrin—just as in the skin. In addition, some mutations in the IL-4R α chain gene increase mouse susceptibility to food allergies.

NON-IgE-MEDIATED RESPONSES

Non-IgE-mediated food hypersensitivities are well described in humans and are recorded in companion animals. They include several different syndromes, of which the most important is gluten-induced enteropathy (celiac disease). This disease is characterized by chronic inflammation of the small intestine, and is triggered by the ingestion of cereal protein, gluten derived from wheat, barley, and rye, in genetically predisposed individuals. As a result, affected individuals develop B cells and cytotoxic

T cells that attack and destroy intestinal epithelial cells. The triggering protein is a major component of gluten, called gliadin, which triggers an innate immune response that increases the permeability of the intestinal epithelial barrier. As a result, the gliadin gains access to the lamina propria. The gliadin also acts on helper T cells that promote B cell responses. These B cells make IgA and IgG antibodies directed against both gliadin and an autoantigen, tissue transglutaminase 2 found in intestinal epithelial cells. The activation of cytotoxic T cells results in the destruction of the epithelial cells and the inflammatory reaction progressively increases in severity, resulting in villous atrophy. Unlike IgE-mediated diseases, the symptoms may be delayed from hours to weeks after ingestion of the offending gluten. Diagnosis is often difficult owing to a lack of non-invasive diagnostic tests.

Gluten-sensitive enteropathy may develop in some Irish Setters in which it is an autosomal recessive disease under the control of a single gene locus. Unlike the situation in humans, this canine gene is not linked to the major histocompatibility complex. The affected dogs usually present with vomiting, dehydration, abnormal or bloody stools, and protracted diarrhea. Pathologic changes include partial villus atrophy in the jejunum resulting in anorexia, poor growth, and weight loss. The disease may be managed by strict avoidance of the offending gluten.

Gluten exposure has also been associated with paroxysmal gluten-sensitive dyskinesia in Border Terriers. These dogs present with neurologic signs (difficulty walking, tremors, and dystonia of the limbs, head, and neck), atopy, the presence of autoantibodies against transglutaminase 2 and anti-gliadin antibodies, and evidence of gastrointestinal disease.

SELECTED HUMAN FOOD ALLERGIES

Four types of food allergies in humans are of special relevance to veterinarians.

Eosinophilic Esophagitis

Eosinophilic esophagitis was scarcely recognized prior to 1990 but has since become increasingly common in humans in the United States. It presents as a characteristic eosinophilic inflammation of the esophagus that improves once cow's milk has been removed from a child's diet. The affected children may have low titers of IgE to cow's milk proteins and other food allergens. On the other hand, they have high titers of IgG4 antibodies to cow's milk proteins. The disease does not improve after treatment with anti-IgE (omalizumab). Eosinophilic esophagitis has rarely been reported in dogs and cats. In one reported canine case, a 4-year-old mixed-breed female dog with a history of allergic skin disease presented with regurgitation, coughing, and dysphagia. The animal had severe diffuse esophagitis. Biopsy showed an eosinophilic ulcerative tissue reaction. Eosinophils constituted 14%–50% of the inflammatory infiltrate. The dog responded well to anti-reflux medications, systemic glucocorticoid therapy, and esophageal bougienage. The underlying cause was suspected to be a food allergy.

Pork-Cat Syndrome

An interesting example of an allergy to other animal proteins is pork-cat syndrome. This syndrome results from an allergy to cat serum albumin that often develops in cat owners (and vets). However, cat albumin cross-reacts with pig albumin. As a result, victims also develop an allergic response after eating lightly cooked pork products. (The allergen is destroyed by high temperatures, so a reaction does not occur every time pork is eaten.) These allergic reactions may range from pruritus to anaphylaxis. The affected individuals also show a positive prick test to both cat dander and pork. This syndrome develops in adults or teens rather than in children.

Alpha-gal Allergy

Approximately 28 million years ago, an ancestral primate underwent a mutation in the gene that encodes the galactosyl transferase that makes galactose alpha-1,3-galactose (alpha-gal)-linked carbohydrates. As a result, this enzyme was functionally inactivated. Ever since then, their

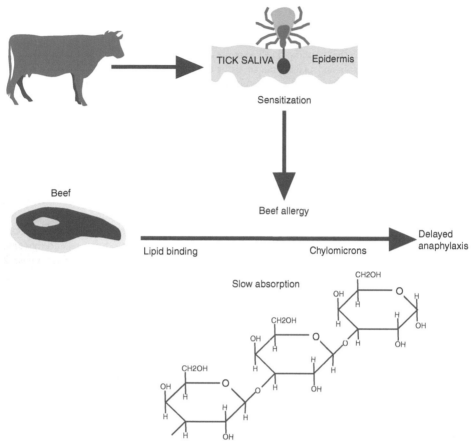

Fig. 11.4 **Mechanisms of alpha-gal allergy where a sensitization to beef is triggered by a tick bite and injection of the allergen via the tick bite lesion.** The origins of the alpha-gal are unclear. It may be synthesized by the tick or be a residue from the tick previously feeding on cattle. When meat is ingested, the alpha-gal is slowly absorbed from the intestine in the form of a glycolipid. Delayed anaphylaxis may result in sensitized individuals.

descendants (including humans, apes, and old-world monkeys) lack the ability to make glycoproteins and glycolipids with alpha-gal side-chains. All other mammals have retained the enzyme. Therefore, alpha-gal is expressed on cell surfaces in non-primates (Fig. 11.4). It is found in skeletal muscle, organs, milk, and gelatin. Most humans make "natural" IgM and IgG antibodies against this foreign oligosaccharide because of continuous exposure to it from the gut microbiota.

Alpha-gal is present in the saliva of some ticks; therefore, some humans make IgE against alpha-gal in response to a tick bite. (This is somewhat unusual because it is the only carbohydrate known to act as a major allergen; all other allergens are proteins.) Alpha-gal allergens have been detected in the salivary glands of two North American tick species, *Amblyomma americanum* and *Ixodes scapularis*. There are three theories as to its origin. It may be produced directly by the tick salivary glands, it may represent residual antigen remaining in ticks that have recently fed on the blood of another mammal, or it may be produced by commensal microbes within the tick. Tick bites preferentially attract large numbers of basophils, which establish a local environment favoring type 2 responses. Thus, the combination of alpha-gal and an environment that promotes type 2 responses may trigger the IgE response. Dogs are an alpha-gal positive species; therefore, alpha-gal allergies are not expected to occur in dogs. However, healthy dogs may develop IgM antibodies to alpha-gal in response to bites of the tick, *I. ricinus*. In this case, it has been speculated that something in the tick saliva might cause a breakdown in tolerance.

When tick-sensitized individuals encounter the alpha-gal oligosaccharide, by eating beef, pork, venison, lamb, goat or rabbit, they may develop delayed onset anaphylaxis. This occurs not only in response to meats but also to vaccines that contain gelatin or drugs ingested in gelatin capsules. Therefore, allergic responses to alpha-gal are unusually common. Although mediated by IgE, the onset of symptoms may be delayed for 4–8 h or longer after ingesting the meat. Approximately 70% of victims develop respiratory distress, urticaria, and possible anaphylaxis. The unusual delay in the allergic response to alpha-gal results from the slow passage of allergenic glycolipids across the intestinal epithelium. These sensitizing molecules will only cross the epithelial barrier when bound to lipids.

Glycoproteins can cross into the bloodstream in 1–2 h; however, it takes 4–5 h for dietary lipids to reach the circulation carried by chylomicrons. Thus, the slower digestion and absorption of the glycolipids cause the delay in the onset of clinical signs.

Bird-Egg Syndrome

Bird-egg syndrome occasionally develops in individuals who keep pet birds, such as budgerigars and parrots. In effect, these individuals become sensitized and often develop signs of respiratory allergies on exposure to these birds. As a result, they can also develop an allergy to eggs and poultry meat. This syndrome is due to cross-sensitization between bird allergens found in feathers, droppings, egg yolk, and poultry meat. Affected individuals develop rhinitis, conjunctivitis, or asthma on exposure to avian aeroallergens. The symptoms associated with egg allergies are digestive, cutaneous (urticaria or angioedema), or respiratory (dyspnea). The offending cross-reactive allergens are alpha-livetins (serum albumin, Gal d 5). The reaction often develops after ingesting soft-boiled egg yolk or chicken or turkey meat. (Duck and goose meat cause milder reactions.) Patients with an allergy to chicken meat may also react unexpectedly to fish and shrimp. Again, this is a response to cross-reactive allergens, probably associated with myosin light chains.

Oral Allergy Syndrome

Some patients develop oral and perioral pruritus and inflammation following ingestion of a food item that cross-reacts with an environmental aeroallergen to which the patient is sensitive. For example, pollens may contaminate many vegetable and fruits. A single canine case has been reported from Japan where a dog, sensitized to Japanese cedar extract, ingested a contaminated tomato. A similar severe allergic response occurs in humans who ingest pancakes or pastries made with flour contaminated by storage mites (*Tyrophagus putrescentiae*) (Chapter 12).

Food Allergic Animals

DOGS

Adverse food reactions likely account for up to 6% of skin disorders observed in a general veterinary practice and up to 50% in specialty veterinary dermatology practices. However, diagnosis is challenging because the clinical signs are indistinguishable from non-seasonal AD. The clinical consequences of food allergies are seen both in the digestive tract and on the skin. While the disease is clearly non-seasonal, it often develops relatively suddenly even after an animal has consumed a specific food for months or even years.

Approximately 10% of dogs with food allergies show only gastrointestinal disturbances. The intestinal reaction may be mild, perhaps showing only as an irregularity in the consistency of the feces or frequent defecation (more than 4–5 times daily) or it may be severe, with vomiting, cramps, and violent, sometimes hemorrhagic, diarrhea occurring soon after feeding.

The cutaneous symptoms of food allergies are indistinguishable from those of AD. Most affected dogs develop dermatitis. The skin reactions are usually papular and erythematous and may involve the feet, eyes, ears, and axillae, or perianal areas. Anal licking and scooting may be common. The skin lesion itself is usually highly pruritic and commonly masked by self-inflicted trauma and secondary bacterial or yeast infections. This pruritus responds poorly to topical corticosteroid treatment. In chronic cases, the skin may be hyperpigmented, lichenified, and infected, leading to pyoderma. Food-allergic dogs are also prone to develop chronic pruritic otitis externa. Analysis of the skin infiltrate in these dogs shows that $CD8^+$ T cells predominate and IL-4 and IL-13 expression are increased.

In general, the first signs of food allergy appear around 6–12 months of age; however, this can vary from 1 to 13 years. Four breeds, German Shepherds, West Highland White Terriers, and Labrador and Golden Retrievers, account for approximately 40% of affected dogs. Most dogs present with unrelenting pruritus affecting the ears, feet, and abdomen. Many cases present with recurrent or chronic bacterial skin infections, hot spots, otitis externa, and AD. It is possible that the only signs of food allergies may be a chronic recurring otitis.

CATS

Feline food allergy is one component of feline atopic syndrome. Food-induced hypersensitivity accounts for approximately 1%–6% of all feline skin diseases. The most common allergens affecting cats are fish and fish-containing foods. Other commonly incriminated foods are beef and dairy products. Allergies to lamb, pork, rabbit, chicken, and eggs have also been reported. There are no sex, age, seasonal, or breed predispositions to food allergies recorded in cats. Food allergies commonly trigger a non-seasonal pruritus of variable severity, primarily involving the anterior third of the body, especially the head, face, neck, and pinnae. However, as in dogs, it cannot be diagnosed based on clinical signs alone. Miliary or exfoliative dermatitis and eosinophilic lesions (plaques and ulcers) are also common. Eosinophilia may be present in 20%–50% of cases.

Cats may overgroom certain areas, and self-inflicted trauma is common and results in symmetrical alopecia. Cats may also present with vomiting or diarrhea. Severe, generalized pruritis without other obvious lesions, conjunctivitis, salivation, flatulence, and hyperactive behavior has also been reported. Published data on cats with allergic reactions to foods is limited. They develop signs later than dogs with a mean age of onset of 3.9 years (range: 4 months to 15 years). Helminth-parasitized cats develop significantly higher levels of antibodies to food allergens than unparasitized cats. Most importantly, they develop higher levels of IgE antibodies, suggesting that the presence of parasitic worms in the intestine provokes food allergies in this species.

ELIMINATION DIET TRIALS

As with other allergic diseases, the effective management of food hypersensitivities is best achieved by allergen avoidance. Therefore, treatment involves eliminating the responsible food after correctly identifying it.

The first step is to remove all currently fed foods and replace them with either a home-cooked or prescription diet (Fig. 11.5). This may be difficult when clients are fed diverse foods and treats. Resolution of the clinical disease should only be expected to occur by feeding a suitable elimination diet for at least 8 weeks. This may then be followed by a provocation trial where recurrence of the clinical signs may occur following feeding either the complete diet or individual suspected components. The recommended procedure to identify food allergy-related AD is to perform an elimination diet trial for 8–12 weeks followed by a 2-week provocation trial with the previous diet.

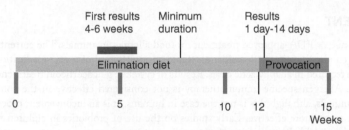

Fig. 11.5 A Suggested time course of elimination diet trials in dogs.

Experience suggests that remission will develop in about 80% of patients by 4–6 weeks, but some animals may take as long as 8–12 weeks to benefit. This type of challenge test takes a very long time to identify the specific allergens. Owners are not always prepared to suffer the inconvenience associated with completion of the program and compliance may be low. The pet should be rechecked frequently to determine both progress and compliance. If the animal improves so that both pets and their owners are satisfied, they may simply continue the new diet. However, a provocation trial provides useful confirmation of the identity of the offending food and a guide to the types of commercial foods that may be appropriate in the future. Experience suggests that clinical signs of the allergy will return in 1–3 days in most dogs following provocation; however, it may take as long as 14 days and it can be as short as 1 h. More than 90% will flare by 14 days. In provoked cats, the signs may return any time between 15 minutes and 10 days, but more than 90% will flare by 7 days.

In seeking to control food allergies, a large market for hypoallergenic diets has developed. These diets generally contain novel ingredients that an average dog likely would not have encountered previously. For example, they may include rabbit and potato or brown rice, venison and potato, or even kangaroo and oats. (Fish and lamb are commonly found in commercial diets and cannot be considered as novel.) Selected baby foods may be used for cats.

However, a review of the literature has found ingredients in these diets that were not listed on the label approximately 45% of the time. Conversely, about 1% of the diets lacked the ingredients listed on the label. Thus, these diets may be mislabeled and may contain unexpected components. These contaminating ingredients may produce incorrect conclusions regarding the elimination diet. Homemade diets may work well if carefully and consistently prepared. Ideally, they should contain one protein and one carbohydrate source. They are, however, often nutritionally inadequate, which may affect young growing animals. They should therefore be carefully supplemented. No other food products such as table scraps or treats such as rawhides should be given while the trial is in process.

In general, if a food allergy is responsible for the pruritus, the severity of the itching should drop visibly by 4–6 weeks. If no response is observed, then several alternatives present themselves. It is possible that the pruritus is not of dietary origin and the animal has a concurrent hypersensitivity, such as a flea allergy. It could also be because owner compliance is poor or that the replacement diet also contains the allergen.

The immune system preferentially responds to large protein molecules. These can be readily captured, processed, and presented to T cells by DCs. If these proteins are extensively hydrolyzed to short-chain peptides (maximum 3–5 kDa) and single amino acids, their allergenicity and ability to bind and cross-link IgE on mast cells is very much reduced. However, the reduction in allergenicity is directly related to the degree of hydrolysis. The hydrolysis of food proteins must be very extensive if allergic responses are to be avoided completely (see Fig. 20.7).

TREATMENT

There is no cure or FDA-approved treatment for food allergies in animals. The current standard of care is allergen identification and avoidance. Rapid administration of rescue medication (epinephrine) may be required in anaphylactic cases. Results of systemic glucocorticoid treatments have been inconsistent. Allergen-specific immunotherapy is not considered effective in the control of food allergies in animals, although this is not the case in humans. It is an inconvenient procedure where avoidance is much more effective. Early studies on the use of probiotics in children with a cow's milk allergy have yielded encouraging but imprecise results.

Milk Allergy in Cattle

In 1903, two French veterinary students, Houllier and Dellanoy, described urticaria in cows that had "retained their milk." Allergy signs developed in those cows that had not been milked for 24 h to make their udders look good when sold. While obviously not a food allergy, it is an interesting observation that many cows make IgE autoantibodies to their own milk. This typically happens during the drying-off period when intramammary pressure rises and milk proteins, especially casein, are forced back into their bloodstream. As a result, the cows mount an IgE response and, on subsequent exposure to milk proteins, may develop allergic reactions. Once sensitized, the condition may recur repeatedly in some animals. Clinically, the animals present with urticaria and respiratory distress. The urticaria varies in severity; however, large edematous plaques may develop on the skin of the face, perineum, and udder. Animals may cough or develop dyspnea and tachypnea. In extreme cases, the animals may die from acute anaphylaxis.

Some of these affected cows have been successfully treated with antihistamines. In other cases, the influx of casein into the bloodstream may be reduced simply by milking the animals to lower the intramammary pressure. These cows may then be "dried off" slowly, or even milking may be continued without a break. In a survey in New York State in 1968, Dr. Gordon Campbell determined that the annual incidence of milk allergies in cows was 0.5%. The disease appears either when the cows are being dried off at the end of lactation or at calving, when their udders are beginning to fill and become engorged. Campbell's survey indicated that milk allergy predominantly occurs in Channel Island breeds. In some Jersey herds, as many as 22% of the cows were affected. Several veterinarians also reported seeing the condition in lactating mares and bitches. In some cases, the appearance of hives coincided with milk let-down prior to milking. Other clinical signs include restlessness, evidence of pruritus with scratching, increased respiratory rate, edema of the eyelids, copious lacrimation, bilateral nasal discharge, excessive salivation, and difficulty swallowing. In terminal cases with severe dyspnea, some animals may become cyanotic. As urticaria develops, some cows pass a large volume of liquid feces. Some farmers believed that the condition caused cows to abort. Urticaria on the udders results in significant edema and very tender teats so that milking becomes difficult. Skin urticaria is revealed by the hair standing upright over an area of skin thickening. These affected areas may be itchy and painful. Angioedema may develop on the ears, muzzle, anus, vulva, and udder. Local hemorrhage may also occur at urticarial and angioedematous sites. Generalized lymphadenopathy may develop. Recovery after milking may be rapid, although the condition frequently recurs.

Campbell also demonstrated that affected cows responded to intracutaneous injection of their own diluted, defatted milk by the development of large wheals. Thus, 0.1 mL of milk diluted to 1:10,000 could elicit a visible reaction. They were equally sensitive to autologous and homologous bovine milk. Hypersensitivity to milk could also be transferred to the skin of an unsensitized cow by serum from a milk-allergic cow. Subsequent studies indicated that the allergen that caused this allergy was α-casein. As Campbell noted, the best way to manage this condition was to establish a milking routine to ensure that milk was never allowed to engorge the udder, preventing an excessive increase in intramammary pressure.

Parasite "Self-Cure"

Large multicellular helminth parasites effectively promote type 2 immune responses. Animals infested with gastrointestinal helminths have elevated serum IgE levels (see Table 2.1). In species such as sheep, these may increase more than 10-fold. In calves, the response is more complex, with animals with light infestations having high IgE levels and those with heavy worm burdens having only moderate increases in IgE. (It is unclear whether the high IgE levels are responsible for the lighter infestations.) There is also a seasonal correlation of IgE levels in calves related to worm burden and parasite developmental stage. Calves exposed during December–February had no detectable IgE response, whereas calves exposed during late spring and summer had the greatest responses. While embedded in the intestinal and abomasal mucosa, worms secrete and excrete multiple antigens that can trigger IgA and IgE responses. IgA is associated with some resistance to parasites because it can reduce worm size and fecundity. However, IgE responses are more important because they play a major role in controlling adult worm populations. This is most evident in the "self-cure" reaction in lambs infected with gastrointestinal nematodes, especially *Haemonchus contortus, Nematodirus* species, *Ostertagia circumcincta*, and *Trichostrongylus colubriformis*.

"Self-cure" is an immediate, histamine-mediated, hypersensitivity reaction that acts on the abomasal and intestinal smooth muscles to increase their tone and motility, causing adult worms to detach from the gut wall and be expelled. The process requires a coordinated response by multiple cell types under the control of T cell-derived cytokines at the time of larval exsheathment. These cells collectively trigger a response that results in mast cell degranulation, acute inflammation in the intestinal wall, and expulsion of the parasites (Fig. 11.6).

The presence of adult worms and their excretory and secretory products in the intestinal wall can trigger PRRs. Some helminth products can activate TLRs, and the mannose receptor is known to bind the excretory/secretory proteins of *Trichuris muris*. If the worms cause tissue damage, this will also trigger the release of the three Th2-stimulating alarmins, TSLP, IL-25, and IL-33, from enterocytes and tuft cells. TSLP activates DC2. IL-25 also stimulates the production of type 2 cytokines by ILC2 cells and facilitates the differentiation of Th2 cells. IL-33 acts on Th2 cells, ILC2 cells, basophils, and mast cells to drive IL-4, IL-5, and IL-13 production. In response to these stimuli, T cells release their own effector cytokines. For example, γ/δ T cells in the intestinal epithelium produce IL-4 and IL-25. Similarly, Th2 cells produce more IL-4 in a positive feedback loop, generating other Th2 cytokines and IL-25. IL-4 causes further differentiation into Th2 cells and suppresses Th1 responses. IL-6 acts with TGF-β to induce Th17 responses. IL-13 promotes goblet cell hyperplasia, enhances mucus production, and together with IL-9, recruits and activates MMC. IL-4 and IL-13 both activate enterocytes, smooth muscle cells, and macrophages. These cytokines also increase intestinal permeability and fluid secretion. Th2 cytokines stimulate Paneth cells and their consequent release of defensins may also damage helminths. The cytokines stimulate goblet cells to produce a resistin-like molecule that interferes with worm feeding. Mucins and other goblet cell products may also promote worm expulsion. IL-4, and IL-13, and IL-9 promote smooth muscle contractility.

Mast cell numbers increase in the intestinal submucosa during helminth infection. They may be activated directly by pathogen-associated molecular patterns via pattern recognition receptors, although it is unclear which parasitic pathogen-associated molecular patterns do this.

The combination of helminth allergens and mast cell-bound IgE triggers mast cell degranulation and the release of histamine, cytokines such as IL-13 and IL-33, chitinases, and proteases. These molecules stimulate vigorous smooth muscle contraction and increase vascular permeability. IL-13 promotes parasite expulsion by stimulating epithelial cell proliferation. Presumably, this rapid epithelial cell turnover acts as an "epithelial elevator" to assist in expelling the parasites.

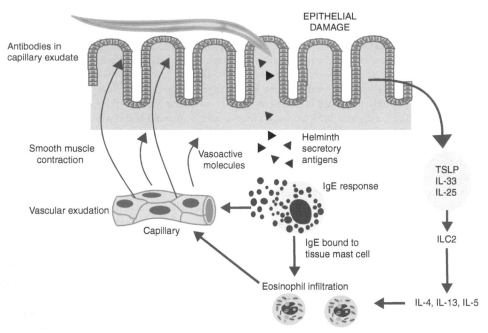

Fig. 11.6 Mechanisms involved in the "self-cure" reaction against intestinal helminths. The animal mounts an IgE-mediated allergic response to the salivary and excretory allergens of attached nematodes. Acute local inflammation and the changes in gut motility cause the worms to detach from the intestinal wall and be expelled in the feces.

Specialized enteroendocrine cells in the intestine called enterochromaffin cells secrete serotonin. The serotonin functions as a neurotransmitter and hormone that among other functions acts on enteric neurons to control gut motility, epithelial secretion, and peristalsis. IL-33 acts directly on enterochromaffin cells via its ST2 receptor and induces them to secrete increased amounts of serotonin, thus increasing gut motility and resulting in worm expulsion.

Mast cell proteases can degrade tight junctions between intestinal epithelial cells, which allow fluid efflux into the intestine and enable intact proteins to penetrate the gut wall and interact with allergen processing cells. Some mast cell products may be directly toxic to helminths. Tissue edema can inhibit parasite attachment. Increased permeability, epithelial cell proliferation, smooth muscle contraction, and mucus production all contribute to worm disengagement, leading to expulsion. This expulsion is accompanied by mucosal mast cell infiltration, intestinal eosinophilia, elevated serum IgE, and elevated parasite-specific IgG1 levels.

Contractions of the intestinal muscles caused by histamine and an increase in the permeability of intestinal capillaries cause an efflux of fluid into the intestinal lumen, resulting in dislodgment and expulsion of many worms. (This has been characterized as "weep and sweep.") In sheep that have just undergone self-cure, IgE antibody levels are high and experimental administration of helminth allergens at this time can cause acute anaphylaxis (Chapter 8). A similar reaction is seen in fascioliasis in calves, where peak IgE antibody titers coincide with expulsion of the parasite.

Suggested Readings

Berin MC. Pathogenesis of IgE-mediated food allergy. *Clin Exp Allergy*. 2015;45(10):1483-1496.

Bexley J, Nuttall TJ, Hammerberg B, Halliwell RE. Co-sensitization and cross-reactivity between related and unrelated food allergens in dogs – a serological study. *Vet Dermatol*. 2017;28(1):31-e7.

Bryce PJ. Balancing tolerance or allergy to food proteins. *Trends Immunol*. 2016;37(10):659-667.

Bunyavanich S, Berin MC. Food allergy and the microbiome: current understanding and future directions. *J Allergy Clin Immunol*. 2019;144(6):1468-1477.

Campbell SG. Milk allergy, an autoallergic disease of cattle. *Cornell Vet*. 1970;60(4):684-721.

Connors L, O'Keefe A, Rosenfeld L, Kim H. Non-IgE-mediated food allergy. *Allergy Asthma Clin Immunol*. 2018;14(Suppl 2)(suppl 2):56-64.

Craig JM. Atopic dermatitis and the intestinal microbiota in humans and dogs. *Vet Med Sci*. 2016;2(2):95-105.

Craig JM. Food intolerance in dogs and cats. *J Small Anim Pract*. 2019;60(2):77-85.

Delgado C, Lee-Fowler TM, DeClue AE, Reinero CR. Feline-specific serum total IgE quantitation in normal, asthmatic and parasitized cats. *J Feline Med Surg*. 2010;12(12):991-994.

Feng T, Elson CO, Cong Y. Treg cell-IgA axis in maintenance of host homeostasis with microbiota. *Int Immunopharmacol*. 2011;11(5):589-592. doi:10.1016/j.intimp.2010.11.016.

Hodzic A, Mateos-Hernandez L, Leschnik M, et al. Tick bites induce anti-α-gal antibodies in dogs. *Vaccines (Basel)*. 2019;7(3):114-130.

Johnston LK, Chien KB, Bryce PJ. The immunology of food allergy. *J Immunol*. 2014;192(6):2529-2534.

Klug C, Hemmer W, Roman-Carrasco P, et al. Gal d 7 – a major allergen in primary chicken meat allergy. *J Allergy Clin Immunol*. 2020;146(1):169-179.

Leyva-Castillo JM, Galand C, Kam C, et al. Mechanical skin injury promotes food anaphylaxis by driving intestinal mast cell expansion. *Immunity*. 2019;50(5):1262-1275.

Lowrie M, Hadjivassiliou M, Sanders DS, Garden OA. A presumptive case of gluten sensitivity in a Border terrier: a multisystem disorder? *Vet Rec*. 2016;179(22):573. doi:10.1136/vr.103910.

Matsui S, Kataoka H, Tanaka JI, et al. Dysregulation of intestinal microbiota elicited by food allergy induces IgA oral dysbiosis. *Infect Immun*. 2020;88:e00741-19. doi:10.1128/IAI.00741-19

Oriel RC, Wang J. Diagnosis and management of food allergy. *Pediatr Clin North Am*. 2019;66(5):941-954.

Platts-Mills TAE, Commins SP, Biedermann T, et al. On the cause and consequences of IgE to galactose-alpha-1,3-galactose: a report from the National Institute of Allergy and Infectious Diseases workshop on understanding IgE-mediated meat Allergy. *J Allergy Clin Immunol*. 2020;145(4):1061-1071.

Plunkett CH, Nagler CR. The influence of the microbiome on allergic sensitization to food. *J Immunol*. 2017;198(2):581-589.

Rupa P, Schmied WBN, BN Wilkie. Porcine allergy and IgE. *Vet Immunol Immunopathol*. 2009;132(1):41-45.

Sampson HA, O'Mahony L, Burks W, Plaut M, Lack G, Akdis CA. Mechanisms of food allergy. *J Allergy Clin Immunol*. 2018;141(1):11-19.

Shaw RJ, McNeill MM, Gatehouse TK, Douch PG. Quantitation of total sheep IgE concentration using anti-ovine IgE monoclonal antibodies in an enzyme immunoassay. *Vet Immunol Immunopathol*. 1997; 57(3-4):253-265.

Suto A, Suto Y, Onohara N, et al. Food allergens inducing a lymphocyte-mediated immunological reaction in canine atopic-like dermatitis. *J Vet Med Sci*. 2015;77(2):251-254.

Thatcher EF, Gershwin LJ, Baker NF. Levels of serum IgE in response to gastrointestinal nematodes in cattle. *Vet Parasitol*. 1989;32(2-3):153-161.

Verlinden A, Hesta M, Millet S, Janssens GP. Food allergy in dogs and cats: a review. *Crit Rev Food Sci Nutr*. 2006;46(3):259-773. doi:10.1080/10408390591001117.

Whibley N, Tucci A, Powrie F. Regulatory T cell adaptation in the intestine and skin. *Nat Immunol*. 2019;20(4):386-396.

Wilson JM, Platts-Mills TA. Meat allergy and allergens. *Mol Immunol*. 2018;100:107-112.

A series of nine papers entitled *Crit Appraised Top Adverse Food React Companion Anim* was published in BMC Veterinary Research between August 2015 and May, 2020: 2015 11:225; 2016 12:9; 2017 13:51; 2017 13:275; 2018 14:244; 2018 14:341; 2019 15:140; 2020 16:158.

CHAPTER 12

Allergies to Arthropods

Allergies are commonly associated with exposure to arthropods and their associated allergens. For example, there are numerous examples of humans developing severe anaphylactic shock in response to insect envenomation or ant bites. Anaphylaxis can also occur in cattle infested with the warble fly (*Hypoderma bovis*) if their subcutaneous pupae rupture and the animal reacts to the released coelomic fluid. In the 1960s, 40% of allergic patients living in New York City were sensitized to cockroach allergens, as shown by skin testing and serum immunoglobulin E (IgE) measurements.

In general, arthropod allergens enter the animal body in three ways. First, salivary allergens may be injected by biting insects such as fleas, mosquitos, and midges. There are many proteins in their saliva that can sensitize animals and result in the development of pruritic dermatitis. Second, arthropod allergens may be injected by stinging insects. Thus, wasp and bee venoms can induce severe allergic reactions, including anaphylaxis. Third, arthropod allergens may be dispersed in dust and inhaled, which occurs with the fecal material of house dust mites (HDMs). These aeroallergens may also be absorbed through skin contact. Mite allergens can cause severe skin or respiratory allergic responses.

Two major types of immune responses occur following exposure to arthropod allergens. One is an IgE-mediated immediate reaction—a typical pruritic allergic response classified as a type I hypersensitivity. The other is a slowly developing reaction that is mainly T cell-mediated and is classified as a type IV hypersensitivity.

Chitin Responses

Chitin, an N-acetyl-D-glucosamine polymer cross-linked by β-(1-4)-glycosidic bonds, is a major structural component of fungal cell walls and the exoskeletons and fecal pellets of arthropods. It is the second most abundant polysaccharide in nature after cellulose. Its extensive cross-linking makes chitin incredibly stable. Mammals cannot synthesize chitin; however, they produce many chitinases and chitin-binding proteins. (Chitinases are chitin-degrading enzymes expressed by epithelial cells and macrophages.)

Chitin is too inert to be directly allergenic; however, it is a very effective pathogen-associated molecular pattern and acts as a potent trigger of type 2 responses (Fig. 12.1). Therefore, it plays a key role in the induction of arthropod-associated inflammatory and allergic diseases. For example, small chitin particles, 1–10 μm in diameter, are readily phagocytosed by macrophages and stimulates them to produce cytokines such as interleukin 12 (IL-12) and tumor necrosis factor-α. Chitin stimulates NK cells to produce gamma interferon. Larger chitin particles can trigger type 2 innate lymphoid cells to release IL-5 and IL-13, resulting in an eosinophilic response in the absence of type 2 helper (Th2) cell activation. Additionally, chitin can act as an adjuvant when administered with an allergen such as ovalbumin. When this mixture is inhaled, it enhances Th2 responses and eosinophilic airway inflammation. The pattern recognition receptors, toll-like receptor 2 (TLR2) and dectin-1, and lung chitinases are required to produce this effect. Chitin also enhances IL-13-induced IL-33 production by dendritic cells (DC2s) in the lung. Chitin particles also activate $\gamma\delta$ T cells and promote local type 17 responses.

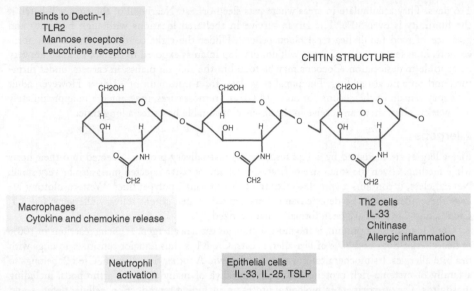

Fig. 12.1 Structure of chitin and the ways by which it can influence type 2 immune responses in animals.

FLEA ALLERGIES

Flea infestations are responsible for the most common allergy of all, flea allergy dermatitis (FAD). There is no breed or gender predisposition to this; however, atopic animals and those exposed to fleas on an intermittent basis experience a more severe disease. Pruritus is a consistent feature. In addition to their characteristic clinical signs, affected animals will react positively to intradermally injected flea allergen. Most sensitive animals will respond within a few minutes; however, up to 30% may also develop a delayed reaction at 24–48 h. Hyposensitization therapy has not been shown to be successful in treating flea allergy. It can only be successfully treated by total flea control.

Biology

Several different species of flea are found on domestic pets in the United States. These include *Ctenocephalides canis, Pulex simulans,* and *Echidnophaga gallinacea.* However, the species that accounts for over 90% of flea allergy cases is the cat flea, *C. felis felis.* There are four subspecies of *C. felis,* all of which parasitize carnivores. Three of the subspecies are restricted to parts of Africa and Asia. However, *C. felis felis* is found worldwide and is the only subspecies to occur in North America. In addition to being responsible for canine and feline dermatitis, the cat flea can spread endemic typhus and serve as an intermediate host for parasites such as the tapeworm *Hymenolepis nana.*

Adult fleas rely on visual and thermal cues to find their hosts. Newly emerged flea larvae will climb plants or move to the top of the carpet pile, where they wait until they encounter a host animal. Once they attach to a host, they feed almost immediately. A blood meal is required for a flea to begin reproducing. Mating occurs after the fleas have fed and egg laying can begin within 48 h after the meal. Fleas lay a lot of eggs, ~40–50 daily at peak production, with an average of 27 eggs daily for 50 days.

Flea eggs are white and about 0.5 mm in length. They readily fall on the floor, into carpets and cushions, or on the ground. Depending on humidity and temperature, they will hatch in

1–6 days. They accumulate in areas where pets sleep or rest. Nearly all of the eggs will hatch if the humidity is over 50%. The larvae survive in sheltered locations with high humidity and a source of food (adult flea fecal blood pellets). Under the right conditions, larvae may form cocoons in as few as 8 days. Larvae will not develop in areas exposed to the hot sun and are very susceptible to desiccation. Cocoons may be found in the soil, on plants, in carpets, under furniture, and on animal bedding. The pupal stage lasts for a minimum of 13 days. However, adult fleas may remain in the cocoon for up to 140 days. In most cases, they emerge in approximately 3–5 weeks. Thus, they can survive in the absence of suitable hosts for a long time.

Allergens

Flea allergies are mediated by a Th2 response against salivary proteins injected into their hosts while feeding. Given the small size of fleas, the volume of saliva injected must also be very small. Nevertheless, it contains a complex mixture of diverse small polypeptides. Western blotting allows these allergens to be detected and characterized. Three potent salivary allergens, Cte f 1, Cte f 2, and Cte f 3, have been formally characterized.*

Cte f 1, an 18 kDa protein, is the most significant cat flea allergen. It elicits reactions in 100% of flea-allergic dogs and 80% of flea-allergic cats. Cte f 1 is thus a major sensitizer in dogs with flea bite allergies. Its biochemical function is unknown. Another flea allergen, Cte f 2, belongs to a family of cysteine-rich proteins found in the saliva of many different arthropods, including mosquitos. They participate in biological processes, including reproduction, cellular defense, and immune evasion. There are numerous other flea salivary proteins with molecular weights ranging from 14 to 62 kDa that have also been identified as allergens but have yet to be characterized. There are also low molecular weight components (<500 Da) in flea saliva that may act as haptens if they bind to skin proteins such as collagen and induce delayed T cell responses. In addition to saliva, other allergenic components derived from fleas include shedding exoskeletons, molting enzymes, and fecal pellets.

Epidemiology

Although adult fleas feed on domestic pets, more than 95% of their life-cycle is spent off the host. Thus eggs, larvae, and pupae may be found in large numbers in the local environment. Simply eliminating adult fleas on the host is inadequate for breaking the flea life-cycle. In addition, grooming efficiency differs greatly between individual animals, especially cats; therefore, the adult flea burden and FAD severity may vary, even within the same household.

Clinical Disease

FAD is the most common dermatological disease of dogs and cats in endemic areas. Dogs may develop FAD in combination with atopic dermatitis (AD); dogs affected with AD are almost four times as likely to suffer from FAD than non-affected dogs. Reflecting the Th2 response to flea allergens, susceptible animals develop an eczematous pruritic skin disease. The intense pruritis results in self-mutilation from persistent licking, scratching, or chewing of the affected areas. Animals develop erythema, papules, and pustules that will often crust. The self-inflicted damage may result in secondary bacterial or fungal infections. In chronic infestations, animals may develop disfiguring hyperpigmented and thickened skin. Flea allergy lesions are restricted to the neck, pinnae, lower back, tail base, and the backs of the legs and ventral abdomen (Figs 12.2 and 12.3). This differs from typical AD lesions that are restricted to areas with thinner skin (see Fig. 9.7). Following repeated exposure to flea saliva, dogs develop an allergic response that occurs in two

---

*Allergens are named according to a standard procedure. This consists of the first three letters of the genus and the first letter of the species of origin. They are then numbered in the order of their discovery.

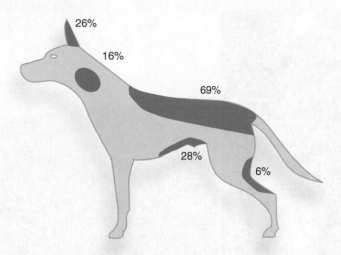

Fig. 12.2 **Characteristic distribution of lesions in dogs with flea bite allergy.** Compare this with Fig. 9.7, which shows the typical distribution of atopic dermatitis lesions. (Data from Bruet V, Bourdeau PJ, Roussel A, Imparato L, Desfontis J-C. Characterization of pruritus in canine atopic dermatitis, flea bite hypersensitivity, and flea infestation and its role in diagnosis. *Vet Dermatol* 2012; 23:487-e93).

phases. An immediate response occurs within the first 15 minutes and a delayed cell-mediated response peaks 14–48 h later.

Dogs chronically infested by fleas may eventually become desensitized, resulting in clinical improvement. Continual exposure of young animals to fleas at an early age also appears to cause desensitization. Conversely, intermittent flea exposure causes the most severe skin responses, whereas continually exposed dogs develop a milder disease and may have low or undetectable levels of flea-specific IgG and IgE in their serum. In some situations, an allergic response may result from inhalation of flea allergens, presumably those found in dried airborne feces. Fleas feed on blood; therefore, if there are enough of them biting for an adequate period, the infested animals may become anemic, especially if they are iron deficient.

FAD is not uncommon in cats and causes miliary dermatitis, alopecia, excoriation, and eosinophilic plaque development. Some cats develop indolent lip ulcers. However, even in a flea-rich environment, only a small fraction of cats become hypersensitive. Given that cat grooming behavior is very effective and cats may actually ingest fleas, it has been speculated that this low level of hypersensitivity might be due to oral tolerance.

Diagnosis

FAD diagnosis is based on history, clinical signs, the presence of fleas and flea "dirt," and the appropriate response to anti-flea treatment. (The flea "dirt" is rich in blood. Thus, if placed in water, it will dissolve into a red paste.) However, the clinical signs of FAD can match many other causes of pruritic dermatitis and may be masked by grooming.

Therefore, reliable allergy tests are required to confirm the diagnosis. However, these may present problems because not all flea-infested dogs mount an IgE response to flea allergens. Likewise, the presence of a flea infestation does not exclude the possibility of other causes of AD. Intradermal skin testing is an obvious approach; however, this may be difficult to interpret, especially in cats. Cats do not generate well-defined wheals and erythema. Another problem is that about a third of healthy, normal cats may respond positively to intradermal testing, and this testing may effectively boost their allergic response. One other problem encountered in serologic and

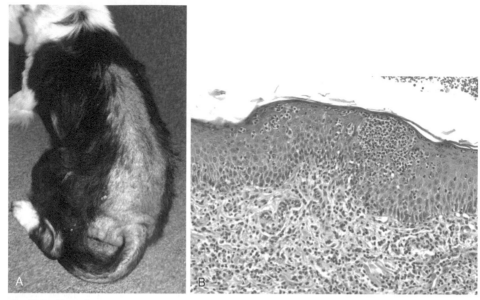

Fig. 12.3 Flea allergy dermatitis. (A) Severe lumbar and tail head dermatitis in a flea-allergic dog. (B) A Section of skin showing the pathology associated with flea bite allergy with superficial dermal inflammation and eosinophilic pustules in the epidermis. [(A) From Medleau L, Hnilica KA. *Small animal dermatology*, 2nd ed. Saunders, 2006; (B) Courtesy of Dr. Aline Rodrigues-Hoffman and Dr. Dominique Wiener.]

intradermal testing is the non-standardized nature of flea allergen extracts. Thus, crude whole flea extracts may contain very little of the relevant salivary allergens. Serologic testing involving a FcεRIα-based assay using purified flea saliva produces the most reliable results (Chapter 20).

Treatment and Control

The two goals of treatment are to eliminate fleas and relieve the discomfort of the animal. Oral or topical flea prevention medication will generally eliminate adult fleas, but there must be environmental flea control also. It is not sufficient to target the adult fleas only but also the eggs and larvae, otherwise they will serve as a source of new adults and the problem will recur. All the other animals in a household and the house and yard must be treated. Thus, vacuuming, treatment of pet bedding by washing in hot water, and drying (over 60°C) is required. There is a great diversity of flea control medications available. Those that target adult fleas such as fipronil, imidacloprid, and selamectin may be administered topically by dropping the fluid on the animal's skin or as a daily or monthly pill. In addition, it is essential to break the flea life-cycle. Because of the length of each of the free-living flea life stages, it is important to persist with treatments rather than simply seek long-term adult control. Juvenile hormone analogs such as methoprene and pyriproxyfen disrupt the flea life-cycle. Lufenuron and cyromazine interfere with the synthesis of chitin and disrupt flea growth. Systemic isoxazolines are especially effective because they kill adult fleas only after they bite an animal but do this rapidly before egg laying begins. Matrix-impregnated vinyl or polyurethane flea collars have been widely employed and are useful in situations where flea infestations are heavy. They may have the added benefit of also killing ticks. Thus, collars may contain both imidaclopid for flea control and flumethrin for ticks. They remain effective for up to 8 months, although it may be difficult to tell when they are no longer effective. Allergen-specific immunotherapy for flea allergies is ineffective (Chapter 16).

BITING FLY ALLERGIES

Bloodsucking insects such as mosquitos, black flies, horseflies, and midges are important causes of allergic diseases in horses, sheep, and cattle. Hypersensitivity to insect bites may cause an allergic dermatitis variously called, according to geographical location, Gulf Coast itch, summer eczema, Queensland itch, or sweet itch. The insects involved include midges (*Culicoides* species), black flies (*Simulium* species), stable flies (*Stomoxys* and *Haematobia*), mosquitos, and stick-tight fleas (*E. gallinacea*). (Some of these species are incriminated because their saliva triggers a positive response in an intradermal skin test, but this may simply be cross-reactivity.) Insect bite hypersensitivity (IBH) is a common pruritic dermatitis primarily caused by types 1 and IV hypersensitivity reactions to allergens in *Culicoides* saliva.

Biology

Culicoides are very small, blood-feeding midges, approximately 1–3 mm in length (Fig. 12.4). (This is about the same size as a cat flea.) As in mosquitos, only the females feed on blood. *Culicoides* midges are smaller than mosquitos, but much more abundant. Similar to mosquitos, they breed in standing water, including salt marshes, ponds, lakes, and even wet manure. They are not strong fliers, so they do not fly long distances and cannot fly against the wind. They prefer still, warm nights, and fly at dawn and dusk when large swarms may be seen. While globally widespread, local environmental conditions affect their prevalence and behavior. There are multiple culicoides species and subspecies found worldwide. *C. obsoletus* is the most common species affecting horses in North America and Europe. *C. nubeculosis* is found in Europe. *C. variipennis* is found in North America. All three of these species can act as vectors for diseases such as bluetongue. Because of their diversity, it is not uncommon for more than one species of *Culicoides* to feed on a single horse. They do not suck blood like mosquitos; they bite. These bites are painful and very annoying. Depending on the species, the lesions may be generalized or mainly ventral. IBH is a multifactorial disease influenced by genetic and local environmental factors. It occurs more frequently in some horse families than in others and its severity is associated with some equine major histocompatibility complex genes. Its heritability

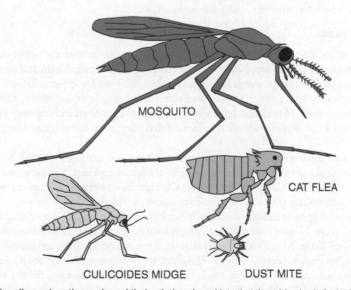

Fig. 12.4 **Major allergenic arthropods and their relative sizes.** Note that the midge is similar in size to the flea.

ranges from 0.08 to 0.30. Its proximal cause is a type 2 immune response to *Culicoides* salivary allergens.

Allergens

There is no evidence for the preexistence of a skin barrier defect in IBH-affected horses. The mouthparts of *Culicoides* midges can easily penetrate the skin barrier. Female midge mouthparts consist of two serrated blades that they push into the skin and cut with a backward stroke. They insert these blades either directly into a capillary or into a pool of extravasated blood. Simultaneously, they inject saliva that is both anticoagulant and vasodilatory and may even have anesthetic properties. Enzymes in the saliva break down epithelial tissue barriers. Some horses react to these injected foreign proteins by mounting antibody and cell-mediated immune responses. Therefore, *Culicoides* hypersensitivity may be a mixture of type I and IV reactions.

The severity of type I hypersensitivity is determined by Th2 cells and the balance between Th2 and regulatory T cell activity. At least 21 salivary allergens have been identified as being relevant to IBH. For example, the saliva of *C. nubeculosus* contains 11 characterized allergens, Cul n 1 to Cul n 11. Four salivary allergens from the blackfly *Simulium vittatum* (Sim v 1–4) are also bound by equine IgE; however, these may simply be from cross-reactions with *Culicoides*. In the Netherlands, the predominant *Culicoides* species is *C. obsoletus*. Of course, not all horses react to all allergens. Their reactivity ranges from 13% to 56%, depending on the allergen tested. On average, each horse reacted to four allergens (range 1–10). Cul n 1 and Sim v 1 share sequence homology with an allergenic protein in wasp venom, and Cul n 2 is a hyaluronidase related to a major allergen in bee venom. A mixture of *C. obsoletus* allergens used in the Netherlands in an ELISA assay had a sensitivity of 92% and a specificity of 85% compared to intradermal skin testing. In contrast, total IgE is not significantly increased in horses affected by IBH compared to healthy control animals.

Epidemiology

Culicoides hypersensitivity may or may not be seasonal depending on the prevalence of the midges. Clinical signs do not usually appear until a horse has reached 2–4 years of age and then gradually worsen. The lesions appear during the summer months when the flies are biting but may improve somewhat over the cooler winter months.

Clinical Disease

The severity of the lesions depends on the disease stage, the intensity of the pruritus, and degree of secondary infection. The initial lesions include many papules, tufted hair, and skin sensitivity (Fig. 12.5). As in flea allergy, intense pruritus is often followed by self-mutilation, resulting in excoriation, erosion, ulceration, hair loss, and skin thickening. In some horses, *Culicoides* bites cause the development of urticaria accompanied by intense pruritus. Itching may provoke self-mutilation with a subsequent secondary infection that may mask the original allergic nature of the lesion.

The preferred feeding sites of the insect are along the dorsal midline at the tail base, the withers, and the mane. Less commonly, they attack the head, ears, and legs. Similarly, some *Culicoides* species may cause ventral midline dermatitis. Chronic lesions result in alopecia with skin lichenification and scaling that may develop into transverse ridges.

The Culicoides hypersensitivity response is induced by a type I reaction mediated by Th2 cells and IgE production. Horses have a relatively high level of IgE in their blood. They average about 84.0 µg/mL (see Table 2.1). This is higher than in humans and has been attributed to the presence of endoparasites, especially worms. However, there is enormous variability in IgE levels between individual horses. Therefore, total serum IgE is not a useful assay for the confirmation of allergic disease. IgE$^+$ cells can be readily detected in biopsies from acute skin lesions. Some

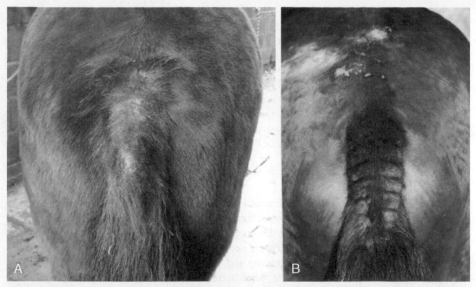

Fig. 12.5 Signs of insect bite hypersensitivity (IBH). (A) Localized hair loss and excoriations at the tail. (B) More severe form of IBH with lichenification of the skin, a "rat-tail," and affected areas on the croup. (From Schaffartzik A et al. Equine insect bite hypersensitivity: What do we know. *Vet Immunol Immunopathol*. 2012. 147: 115.)

evidence suggests that *Culicoides*-specific IgG3 and IgG5 are present in affected horses and may also contribute to disease pathogenesis. Key mediators of these IBH reactions are histamine, which may be largely responsible for pruritus, leukotrienes, platelet-activating factor, and IL-31. Infiltrating eosinophils and neutrophils also contribute to the development of itch. Histamine can be detected in the plasma of horses with acute lesions. Intradermal injection of platelet-activating factor results in the development of lesions similar to those induced by *Culicoides*. Experimentally, leukotrienes and histamine can be released from *Culicoides*-stimulated equine leukocytes. Thus, 78% of allergic horses and 3% of controls released leukotrienes after their leukocytes were exposed to *C. nubeculosus* allergens.

Measurement of IL-31 in skin punch biopsies of insect bite hypersensitive horses and allergen-stimulated mononuclear cells in vitro demonstrated its presence in significant amounts. Vaccination against equine IL-31 using the cytokine coupled to virus-like particles successfully induced autoantibodies against IL-31 and reduced the IBH severity lesion scores as determined by double-blind, placebo-controlled studies.

Several studies have detected a T cell-mediated delayed hypersensitivity response to injected allergens in IBH. However, results are inconsistent, and its possible significance remains unclear. Lesional skin of IBH-affected horses contains large numbers of CD4[+] T cells and few CD8[+] cells.

On histopathology, the lesions consist of a perivascular dermatitis and subepidermal edema. The cellular infiltrate consists of mononuclear cells; however, this is often associated with a perivascular or diffuse eosinophil infiltration, especially in acute cases. Tryptase-positive mast cells may accumulate at the dermoepidermal junction. Langerhans cells also accumulate here. Some horses may develop an eosinophilic folliculitis, epidermal pustules, or eosinophilic granulomas. Old lesions show epidermal hyperplasia, hyperkeratosis, lichenification, and dermal fibrosis.

As in so many allergic diseases, more than one allergic response may develop simultaneously in a single individual. For example, IBH may be accompanied by severe equine asthma syndrome (Chapter 13). In general, IBH development precedes the development of severe asthma in a manner reminiscent of the human "allergic march." The immunological challenge presented by IBH might redirect the immune system as a whole to alter its normal balance and move toward a Th2-biased state. Studies on horses with IBH have shown that their pO_2 is lower than normal horses even in the absence of overt respiratory disease. There is an association between IBH and equine asthma; however, this might not be IgE-mediated. Thus, horses affected by both IBH and asthma do not have higher IgE concentrations than horses affected by each condition alone. However, the measurement of IgE levels alone is of limited value because it does not take IgE specificity and affinity into account.

Diagnosis

Diagnosis of equine IBH is based on clinical signs, history/seasonality, lifestyle (pasture close to standing water), and absence of fly control. Skin testing using whole *Culicoides* extracts may be useful; however, even clinically healthy horses may give positive results in in vivo and in vitro testing. These crude, whole-body extracts are not standardized and the amount of salivary allergens in them may be minimal. False-positive and -negative results are common. IgE detection denotes exposure, not necessarily disease. Some horses may not have detectable IgE levels if they mount a cell-mediated, type IV hypersensitivity response.

Treatment and Control

Treatment involves avoidance. This is the only safe and effective method of prevention. There are many different fly repellent products available in the form of sprays, wipes, and spot-on products. These usually contain pyrethrins or permethrin. Piperonyl butoxide and perfumes such as citronella oil may also be added. Lightweight blankets are the easiest and most common protection methods. They should be put on prior to dusk and removed well after dawn. It is difficult to insect-proof stables. Reduction of the acute inflammation and pruritus through the use of topical or systemic steroids may make animals much more comfortable. Immunotherapy has yet to yield significant positive benefits, probably because only crude midge extracts are available.

MOSQUITO ALLERGIES

There are over 3000 different mosquito species worldwide. Allergic reactions to mosquito bites are of growing concern in humans. Members of many different genera can cause these reactions, especially *Aedes*, *Culex*, and *Anopheles*. Some of these reactions can be severe, including generalized urticaria and anaphylaxis. Allergic responses to mosquito bites may be mediated by IgE, IgG, or T cells.

Allergens

To feed, mosquitos first probe the skin to find a blood vessel. They make several attempts before they are successful. Then, they draw the blood from the opened blood vessel or the surrounding hematoma. As they probe and feed, female mosquitos inject saliva. Mosquito saliva consists of a complex mixture of at least 70 proteins. Many of these are anticoagulant, vasodilatory, and anti-inflammatory. Many are also highly allergenic. Some of these allergens are shared between mosquito species, while others are species specific. Their number and significance vary between species. When injected into sensitized animals, these will induce significant cellular infiltration and inflammation.

Epidemiology

Some cats are predisposed to developing allergic responses to mosquitos. Feline mosquito bite hypersensitivity shows significant regional and seasonal variation. It occurs in cats with outdoor access, especially at dawn and dusk. Cats of any age can be affected.

Clinical Disease

Feline mosquito hypersensitivity causes a pruritic dermatitis, usually located on the pinnae and bridge of the nose (Fig. 12.6). The lesions develop less commonly on the eyelids, lips, chin, or skin around the nipples and footpads. The response results in the development of erythematous papules that undergo ulceration and crusting. These lesions are very pruritic. Alopecia, depigmentation, edema, and lymphadenopathy may develop. In severe cases, fever and an eosinophilia may also occur. The lesions consist of a perivascular and interstitial eosinophilic dermatitis with furunculosis and folliculitis.

Canine eosinophilic furunculosis is a rapidly developing skin disease that resembles feline mosquito bite allergy. The lesions, nodules, ulceration, and crusting are usually confined to the face, especially the nose and muzzle. It may be intensely pruritic. A skin biopsy shows acute inflammation accompanied by a marked eosinophilic infiltration. It is believed to be an acute hypersensitivity response to biting or stinging arthropods encountered by curious dogs.

Diagnosis

Other causes of eosinophilic dermatitis, including pemphigus, AD, flea bite sensitivity, dermatophytosis, and mange, must be excluded. Intradermal skin testing is of limited usefulness in cats because of the elasticity of their skin.

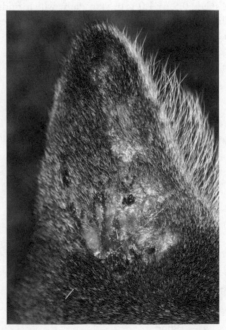

Fig. 12.6 Mosquito bite hypersensitivity in a cat. Note the alopecia and crusts on the ear pinna. (From Medleau L, Hnilica KA. *Small Animal Dermatology*, 2nd ed. Saunders; 2006.)

Treatment and control

Treatment consists of keeping cats indoors, especially during the early morning and late evening when mosquitos are present. Systemic glucocorticoid therapy may be required. Some mosquito repellants are toxic for cats and should be avoided.

Inhalant Allergies

HOUSE DUST MITE (HDM) ALLERGIES

HDMs are a major cause of atopic sensitization and allergic disease in humans and their pets. HDM hypersensitivity rates have been reported to range from 20% to 100% in dogs.

Biology

HDM are eight-legged arachnids of the family Pyroglyphidae. The most important of these are *Dermatophagoides pteronyssinus* (the European HDM) and *D. fariniae* (the American HDM). Both are translucent and pale amber in color, and globular in shape, with a striated cuticle (Fig. 12.7). (Despite their common names, both species are found on both continents.) They occur worldwide but prefer regions of high humidity. Adult mites are 0.2–0.3 mm long and barely visible to the naked eye. However, they are easily seen under a low power light microscope. Dust mite allergens have been detected in approximately 85% of US homes and about 68% of European homes. Unlike scabies or demodex mites, HDMs are not parasitic and do not burrow into the skin. Other important dust mite species include *Euroglyphus maynei* and *Blomia tropicalis*. The latter is a major source of mite allergen in tropical environments. *D. pteronyssinus* and *D. fariniae* are found throughout the United States, whereas *B. tropicalis* and *E. maynei* are restricted to the southern states (Box 12.1).

The average human sheds 0.5 to 1.0 g of skin daily, which finds its way into upholstered furniture, carpets, bedding, and stuffed toys. HDMs feed on this desquamated skin and some molds, and thus enjoy a high-keratin diet.

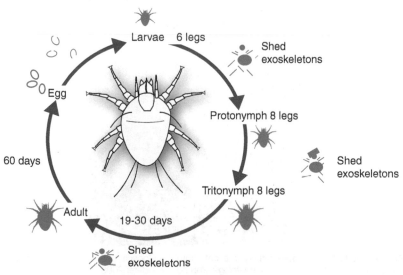

Fig.12.7 House dust mite and its life-cycle.

> ### BOX 12.1 ■ Sarcoptic Mange
>
> Sarcoptic mange is an intensely pruritic inflammatory skin disease caused by the burrowing mite *Sarcoptes scabei*. As with other arthropods, the skin response shows features of types I and IV hypersensitivity. Similar to other parasitic arthropods, *S. scabei* can trigger a type 2 immune response and generate specific IgE and IgG antibodies to the major scabies allergens. Among these major allergens are the muscle proteins tropomyosin (Sar s 10) and paramyosin (Sar s 11). In general, these invertebrate muscle proteins are conserved across multiple species. Thus, *Sarcoptes* muscle allergens cross-react with tropomyosin and paramyosin from HDMs. However, these immune responses to scabies mites are ineffective in controlling infestations.
>
> ---
>
> Bhat SA, Mounsey KE, Liu X, Walton SF. Host immune responses to the itch mite, *Sarcoptes scabei*, in humans. *Parasit Vectors.* 2017; 10:385. doi:10.1186/s13071-017-2320-4

Dust mites have a life-span of 65–100 days. They go through several life stages, including egg, larva, two nymphal stages, and an active adult stage (Fig. 12.7). They take 19–30 days to complete their life-cycle, depending on temperature and humidity. Mated females live for approximately 60 days. A female mite can lay 60–100 eggs over 5 weeks. As they go from one life stage to another, the mites shed their exoskeletons, which serve as major sources of chitin and mite allergens.

HDMs thrive at temperatures around 24°C. They dehydrate below 50% humidity and eventually die; therefore, they are critically dependent on ambient water vapor to survive. They prefer humidity of 70%–80% and are comfortable in most Western homes. Mites will survive home refrigeration but will die in home freezers at −17°C. Eggs can only be killed by deep freezing at −70°C.

Allergens

More than 80% of mite allergens are found on particles >10 μm in size and are undetectable in the air of undisturbed rooms. They only become airborne after disturbances of the soft furnishings where mites thrive. In addition to aeroallergens stimulating type 2 responses, many mite components bind and activate pattern recognition receptors. These include chitin and mite DNA, bacterial DNA, and endotoxin. Most exposure occurs during the day when persons and their pets are moving around. Animals inhale mite-derived particles where they settle in the nose and throat.

Mite Feces. Each mite will produce approximately 1000 fecal pellets and partially digested fecal particles. Each fecal pellet is surrounded by a peritrophic membrane that contains proteases. These enzymes continue to digest the fecal material so that the mites can indulge in coprophagia. More importantly, the peritrophic membrane is a source of potent allergens. Living on a keratin-rich diet, the mite gut must contain proteases. These are shed in the fecal pellets and act as major allergens. When mites die, their body parts and debris serve as allergens. A total of 28 allergens have been characterized in *D. fariniae*. These are named Der f 1–33 (several are missing) and 20 for *D. pteronyssinus*, 14 for *B. tropicalis*, and 5 for *E. maynei*. Humans and dogs do not typically produce IgE against all of these.

The most potent HDM allergens in humans are the cysteine proteases Der p 1 and Der f 1 (Fig. 12.8). Other allergens such as Der p 3, p 6, and p 9 are serine proteases. All are very effective in degrading keratins. Therefore, these allergens have direct effects on epithelial surfaces. They break tight junctions between cells, and can disrupt the epithelial barrier. They can penetrate as far as the dermis and bind to dendritic cells. They can act directly on mast cells and basophils via protease-activated receptors such as MRGPRB to cause IL-4 release. They can inhibit Th1 responses by destroying the IL-2 receptor. Thus, they preferentially stimulate type 2 responses. In addition, they activate protease-activated receptor-2 (PAR₂) on keratinocytes and dermal nerves,

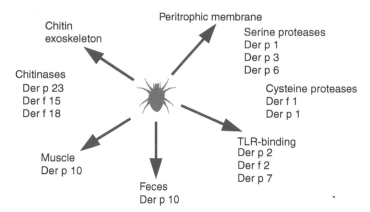

Fig. 12.8 Major house dust mite allergens.

and trigger pruritus. PAR_2 interacts with TLR4 to stimulate the release of IL-33 and thymic stromal lymphopoietin. Der p 1 also cleaves IL-33 into active peptides and enhances its activity. This can also delay the healing and recovery of skin epithelial barrier function. In cases of atopic asthma, the inhaled enzymes activate protease-activated receptors in the bronchial epithelium, causing the release of cysteinyl leukotrienes and hypertrophy of bronchial smooth muscle.

A second group of mite allergens such as Der f 2 and Der p 2 has sequence homology with MD2, a ligand for TLR4, the lipopolysaccharide-binding toll-like receptor. These enhance the effects of bacterial endotoxins on lesion development and directly activate human B cells. These group 2 allergens are important in humans; however, their significance in dogs is unclear. They are minor allergens in European and American dogs but are much more important in Japanese dogs.

Der p 10 is a muscle allergen and cross-reacts with other invertebrate tissues such as those from shrimp. Der p 11 is present in dust mite bodies and is a significant allergen in human AD.

In contrast to humans, the primary allergens that sensitize dogs are the high molecular weight molecules, Der f 15 chitinase and Der f 18, a chitin-binding protein. While found in the mite gut, they are not present in mite feces. Another major Der f allergen is Zen-1. (This is the provisional designation of a novel protein of 188 kDa.) IgE seropositivity against this allergen has been reported to be as high as 85% in atopic HDM dogs.

Chitin in mite exoskeletons triggers innate immunity via pattern recognition receptors, including TLR2 and C-type lectins and contributes to these Th2 responses. Der p 23 is a chitinase and a major allergen.

Epidemiology

In a study of California horses, 34 of 44 horses (77%) tested positive by intradermal skin testing to *D. fariniae*. This sensitization level is similar to that seen in dogs in the same region. Therefore, HDMs may also be prevalent in stables or barns, and are present in horse rugs. It is possible that cross-reactions may occur between mites and other arthropods, and storage mites are likely to be present in stored horse feed.

Clinical Disease

Contact of dust mite particles with epithelial surfaces in the eyes, nose, airways, skin, and intestine can induce sensitization and allergic responses. When fecal particles contact a moist epithelial surface, such as when inhaled, the pellets fall apart, releasing proteases. House dust mites (HDMs) are the most common trigger of non-seasonal allergies and asthma in humans and pets.

In humans, mite sensitization and exposure result in rhinitis, sinusitis, conjunctivitis, asthma, and AD. In dogs, these allergies are expressed as AD accompanied by pruritus, recurrent otitis, and seborrhea. The ingestion of food contaminated by house mite antigen (Der p 1) may result in a chronic enteropathy in dogs. Cats may develop eosinophilic granulomas, pruritus, chin acne, recurrent otitis, and plasma cell pododermatitis.

Diagnosis

In intradermal skin testing, 30%–80% of atopic dogs and cats may test positive to dust mite extracts. Cross-reactions occur between mite and other arthropod allergens, including fleas, black ants, black flies, and cockroach allergens. Diagnosis requires the exclusion of other allergies such as food and flea allergies. Concomitant *Toxocara* infestation might increase the sensitization to Der f allergens in dogs, although such dogs have lower skin lesion scores. These allergies will also respond positively to glucocorticosteroid treatment, and immunotherapy may have beneficial effects.

Treatment and Control

Allermune HDM (Nippon Zenyaku Koygo–Zenoaq: Fukushima, Japan) is an immunotherapy formulation that contains high doses of recombinant Der f 2 conjugated with polymers of the maltose pullulan. Administration is claimed to lead to rapid improvement in the pruritus and skin lesions associated with HDM sensitivity.

Dust Mite Control. While complete dust mite elimination may not be possible, their numbers may be reduced by aggressive cleaning. Dust mites prefer a warm, dark, humid environment. They thrive in mattresses, bedding, upholstered furniture, and carpets. Given how skin squames are shed in bed, it is expected that the population of mites will be greatest in bedrooms and on the floor around beds. They are especially fond of old mattresses. Therefore, mattresses and pillows should be covered in zippered, dust- and mite-proof covers. These can exclude both mites and their feces. Plastic or vinyl mattress covers may also help. They may be marketed as "allergen impermeable." Sheets and blankets should be washed weekly in water hotter than 130°F. It makes sense to do exactly the same with pet sleeping material. Subsequent hot tumble drying for at least 20 minutes will help finish the job. Vacuuming is usually insufficient to get rid of all mites and their waste. However, it should be performed regularly to reduce dust levels. For example, many mites may live deep within the stuffing of pillows, mattresses, and pile carpeting. Keeping the humidity below 50%, using a dehumidifier or air conditioner, also helps considerably. Animals should be groomed regularly to minimize shedding.

Storage Mite Allergies

Storage mites are another significant source of aeroallergens. Storage mites live in dry food items such as hay, flour, grains, dried fruits, and cereals. Three species, *Tyrophagus putrescentiae*, *Lepidoglyphus destructor*, and *Acarus siro*, thrive in environments with high humidity or moisture. They may be found in bags of dry dog and cat food, especially those rich in protein and fat. Dry pet food contains about 10% moisture, which is enough to permit storage mite contamination, especially if stored under suboptimal conditions. Storage mites can also live in association with HDMs and can be detected in similar dark, humid habitats. Dogs exposed to storage mites such as *A. siro* through the ingestion of infested food, inhalation, or absorption through the skin can develop AD. These reactions are non-seasonal and include pruritus, erythema, and recurrent otitis. Given their association with foods, they may be misdiagnosed as food allergies. These mites can also cause anaphylaxis when ingested. Thus, flour contaminated with storage mites can cause "pancake syndrome" or "baker's lung." Patients develop symptoms of allergic hypersensitivity, sneezing, urticaria, angioedema, and dyspnea after eating beignets, pancakes, tempura, pizzas, or other cakes made with mite-infested flour. Baking the food does not solve the problem because the mite allergens are heat stable.

It is a misconception that dry pet food comes already contaminated from the manufacturer. In most cases, mites invade via defective seals while the food is stored at the owner's home. Dry pet food should not be stockpiled; simply purchase sufficient for a 30-day supply. Store pet foods in airtight containers in a cool, dry place. If possible, divide the pet food into weekly portions and store the unused portions in a freezer until needed. Pet storage containers should be washed regularly in hot water and dried thoroughly before refilling. They should be sealed to prevent contamination.

COCKROACH ALLERGIES

There are three different species of cockroach found in the United States; the German cockroach (*Blattella germanica*), the American cockroach (*Periplaneta americana*), and the Oriental cockroach (*Blatta orientalis*). The commonest of these is the German cockroach, an indoor-living species. All may serve as potent sources of allergens and they are a major risk factor for asthma in children in inner-city neighborhoods. Dogs may also become sensitized to cockroach allergens. Exposure results from the inhalation of dust containing roach feces, secretions, exoskeletons, body parts, and saliva. The major allergens are Bla g 1 and Bla g 2. There is an inverse relationship between cockroach allergies and the presence of household cats, with the suggestion being that the cats eat the critters. As with HDM allergen preparations, cockroach allergen solutions contain high levels of proteases and must be treated accordingly.

Allergies to Insect Venoms

Insect stings account for many human deaths each year as a result of acute anaphylaxis following sensitization to venom. It is estimated that about 3.3% of adults in the United States are allergic to insect stings. Therefore, insect venoms may result in severe life-threatening allergic responses. These reactions develop from being stung by honeybees and bumblebees (Apoidea); yellow jackets, wasps, and hornets (Vespidae); or by ants, especially fire ants (Formicidae). Extensive cross-reactivity occurs among the vespid venoms. The allergens that affect animals are the same as those that sensitize humans. Bee venoms contain a complex mixture of peptides such as the mast cell degranulating agent melittin, enzymes such as phospholipase A2 that cause cell lysis, and hyaluronidase that disrupts connective tissue and permits venom spread. Wasp venoms contain a complex mixture of compounds similar to bee venoms; however, they lack melittin. Fire ant venoms contain hyaluronidase and phospholipase in a suspension of alkaloid toxins, which induce the sterile nonimmunologic pseudopustule associated with fire ant bites as well as tissue destruction and vesicle formation.

Anaphylactic reactions to insect venoms in dogs and cats are not common, nor is there any evidence that dogs with AD are more prone to develop these severe reactions. Certain dog breeds such as Boxers and Staffordshire Bull Terriers might be more susceptible to developing severe reactions to insect stings. Clinical signs in dogs after a hymenopteran sting can vary from local reactions to acute, life-threatening anaphylaxis. Urticaria may be a prominent feature in addition to angioedema, gastrointestinal upsets, hypotension, and dyspnea (Fig. 12.9). They usually develop within a few minutes of the animal being stung. Diagnosis is based on history, especially if the sting has been witnessed.

Sensitized dogs should be kept away from flowering areas as much as possible. Likewise, owners should avoid situations where wasps are present and scented objects that may attract hymenoptera. First aid involves the use of ice packs and administration of H1 antihistamines if available. Should signs of anaphylaxis develop, epinephrine must be administered as described in Chapter 8. Sensitized animals may be identified by an appropriate collar tag.

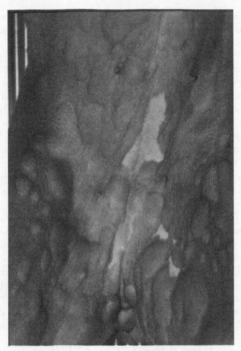

Fig. 12.9 Urticaria in a Boxer stung by a wasp. (Courtesy of Dr. Gwen Ellisalde.)

Suggested Readings

Arlian LG. Arthropod allergens and human health. *Annu Rev Entomol.* 2002;47:395-433.

Arlian LG, Schumann RJ, Morgan MS, Glass RL. Serum immunoglobulin E against storage mite allergens in dogs with atopic dermatitis. *Am J Vet Res.* 2003;64(1):32-36.

Bruet V, Bourdeau PJ, Roussel A, Imparato L, Desfontis JC. Characterization of pruritus in canine atopic dermatitis, flea bite hypersensitivity, and flea infestation and its role in diagnosis. *Vet Dermatol.* 2012;23(6):487-e93.

Calderon MA, Kleine-Tebbe J, Linneberg A, et al. House dust mite respiratory allergy: an overview of current therapeutic strategies. *J Allergy Clin Immunol Pract.* 2015;3(6):843-855.

Komi DE, Sharma L, Dela Cruz CS. Chitin and its effects on inflammatory and immune responses. *Clin Rev Allergy Immunol.* 2018;54(2):213-223.

Laffort-Dassot C, Carlotti DN, Pin D, Jasmin P. Diagnosis of flea allergy dermatitis: comparison of intra-dermal testing with flea allergens and a FceRIa-based IgE assay in response to flea control. *Vet Dermatol.* 2004;15(5):321-330.

Lanz S, Brunner A, Graubner C, Marti E, Gerber V. Insect bite hypersensitivity in horses is associated with airway hyperreactivity. *J Vet Intern Med.* 2017;31(6):1877-1883.

McDermott MJ, Weber E, Hunter S, et al. Identification, cloning, and characterization of a major cat flea salivary allergen (Cte f 1). *Mol Immunol.* 2000;37(7):361-375.

Miller JD. The role of dust mites in allergy. *Clin Rev Allergy Immunol.* 2019;57(3):312-329. doi:10.1007/s12016-018-8693-0.

Naz S, Desclozeaux M, Mounsey KE, Chaudhry FR, Walton SF. Characterization of *Sarcoptes scabei* tropo-myosin and paramyosin: immunoreactive allergens in scabies. *Am J Trop Med Hyg.* 2017;97(3):851-860. doi:10.4269/ajtmh.16-0976.

Olivry T, Dunston SM, Favrot C, Prelaud P, Tsukui T. The novel high molecular weight *Dermatophagoides farinae* protein Zen-1 is a major allergen in North American and European mite allergic dogs with atopic dermatitis. *Vet Dermatol.* 2017;28(2):177-e38.

Olomski F, Fettelschoss V, Jonsdottir S, et al. Interleukin 31 in insect bite hypersensitivity – alleviating clinical symptoms by active vaccination against itch. *Allergy.* 2020;75(4):862-871.

Pali-Scholl I, Blank S, Verhoeckx K, et al. AAACI position paper: comparing insect hypersensitivity induced by bite, sting, inhalation or ingestion in human beings and animals. *Allergy.* 2019;74(5):874-887.

Patel S, Goyal A. Chitin and chitinase: role in pathogenicity, allergenicity and health. *Int J Biol Macromol.* 2017;97:331-338.

Peeters LM, Janssens S, Godderis BM, et al. Evaluation of an IgE ELISA with *Culicoides* spp. extracts and recombinant salivary antigens for diagnosis of insect bite hypersensitivity in Warmblood horses. *Vet J.* 2013;198(1):141-147.

Randall TA, Mullikin JC, Mueller GA. The draft genome assembly of *Dermatophagoides pteronyssinus* supports the identification of novel allergen isoforms in *Dermatophagoides* species. *Int Arch Allergy Immunol.* 2018;175(3):136-246.

Ribeiro JM, Assumpção TC, Ma D, et al. An insight into the sialotranscriptome of the cat flea, *Ctenocephalides felis. PLoS One.* 2012;7(9):e44612. doi:10.1371/journal.pone.0044612.

Schaffartzik A, Hamza E, Janda J, Crameri R, Marti E, Rhyner C. Equine insect bite hypersensitivity: what do we know. *Vet Immunol Immunopathol.* 2012;147(3-4):113-126.

Takahashi K, Yanuma N, Hirokawa M, et al. Presence of the house dust mite allergen in the gastrointestinal tract of dogs with chronic enteropathy: A potential inducer of interleukin-1β. *Vet Immunol Immunopathol.* 2020. doi:10.1016/j.vetimm.2020.110150.

Van der Meide NM, Roders N, Oldruitenborgh- Oosterbaan MM, et al. Cloning and expression of candidate allergens from *Culicoides obsoletus* for diagnosis of insect bite hypersensitivity in horses. *Vet Immunol Immunopathol.* 2013;153(3-4):227-239.

Verdon M, Lanz S, Rhyner C, Gerber V, Marti E. Allergen-specific immunoglobulin E in sera of horses affected with insect bite hypersensitivity, severe equine asthma or both conditions. *J Vet Intern Med.* 2019;33(1):266-274.

Wilson AD, Harwood L, Torsteinsdottir S, Marti E. Production of monoclonal antibodies specific for native equine IgE and their application to monitor total serum IgE responses in Icelandic and non-Icelandic horses with insect bite dermal hypersensitivity. *Vet Immunol Immunopathol.* 2006;112(3-4):156-170.

CHAPTER 13

Allergic Respiratory Disease

Potential allergens in the form of fine particles suspended in inhaled air enter the respiratory tract with every breath. Large particles are usually trapped in the nasal passages, while progressively smaller particles are trapped within the trachea and bronchi. Only the very smallest can penetrate as far as the lungs. One of the commonest forms of allergic disease in humans is "hay fever," an allergic conjunctivitis and rhinitis generally triggered by relatively large particles, such as pollen grains. Asthma, a chronic allergic bronchitis triggered mainly by aeroallergens, is a major debilitating disease in many human populations, especially in children and young adults, and is the most common chronic disease of childhood in North America.

Asthma in Humans

Asthma is a chronic inflammatory syndrome characterized by airway narrowing, resulting in obstruction and airway hyperresponsiveness. These lead to recurrent episodes of wheezing, breathlessness, chest tightness, and coughing. Asthma is not a single disease. It is a syndrome caused by a heterogeneous group of diseases that affect approximately 300 million people worldwide and account for more than 250,000 deaths each year. Recent analysis has shown that asthma is even more complex than previously thought. Multiple asthma phenotypes can be subdivided into many diverse endotypes. These endotypes differ with respect to genetic background, environmental risk factors, age of onset, pathogenesis (the presence or absence of IgE, eosinophils, or neutrophils), clinical course, and response to treatment.

Many endotypes are classified based on their clinical features, age of onset, and so on; however, it is appropriate to classify asthma phenotypes based on their pathogenesis. The syndrome is associated with chronic lung inflammation mediated by four distinct cell types: type 2 helper (Th2) cells, type 2 innate lymphoid (ILC2) cells, eosinophils, and Th17 cells. These cells can act singly or in combination with genetic and environmental factors. However, for simplicity, we will consider there are four major pathogenic asthma types. The most important and prevalent is type 2 hypersensitivity to inhaled aeroallergens. A second type is eosinophilic asthma characterized by bronchial and lung infiltration with eosinophils. A third, non-allergic type is mediated by ILC2 cells. The fourth type is a neutrophilic asthma, largely mediated by Th17 cells. However, many patients suffer from mixed phenotypes, currently termed overlap syndromes.

Th2-HIGH ASTHMA

Most affected children and about half of affected adults suffer from allergic asthma that results from chronic type 2 immune responses against inhaled particulate allergens, such as house dust mite fragments, animal danders, fungal spores, and plant and tree pollens, or dust from foods such as peanuts.

Pathogenesis

As in the skin, Th2-mediated allergic responses in the upper airways are initiated by epithelial barrier dysfunction, which may be inherited or triggered by inhaled allergens or pollutants. Thus,

---

BOX 13.1 ■ Soluble Pattern Recognition Receptors

It has generally been believed that the production of the three master cytokines, IL-33, TSLP, and IL-25, by airway epithelial cells is triggered by cell damage. However, evidence is accumulating that this cytokine production and consequent allergic responses are also triggered when allergens interact with soluble pattern recognition receptors (PRRs) secreted by airway epithelial cells. These cells normally express numerous PRRs on their surface whereby they recognize microbial proteins and nucleic acids. However, many are actively secreted by epithelial cells, and innate and adaptive immune cells. These secreted PRRs include some pentraxins, mannose-binding proteins, C-reactive protein, surfactant proteins, serum amyloid A, and complement components.

The acute-phase protein, serum amyloid A (SAA), is especially important during this process. SAA can bind house dust mite allergens such as Der p 13. Once bound, the allergen-SAA complex will bind to formyl-peptide receptors on epithelial cells and trigger their production of the master regulator, IL-33, which will trigger type 2 and ILC2 cell responses and promote allergic airway disease. Other soluble PRRs such as the complement component C3a, mannose-binding lectin, and surfactant proteins A and D may serve a similar function.

Smole U et al. Serum amyloid A is a soluble pattern recognition receptor that drives type 2 immunity. *Nat Immunol* 2020; 21:756-765

---

inhaled detergents, tobacco, or e-cigarette smoke, micro- and nanoparticles, and microplastics may all induce epithelial damage. Inhaled proteases in allergens such as those from house dust mites, fungi, and pollens are especially effective in degrading tight junctions. They may also damage respiratory epithelial cells and trigger the release of the three master cytokines, interleukin 33 (IL-33), thymic stromal lymphopoietin (TSLP), and IL-25 (Box 13.1). These cytokines can activate Th2 cells. IL-4 and IL-13 may actually promote barrier dysfunction by inhibiting the expression of tight junction proteins such as occludins and E-cadherin. Epithelial barrier damage also permits inhaled allergens to penetrate the barrier and trigger Th2 responses in the underlying nasal and bronchial mucosa. Th2 cells activate B cells and induce IgE production (Fig. 13.1). The IgE binds to mast cells lining the airways. On inhalation of airborne allergens, the IgE binds the allergens and the mast cells degranulate. The release of mast cell mediators, especially histamine and prostaglandin D_2, results in bronchiolar smooth muscle contraction, acute inflammation, and mucus hypersecretion leading to severe dyspnea. Under the influence of IL-13, bronchial epithelial cells can secrete stem cell factor and promote further mast cell activation. Excessive IL-13 production induces airway hyperresponsiveness and chronic airway changes. Eosinophils may be activated as part of this inflammatory cascade.

As a result of repeated allergic attacks, the bronchial smooth muscle cells eventually become hypersensitive and overreact to stimuli, such as cold air or exercise. When prolonged, these attacks eventually cause persistent changes in the airways, including subepithelial fibrosis, goblet cell hyperplasia leading to changes in the properties of the mucus (see Box 13.2), epithelial injury, smooth muscle hypertrophy, and angiogenesis. These all ultimately result in the thickening of the airway walls and narrowing of the airways. The IL-9-producing subpopulation of Th2 cells (Th9 cells) also contributes to the development of this form of asthma. In humans with severe asthma, the numbers of regulatory T (Treg) cells in the blood and sputum are low, and their suppressive effects are reduced.

Clinical Disease

The symptoms of allergic asthma include mucus overproduction, shortness of breath, chest tightness, cough, and reduced lung function. Exacerbation by respiratory infections or air pollutants

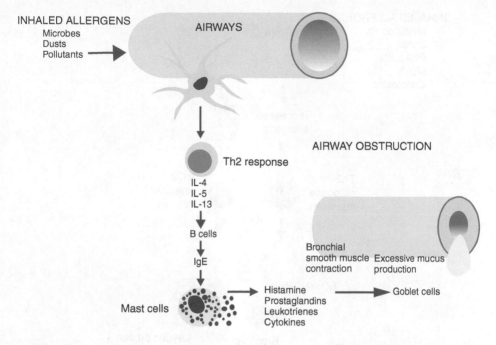

Fig. 13.1 Simplified view of the pathogenesis of type 2 helper (Th2) cell-mediated allergic asthma, which is a type 2 immune response to inhaled allergens.

can worsen the disease and result in respiratory failure. The disease in children starts with allergic sensitization in the first years of life, resulting in the development of eczema. This eventually transitions to allergic rhinitis and then to asthma. This progression has been called the "atopic march." Thus, up to half of the children who develop eczema in early life develop asthma. Up to 80% of patients with allergic asthma also have rhinitis. The atopic march has not been observed in domestic animals.

The most important evidence for an essential role of IgE in this form of asthma is the clinical effectiveness of treatment with the monoclonal antibody omalizumab directed against the constant region of IgE. Omalizumab blocks IgE from binding to its high-affinity receptor FcεRI and effectively "disarms" mast cells and basophils. It also blocks the effects of IgE on dendritic cells (DCs). Th2-high asthma is usually responsive to inhaled corticosteroids.

Th2-HIGH (EOSINOPHILIC) ASTHMA

Approximately half of human asthma cases are associated with eosinophilic airway inflammation. In these cases, bronchoalveolar lavage fluid (BALF), bronchial biopsies, and sputum all contain large numbers of eosinophils. These cases are mediated by Th2 and ILC2 cells. Th2 cells produce IL-4, while both cell types produce excessive amounts of IL-13 and especially IL-5. Kinetic studies suggest that ILC2 cells initiate the response while Th2 cells are responsible for maintaining it (Fig. 13.2).

Eosinophilia in the respiratory tract is driven initially by the release of the master cytokines IL-33, TSLP, and IL-25 from damaged bronchial epithelial cells. These activate ILC2 cells that

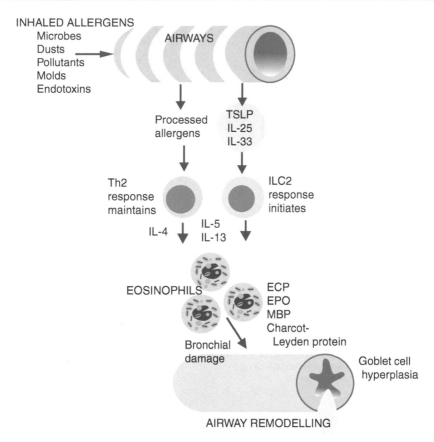

Fig. 13.2 **Probable pathogenesis of eosinophil-mediated asthma.** This can be triggered by either Th2 or ILC2 cells. ILC2 cells are likely responsible for its initiation, whereas Th2 cells are responsible for its persistence. ECP = eosinophil cationic protein. EPO = eosinophil peroxidase. MBP = major protein.

produce large amounts of IL-5, the main driver of eosinophil production. They also release eotaxins that attract more eosinophils. IL-13 from ILC2 cells promotes the release of eosinophil chemoattractants. The early ILC2 response is followed by a Th2 cell response that maintains the influx of eosinophils. When the eosinophils arrive and release their granules, enzymes such as eosinophil peroxidase then cause irritation and bronchial hyperreactivity. They also contribute to airway remodeling and basement membrane thickening via their release of TGF-β. Eosinophils may also undergo cytolysis and release DNA nets containing their granules. Eosinophil NETosis is a feature of the most severe asthma cases. (NETosis is the release of cellular DNA strands that can trap invaders but which can also bind to blood vessel walls to trigger thrombosis.) Depletion of Th2 cells in a mouse asthma model reduces airway eosinophilia but not airway remodeling; therefore, Th2 cells may be responsible for eosinophilia, whereas ILC2 cells are responsible for the remodeling.

Eosinophils directly interact with sensory and autonomic nerve fibers in the airways of patients with asthma. They are found close to these nerves and bind to them using intercellular adherence molecules. By acting on these neurons, their granule contents contribute directly to airway hyperexcitability and bronchoconstriction.

Given the perceived importance of eosinophils in asthma, two monoclonal antibodies against human IL-5 have been developed—mepolizumab and reslizumab. Both block the binding of IL-5 to its receptor. In previous studies on mildly affected patients, encouraging results were obtained; however, there was no objective clinical improvement in formal clinical trials. The importance of eosinophils in these cases is now being reconsidered.

Th2-LOW (ILC2-MEDIATED) ASTHMA

Approximately half of human asthmatics develop the disease in the absence of IgE. This is probably a function of lung ILC2 cells (Fig. 13.3). These cases may develop as a result of epithelial barrier damage and a breakdown of the tight junctional complexes that bind epithelial cells together. These tight junctions may be degraded by inhaled pollutants such as those found in dust and smoke and by allergenic proteases such as those found in pollen grains, mold spores, or arthropod extracts. In this way, inhaled allergens can more readily gain access to DCs and ILC2 cells. Like Th2 cells, ILC2 cells are activated by the cytokines released from damaged bronchial epithelial cells. In turn, they secrete IL-5, IL-9, and IL-13 and promote the activation of other immune cells and allergic inflammation. IL-33 and TSLP directly activate mast cells. Protease-containing allergens such as those from house dust mites and some pollens and molds not only break down tight junctions but also directly activate ILC2 cells through protease-activated receptors. The IL-33 released because of this damage can then induce eosinophilia and bronchial hyperreactivity. ILC2 cells can respond to damage caused by respiratory viruses such as influenza

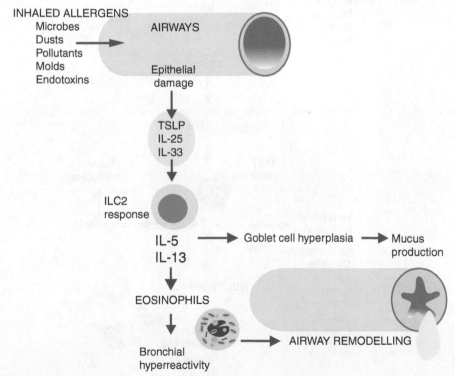

Fig. 13.3 Suggested pathogenesis of non-allergic ILC2-mediated asthma. It is triggered by bronchial epithelial damage and the subsequent release of the three master regulatory cytokines.

and rhinoviruses by suppressing Th1 responses. This may explain how some viral infections may trigger or exacerbate asthma attacks.

TSLP plays a key role in some asthma endotypes. It is produced by damaged bronchial endothelium and activates DCs to produce chemokines such as CCL17 and CCL22 that attract T cells. TSLP regulates DC functions so that they differentiate into DC2 cells and release Th2-inducing cytokines. It also activates mast cells.

Th2-LOW (Th17-MEDIATED) ASTHMA

Many human asthmatics have a neutrophil-dominated disease with elevated IL-17 levels and a neutrophil infiltration in the absence of Th2 cytokines and eosinophils. This IL-17-high phenotype is likely triggered by infections, environmental exposure to endotoxins and air pollutants, including smoking and ozone (Fig. 13.4). Neutrophil dominance occurs in patients with late-onset disease and is more severe, with less reversible airway obstruction and a different mix of cytokines in bronchoalveolar lavage fluid. The fluid contains both Th1- and Th17-type cytokines, including IL-17 and IL-22. IL-22 may also contribute to airway inflammation. Exposure to diesel exhaust fumes exacerbates asthma symptoms and increases blood levels of IL-17. IL-17 contributes to airway remodeling by promoting fibroblast proliferation and counteracting the effects of Treg cells. IL-17 can be derived from Th17, NKT, or ILC3 cells. IL-17 mediated

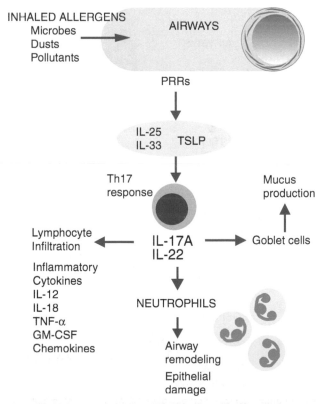

Fig. 13.4 Pathogenesis of Th17 cell-mediated asthma.

asthma also involves the release of tumor necrosis factor (TNF). Neutralization of TNF-α reduces the neutrophil infiltration in the lung, although this has no apparent effect on airway hyperresponsiveness.

OVERLAP SYNDROMES

Eosinophilic asthma is considered a Th2/ILC2 disorder and neutrophilic asthma is a Th17 disorder; however, the boundaries between the two are blurred. Many clinical cases overlap between the two. In experimental mice, very high levels of an allergen challenge can cause a switch from a Th2 response to a Th1 or a Th17 response. Certain allergens also affect this polarization. For example, the Th1 cytokine, gamma interferon (IFN-γ), contributes to the pathogenesis of both eosinophilic and neutrophilic asthma. IL-18 can also drive the activation of Th1 cells to produce IL-13 and airway hyperreactivity.

Genetics and Asthma

Genomic studies in humans have linked asthma susceptibility to inherited defects in skin barrier proteins such as filaggrin or genes affecting the epithelial cytokines such as TSLP or the IL-33 receptor.

Microbiota and Asthma

The healthy microbiota in both the upper and lower respiratory tracts plays an important role in maintaining homeostasis in the airways. Early life dysbiosis in the gut and airways is an important predisposing factor for the subsequent development of allergic diseases. Healthy lungs contain their own microbiota, generally acquired by aspiration and controlled by pulmonary defenses such as alveolar macrophages and mucociliary transport. The normal equilibrium of this resident population is disrupted in diseases such as asthma. For example, a strong local type 2 immune response will reduce the number of resident bacteria. Early childhood respiratory tract infections increase the risk of developing asthma and asthma flares. There are clear connections between the upper respiratory tract microbiota and asthma; but the specific mechanisms involved are unclear. The existence of the gut-lung axis ensures that changes in the intestinal microbiota and the composition of its immune cell populations are reflected in alterations in immunity within the respiratory system and predict the development of allergen-specific Th2 responses (see Fig. 7.9). One such mechanism acts through the production of bacterial products such as short-chain fatty acids in the gut that are then absorbed into the bloodstream. Butyrate has been shown to ameliorate Th2 responses in the airways by limiting eosinophil trafficking and survival, suppressing mast cell degranulation, and reducing type 2 cytokine production by ILC2 cells in the bronchoalveolar fluid. Other pathways include the migration of antigen-presenting cells from the gut to the respiratory tract.

Several comparative studies have been conducted on the microbiota of healthy and asthmatic horses. The fecal microbiota of healthy horses is similar to that of asthmatic horses; however, it does not respond in exactly the same way to changes in diet and environment. Studies on the microbiota of the trachea in asthmatic horses showed a lower bacterial load compared to healthy horses. It is unclear whether this was a cause or consequence of asthma.

Chronic Obstructive Pulmonary Disease (COPD) and Asthma

COPD is an inflammatory disease in smokers that shares several features with some asthma endotypes, termed asthma–COPD overlap. Some COPD patients may show an increase in sputum eosinophils. These have been classified as eosinophilic COPD. Of course, these patients may simply be suffering from both diseases.

Respiratory Allergies in Animals

CANINE ASTHMA

While common in humans, nasolacrimal urticaria is rarely seen in respiratory allergy in dogs and cats. Aeroallergens encountered by humans usually provoke rhinitis and conjunctivitis characterized by a profuse watery nasal discharge and excessive lacrimation. When dogs develop allergic disease, it usually presents as atopic dermatitis or otitis. Natural allergic asthma has been reported in dogs, but is uncommon and has not been studied in detail. However, several dog models have been created to study asthma. These models generally use dogs that have been sensitized to helminth-derived allergens, for example, extracts of *Ascaris suum*, either naturally or by injection, and are Th2 cell-mediated. Many dogs are naturally sensitized to *A. suum* because its allergens cross-react with those of the common canine roundworm, *Toxocara canis*.

In the 1960s, a line of dogs was generated by crossing Basenjis with Greyhounds for transplantation research purposes. Before being discarded, the dogs were tested for sensitivity to allergens. Three female dogs in the colony were found to be hyperreactive to aerosolized allergens. These animals were selectively bred to produce highly atopic dogs with non-specific airway hyperactivity. In addition to this airway hypersensitivity, the dogs were prone to developing atopic dermatitis reflecting their extreme sensitivity to allergens. When challenged by *A. suum* aerosols, the dogs developed increased airway resistance because of severe bronchoconstriction. These *Ascaris*-sensitive dogs also exhibited an allergen-specific, dose-dependent release of histamine after aerosol challenge.

A non-seasonal, chronically relapsing, intensely pruritic dermatitis also develops in these airway-sensitized dogs following immunization and allergen challenge. It presents as lichenified plaques, especially on the limbs, as well as inflammatory nodules developing in the interdigital spaces and edematous papules on the chin. The dermatitis flares follow each aerosol challenge with the *Ascaris* allergen. Biopsies of the skin lesions show changes consistent with self-inflicted scratching with epidermal hyperplasia and dermal fibrosis as well as a dense inflammatory infiltrate that is predominantly lymphohistiocytic. When these dogs are challenged, there is a marked increase in neutrophil numbers but not eosinophils in their bronchoalveolar lavage fluid (BALF).

Similar findings have been reported in Beagles experimentally sensitized to *Ascaris*. They also develop acute bronchoconstriction and a late-phase reaction after bronchial allergen challenge. The response is associated with increased bronchial histamine and prostaglandin D_2.

Another dog model is the ragweed-sensitized Beagle. In this model, Beagle puppies are injected with ragweed allergen in an alum adjuvant intraperitoneally within 24 h of birth and subsequently boosted. Dogs treated in this way develop high levels of specific IgE against ragweed and an eosinophilia. They have high levels of eosinophils in their BALF. Their airways are hypersensitive to histamine. After several challenges, these animals remain sensitized for at least 5 months.

Canine Eosinophilic Bronchopneumopathy

Infiltration of the lungs and airways with eosinophils can develop into an eosinophilic pneumonitis (EP) in dogs as a consequence of parasitic, fungal, or neoplastic diseases. However, many cases are idiopathic. They generally manifest themselves as a progressive cough with respiratory distress accompanied by anorexia, leading to weight loss and lethargy. Dogs with eosinophilic bronchitis may show minimal changes on radiology. Mucosal biopsies show inflammation with increased infiltration of eosinophils (Fig. 13.5).

Dogs may also develop much more severe disease with eosinophilic pulmonary granulomas, where multiple masses develop in the lungs. These pulmonary granulomas contain not only

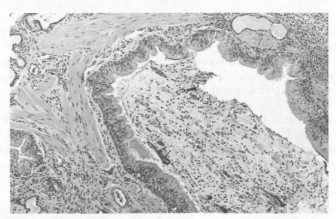

Fig. 13.5 Canine eosinophilic bronchopneumopathy. Note the large number of eosinophils and excessive mucus in the bronchiolar lumen. Smooth muscle hypertrophy and an increased number of submucosal inflammatory cells are also evident. (Courtesy Dr. Brian Porter.)

epithelioid cells and macrophages but also large numbers of eosinophils. Similar granulomas may also be found in the liver or kidneys. Some, but not all, cases are associated with occult heartworm disease.

The causes of EP are unclear, although it may result from allergies to aeroallergens. However, intradermal skin testing of affected dogs has not confirmed this. Total IgE levels have yet to be measured in these dogs. The affected animals show an increase in $CD4^+$ cells and a decrease in $CD8^+$ cells, a phenomenon also observed in some human asthmatics. There is increased expression of transcripts for eotaxins 2 and 3 and macrophage chemotactic protein-3. All three of these molecules are chemoattractants for eosinophils.

Young adult dogs, 4–6 years of age, are primarily affected by EP. One study suggested that Siberian Huskies and Alaskan Malamutes were predisposed to the disease; but further studies failed to confirm this. In general, it affects both large (Labradors and German Shepherds) and small breeds such as Terriers and Dachshunds. There may be a bias toward females.

A persistent, harsh cough is the most common presentation. Dogs may show dyspnea, exercise intolerance, and a nasal discharge. Occasional pruritis has been reported. Diagnosis depends on radiologic and bronchoscopic findings. There may be a preponderance of eosinophils in their BALF. The most common radiographic pattern shows peribronchial cuffing and thickening of the bronchial walls. Eosinophils may constitute as many as 50%–60% of their blood leukocytes. An absence of eosinophilia does not exclude a diagnosis of EP. Airway sampling by bronchoalveolar lavage is required to confirm the diagnosis. Eosinophils constitute <5% of the BALF in healthy dogs. However, in EP, this percentage may exceed 50%. Cytology may also rule out parasitic eggs or larvae or cancer cells. It is essential to run a heartworm test on these dogs in endemic areas and perform a fecal examination for intestinal parasite ova. Treatment with an anthelmintic such as fenbendazole, thiabendazole, or levamisole is prudent. Oral corticosteroid therapy is the treatment of choice. Once the clinical disease is controlled, then the dose may be reduced to maintenance levels.

FELINE ASTHMA

Asthma is a common, chronic, and progressive allergic respiratory disease of cats. It has been estimated to affect approximately 1% of cats. A component of feline atopic syndrome, feline asthma appears to be triggered predominantly by aeroallergens. Common symptoms include coughing and wheezing, dyspnea (rapid open-mouth breathing), and possibly severe broncho-constriction. Animals may produce excess mucus that can cause coughing and wheezing fits. Affected animals may have a moderate increase in total serum IgE levels (see Fig. 20.2). However, investigations into cats with airway eosinophilia found that some possessed IgE antibodies to respiratory aeroallergens, especially house dust mites. However, the percentage of positive animals did not differ significantly from healthy control cats. More research is required on this topic.

Other possible causes of feline asthma include lungworms, respiratory infections, cardiomyopathy, and stomatitis. Pulmonary radiographs and a positive response to steroids help confirm the diagnosis. It may be necessary to sample airway fluid through bronchoalveolar lavage. Recommended treatments include the use of bronchodilators for mild cases and bronchodilators with glucocorticosteroids for more severe cases. Inhaled steroids generally take 10–14 days to elicit significant improvement.

As with many allergic diseases, feline asthma is better avoided than treated. Thus, owners should take steps to minimize allergen exposure. These include pollens, molds, and dusty cat litter. Dry air may also be an issue; therefore, humidity maintenance is beneficial. Siamese and Himalayan breeds and their crosses are more prone to developing asthma. Female cats may be more susceptible than males. An experimental Th2-high model of asthma has been developed in cats by repeatedly exposing them to an *A. suum* aerosol. These cats, when challenged, showed an increase in bronchial smooth muscle thickness, epithelial shedding, eosinophil infiltration, and hyperplasia of goblet cells and submucosal glands. There is a concordance between asthma in cats and their owners, suggesting the involvement of similar allergens. Oral and inhaled glucocorticoids are effective treatments. Intradermal skin testing followed by allergen-specific immunotherapy is another possible treatment modality for selected animals.

BOVINE ASTHMA

A familial allergic rhinitis characterized by extreme nasal pruritus, violent sneezing, dyspnea, mucoid nasal discharge, and excessive lacrimation has been reported in cattle. Depending on the allergen, it may be seasonal. The allergens involved are inhaled and come from a variety of plant and fungal sources. Diagnosis may be confirmed by skin testing.

Nasal granulomas in cattle occur in certain areas of Australia and New Zealand. They occur sporadically in North America. Some are due to fungal infections (mycetomas), whereas others are caused by nasal Actinobacillus infection. However, the great majority of cases are of unknown etiology. This enzootic nasal granuloma occurs predominantly in dairy cattle, with the highest prevalence in Jerseys and Guernseys and smaller numbers in Friesian/Holsteins, Shorthorns, and Ayrshires.

The disease has a gradual onset. The affected animals show evidence of nasal irritation and rub their nostrils against objects or even push their nostrils over plant stems in an attempt to scratch the nasal mucosa. Animals become dyspneic, especially if their nasal passages are blocked by twigs. Gross lesions are generally restricted to the anterior half of the nasal passages. In some cases, these may occupy the entire nasal passages and the larynx and trachea. The lesions are bilateral and often symmetrical. They consist of numerous polypoid nodules, 1 to 4 mm in diameter, situated in the anterior nasal mucosa. On histology, the nodules show squamous metaplasia, goblet cell hyperplasia, and a dense eosinophil infiltration of the epithelium. The lamina propria is edematous and infiltrated with eosinophils, plasma cells, and lymphocytes. In well-developed nodules, their cores consist of connective tissue blood vessels, fibroblasts, and a mixed infiltrate of granulocytes, lymphocytes, and mast cells. No infectious agents have been consistently isolated from these lesions, although yeasts and other fungi are occasionally found.

The cause of this disease is unknown, but it may be a form of allergic rhinitis. Thus, repeated exposure to an inhaled allergen may result in the development of these chronic lesions. Mold spores are the primary suspects. Similar lesions can be reproduced experimentally by repeatedly applying ovalbumin to the nasal mucosa of sensitized cattle. The reaction might also be triggered by an infectious agent such as infectious rhinopneumonitis virus.

SHEEP ASTHMA

In sheep that are naturally sensitized to roundworms, immediate bronchoconstriction occurs on aerosol exposure to a nematode allergen such as *A. suum* extract. When sensitized sheep are challenged, their response conforms to two patterns. Some sheep are acute responders and develop immediate bronchial resistance. Other sheep develop both an acute and a delayed response. The delayed response develops 6–8 h after the challenge. This delayed response is mediated in large part by platelet-activating factor.

PIG ASTHMA

Pigs experimentally sensitized with *A. suum* allergen in alum develop acute bronchoconstriction following aerosol challenge. Weanling pigs may also be sensitized to ovalbumin and, if subsequently challenged with an ovalbumin aerosol, will also develop bronchoconstriction. However, because of their endogenous steroid production, pigs must be treated with the steroid inhibitor metapyrone to elicit a clinical response. There is a marked eosinophil infiltration into their lungs after 8 h.

EQUINE ASTHMA SYNDROME

Asthma in humans consists of several distinctly different endotypes depending on the role of Th2 responses in their pathogenesis (Table 13.1). Some endotypes are associated with high

TABLE 13.1 ■ The Two Major Forms of Equine Asthma Syndrome

	SEVERE (Recurrent Airway Obstruction)	MILD (Inflammatory Airway Disease)
At Rest	Respiratory distress Labored breathing	No respiratory distress Breathing normal
Major signs	Chronic cough Increased breathing effort Airway obstructive episodes Severe respiratory distress	Coughing Underperformance Exercise intolerance
Other important signs	Nasal discharge Thick, viscous mucus Obvious heave line Anorexia	Nasal discharge Excessive mucus production
Pathogenesis	Primarily type 2 and type 17 responses Severe bronchoconstriction Bronchiolitis and bronchitis Emphysema Increased airway muscle mass Airway remodeling	Primarily a type 1 response
Cellular Infiltrate	Neutrophilic	Neutrophilic, mastocytic eosinophilic, or mixed

eosinophil counts in bronchoalveolar washes, whereas others are characterized by high neutrophil counts. Some human cases have both neutrophils and eosinophils, while others have neither. Some are IgE -associated, while others are not. A similar spectrum and complexity occur in equine asthma.

Several forms of obstructive respiratory disease can develop spontaneously in horses and are collectively called equine asthma syndrome (EAS). Severe EAS has been reported to affect 10%–20% of adult horses, whereas mild or moderate EAS may affect up to 30% of horses depending on location and environment. EAS is most conveniently divided into two phenotypes: a severe phenotype called recurrent airway obstruction (RAO) or "heaves," and a milder phenotype called inflammatory airway disease (IAD). Both phenotypes result from chronic exposure to the complex mixture of environmental aeroallergens found in dusty stables.

Recurrent Airway Obstruction (RAO)

RAO (or severe EAS) is an inflammatory disease that resembles severe asthma in humans. The affected animals suffer from episodes of acute respiratory distress triggered by the inhalation of airborne dusts, even while at rest. During these episodes, horses develop airflow obstruction from bronchospasm, increased mucus production, airway hyperplasia and hyperresponsiveness.

Epidemiology. RAO occurs in horses that are housed in poorly ventilated, dusty stables for a long time. It may occur in two forms: a winter form that develops in horses housed indoors and exposed repeatedly to dust from hay, and a summer pasture-associated form where horses are exposed to large quantities of grass pollens. It may also be triggered by respiratory viral infections. RAO is usually seen in horses over 9–12 years of age. There is also some evidence for a genetic predisposition, perhaps involving the gene encoding the IL-4 receptor. The prevalence of RAO is increased 3-fold when one parent is affected and 5-fold when both parents are affected.

Clinical Disease. RAO is a severe disease characterized by dyspnea, coughing, and an increased breathing effort due to diffuse bronchoconstriction. RAO presents with periods of airway obstruction followed by apparent remission. During the obstructive episodes, horses develop breathing difficulty due to bronchospasm throughout the lungs, together with increased mucus production and a nasal discharge that develops into airway hyperplasia and hyperresponsiveness. Horses develop a chronic cough and reduced working or athletic ability.

Characteristically, horses with RAO suffer from labored breathing, even at rest, and they may develop hyperplastic external abdominal muscles, resulting in the appearance of a "heave line." Anorexia may also cause significant weight loss. Affected horses produce large amounts of thick, viscous mucus that may form mucosal plugs due to goblet cell hyperplasia (Box 13.2). This mucus may form spirals of dense material (Curschmann's spirals) visible in the BALF. Alveolar emphysema occurs in approximately 70% of affected horses. RAO is an economically important disease because it significantly reduces the performance of animals used for recreation or sports, or draught animals. It will worsen over time unless changes are made in the management of the animal.

Pathogenesis. Animals suffering from RAO develop bronchitis and bronchiolitis with characteristic changes in airway mucosa and muscularis. Affected animals usually have large numbers of neutrophils in their small bronchioles and high titers of antibodies to equine influenza in their bronchial secretions. The significance of the latter is unclear. Continuous, prolonged activation of bronchoalveolar epithelial cells by dust particles and airborne endotoxins might lead to excessive production of neutrophil-attracting chemokines. These neutrophils then cause damage by producing proteases, peroxidases, and oxidants such as reactive oxygen species and nitric oxide.

BOX 13.2 ■ Problems with Mucus?

The major constituents of airway mucus are heavily glycosylated proteins called mucins. These exist in two forms. One form remains tethered to epithelial cell surfaces, whereas the second form is secreted and forms the fluid mucus in the airways. The most important of these secreted mucins are MUC5B and MUC5AC. MUC5AC is normally produced by goblet cells, whereas MUC5B is produced in the submucosal glands. MUC5B is the predominant mucin produced by healthy individuals. The MUC5B-rich gel is fluid and readily moved by ciliary action. It is a component of the mucociliary escalator and plays a key role in maintaining airway health.

However, in asthma cases, MUC5AC production is enhanced by inflammatory mediators such as histamine or IL-13, whereas MUC5B production is reduced. In addition, the newly produced MUC5AC is not released into the mucus layer but remains tethered to the epithelial cell surfaces, and the tethered MUC5AC molecules impair ciliary function and impede mucociliary transport. Thus, MUC5AC is a major contributor to the excessive mucus accumulation and development of mucus plugs in allergic airway disease.

Similar studies have been undertaken on airway mucus in horses. In healthy horses, MUC5B predominates and contains small amounts of MUC5AC. The amounts of both mucins are significantly increased in horses with obvious mucus accumulation in their airways. This mucus accumulation correlates with the numbers of bacteria detected in the airways.

Bonser LR, Erle DJ. Airway mucus and asthma: The role of MUC5AC and MUC5B. *J Clin Med* 2017; doi:10.3390/jcm6120112

Rousseau K, Cardwell JM, Humphrey E, Newton R, Knight D, Clegg P, Thornton DJ. Muc5b is the major polymeric mucin in mucus from thoroughbred horses with and without airway mucus accumulation. *PLoS ONE* 2011; doi:10.1371/journal.pone.0019678

Some cases of RAO result from a Th2 reaction to inhaled allergens, especially molds in stable dust. Thus, affected horses may show positive skin test responses to intradermal inoculation of diverse actinomycete and fungal extracts (such as *Rhizopus nigricans, Candida albicans, Saccharopolyspora rectivirgula, Aspergillus fumigatus,* or *Geotrichum deliquescens*). Affected horses may develop dyspnea on aerosol challenge with extracts of these organisms. However, there is little correlation between intradermal skin test results and disease severity. Screening of horses suffering from severe asthma syndrome using an allergen-specific IgE microarray has demonstrated that they react to a diverse mixture of proteins derived from pollens, bacteria, and arthropods. This same survey demonstrated that many horses were reactive to natural latex allergens derived from the rubber tree, *Hevea brasiliensis*, including Hev b 11, Hev b 5, and Hev b 3. Horses are exposed to many rubber products, and some synthetic track surfaces may contain recycled tires.

Airway biopsies show significant increases in the inflammatory cytokines, IL-1β, IL-8, TNF-α, TGF-β1, as well as TLR4 and NF-κB transcripts. Similar but less marked trends occur in IL-17 and IFN-γ. High concentrations of the chemokine CXCL8 (IL-8) are found in the bronchoalveolar washings of affected animals. In vitro exposure of cultured equine bronchial epithelial cells to hay dust or lipopolysaccharide also increases IL-8, CXCL2, and IL-1β production. The percentage of CD4$^+$ Treg cells increases in the bronchoalveolar washings of horses with RAO, suggesting these may influence the course of the disease. Neutrophil immigration precedes the development of airway obstruction. Circulating neutrophils in these horses show impaired antibacterial activity against organisms such as *Streptococcus zooepidemicus*. This may, in part, explain their increased susceptibility to infections.

Histopathology. The principal lesion in RAO is a bronchiolitis characterized by neutrophilic infiltration and smooth muscle remodeling (Fig. 13.6). The remodeling involves changes in the

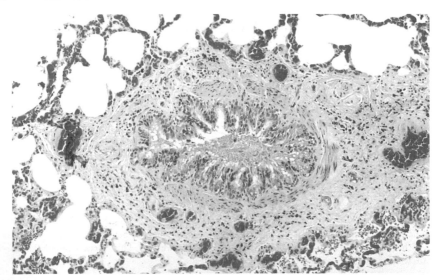

Fig. 13.6 **Bronchiole from a horse with recurrent airway obstruction.** Note the reduction in the size of the airway as a result of intraluminal mucus and epithelial hyperplasia. Also note the smooth muscle hypertrophy and increased number of submucosal inflammatory cells. (Courtesy Dr. Brian Porter.)

epithelium and submucosa. Thus, in the epithelium, there is goblet cell hyperplasia and an increase in stored mucin. In the submucosa, there is subepithelial fibrosis, hyperplasia of smooth muscle cells, enlarged submucosal glands, and increased vascularity. Neutrophils readily migrate into the equine lungs in response to inflammatory stimuli or antigenic challenge. They can be detected in the airway lumen within 4–6 h, followed by mucus hypersecretion and airway obstruction. Peribronchiolar infiltration of lymphocytes is followed by intraluminal accumulation of neutrophils, perhaps under the influence of IL-8, suggesting that animals may have a coexisting type III hypersensitivity response. Chronic activation of innate immunity is characteristic of neutrophilic asthma. Thus, Th17 cells can directly recruit neutrophils into the airways by producing IL-17 and IL-8, CXCL1, and GM-CSF. IL-8 can also promote the development of neutrophil extracellular traps, which have been identified in asthma-affected horses but not in horses in remission. While key participants in innate immunity, neutrophils with their rich content of proteases and oxidants can cause significant tissue damage and contribute directly to bronchoconstriction, mucus production, and airway remodeling. Eosinophils are not normally present in the airway walls of horses affected by RAO.

Another prominent feature of RAO is increased airway smooth muscle mass. In one study, horses with heaves had nearly triple the airway smooth muscle mass of control animals due to increased myocyte proliferation. This remodeling prevents the complete opening of the airways, reduce the elastic properties of the lung parenchyma, and prevent animals from rapidly returning to normal after leaving the dusty environment.

Treatment. The removal of clinically affected horses to a dust-free environment results in improvement of the disease; however, this is reversed if the horses are returned to dusty stables. In some cases, RAO may persist even when horses are moved to low-dust environments, probably because of their chronic airway remodeling.

Diagnosis is based on bronchoscopy, radiography, blood analysis, intradermal skin testing, and bronchial biopsy. The identification of biomarkers in the blood is a potential diagnostic aid for

RAO. Thus haptoglobin, secretoglobin, and surfactant protein D have been examined. Their levels were increased over those in control horses. When all three were used as biomarkers, they had a specificity of 100% and a sensitivity of 45%. Thus, there were no false-positives, but many false-negative results.

Therapy includes the use of systemic and inhaled corticosteroids and bronchodilators. Histamine, serotonin, and leukotrienes mediate equine airway contraction in horses. However, this also means that histamine antagonists have a low efficacy compared to the broader anti-inflammatory effects of glucocorticoids. Inhalation therapy is more effective than systemic therapy. (Fluticasone propionate or beclomethasone dipropionate both work well.) Bronchodilators may be administered by aerosol but should only be used in conjunction with anti-inflammatory therapy. However, inhalation therapy may not be feasible or affordable in many stables.

Summer Pasture-Associated EAS

Horses living in the southeastern US, California, or parts of the UK may develop severe EAS with respiratory signs when grazing on late summer pastures in a warm humid climate. This is a form of RAO that likely results from a Th2 response to airborne molds and grass pollens. Horses should avoid using such pastures during the pollen season. In humans in these regions, peak prevalence of asthma is during the third week of September. This is also the peak of the pollen season.

Inflammatory Airway Disease (IAD)

IAD is a mild form of EAS that can occur in horses of any age. Like RAO, it is associated with chronic exposure to high levels of inhaled airborne particulates in dusty stables.

Epidemiology. IAD affects up to 30% of young horses (<5 years old) in training. Although commonly linked to bacterial or viral infections, in many cases, no infectious agent can be isolated. Affected horses are often housed in poorly ventilated stables where high levels of dust and ammonia can trigger lung inflammation and respiratory damage. Endotoxins and dust particles likely act together to trigger the disease. It may also be triggered by respiratory viral diseases such as equine herpesvirus infections.

Clinical Disease. Affected animals do not look sick. The clinical signs may be very mild, as affected animals do not display dyspnea. The owners generally report coughing, underperformance, and exercise intolerance. Excessive airway mucus production may also be apparent. No labored breathing is seen at rest. Horses develop a neutrophilic inflammation resulting in hypoxia during exercise. Endoscopy is the best method to assess the state of the bronchi and the degree of mucus accumulation. Radiographs and ultrasound do not generally detect the IAD lesions.

Pathogenesis. Its detailed pathogenesis is unknown, but like RAO, IAD is associated with the inhalation of organic dusts and aeroallergens and may be seasonal. Horses affected by insect bite hypersensitivity also show increased airway reactivity, even when they have no overt respiratory signs (Chapter 12). Feeding hay may play a role in the development of EAS due to the release of dust-containing particulate allergens from hay bales. Thus, horses fed hay from round bales are more likely to develop airway inflammation compared to those fed hay from much smaller (and drier) square bales, as there are greater numbers of thermophilic actinomycetes growing in round, dense bales. When eating from these bales, horses keep their nostrils immersed in the bale, thus inhaling the allergens. Air pollution due to nearby road traffic has also been associated with EAS development.

Stable dust is ubiquitous and likely accounts for a high prevalence of IAD in stabled animals. Similarly, seasonal differences in humidity and temperature will affect the degree of hydration of bronchial epithelium. Cold dry air may trigger asthma attacks in humans and horses. A dehydrated airway may cause an increase in IL-4, IL-5 and IL-10 levels and the proinflammatory cytokines IL-1, IL-6, and IL-8, and an increase in BALF neutrophil counts.

Horses are more likely to eat round bale hay during the winter months. It is important to avoid moisture accumulation in bedding to ensure that mold and ammonia levels remain low.

Treatment. Treatment first involves changing the environment to reduce the dust burden. Hay should be fed from the ground on a tarpaulin. Management should change to low-dust feed and bedding. Subsequent treatment may require corticosteroid therapy.

Bronchoalveolar Lavage Fluid. As part of a diagnostic work-up of asthmatic horses, it is usual to harvest BALF from the animal's airways. Cytology and differential cell count using this fluid may provide useful information regarding the disease etiology and pathogenesis (Fig. 13.7).

When harvesting BALF, horses are first sedated. Subsequently, a cuffed catheter is passed nasotracheally until it lodges in a secondary or tertiary bronchus. Approximately 300 mL of warmed saline is repeatedly infused and reaspirated. The pooled washings are then subjected to cytological analysis, including a differential cell count.

IAD has been subcategorized based on the cytological evaluation of bronchoalveolar lavage fluid. Depending on their predominant cell type, BALFs may be classified as neutrophilic, eosinophilic, mastocytic, or mixed. Results from normal horses suggest that mast cells normally constitute less than 2% of the BALF cells. Counts above 2% are appropriate for defining mixed responses, but above 5% are required for diagnosing a mastocytic response. BALF from affected horses shows mild neutrophilia (>5%), eosinophilia (>0.5%), and mast cells (2%). Some horses may have mastocytosis/eosinophilia, whereas others may have neutrophilic inflammation. Cytokine transcripts show elevated IL-1β, IL-5, IL-6, IL-8, IL-10, IL-17, and IL-23, and TNF-α and IFN-γ in BALF from affected horses. However, these differences are influenced by the cells present. For example, in washes with high neutrophil numbers, IL-17 was also elevated, whereas IL-4 was depressed com-

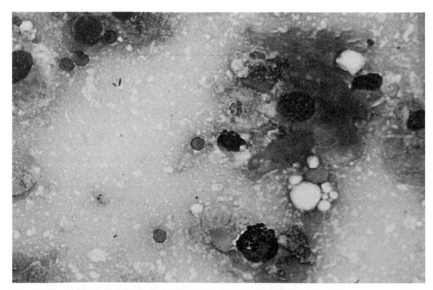

Fig. 13.7 Equine bronchoalveolar lavage smear showing extracellular bacterial rods, an eosinophil, and several erythrocytes. (Courtesy Dr. MC Johnson.)

pared to high mast cell numbers. Therefore, both Th2-high and -low endotypes occur. Mastocytic and eosinophilic BALF represent a Th2-high phenotype, whereas a neutrophil predominance likely reflects a Th2-low phenotype. Only horses with mastocytic or mixed subgroups have detectable IgE in their BALF.

Suggested Readings

Arrieta MC, Arevalo A, Stiemsma L, et al. Associations between infant fungal and bacterial dysbiosis and childhood atopic wheeze in a nonindustrialized setting. *J Allergy Clin Immunol.* 2018;142(2):424-434.

Aun MV, Bonamichi-Santos R, Arantes-Costa MF, Kalil J, Giavina-Bianchi P. Animal models of asthma: utility and limitations. *J Asthma Allergy.* 2017;10:293-301.

Barcik W, Boutin RC, Sokolowska M, Finlay BB. The role of the gut and lung microbiota in the pathology of asthma. *Immunity.* 2020;52(2):241-255.

Bond S, Leguillette R, Richard EA, et al. Equine asthma: integrative biological relevance of a recently proposed nomenclature. *J Vet Intern Med.* 2018;32:2008-2098.

Butler MC, Johnson LR, Outerbridge CA, Vernau W, Wdite SD. Serum immunoglobulin E responses to aeroallergens in cats with naturally occurring airway eosinophilia compared to unaffected control cats. *J Vet Intern Med.* 2020;34(6):2671-2676.

Calzetta L, Roncada P, di Cave D, et al. Pharmacological treatments in asthma-affected horses: a pair-wise and network meta-analysis. *Equine Vet J.* 2017;49(6):710-717.

Caminati M, Pham DL, Bagnasco D, Canonica GW. Type 2 immunity in asthma. *World Allergy Organ J.* 2018;11(1):13. doi:10.1186/s40413-018-0192-5.

Carbonell PL. Bovine nasal granulomas: gross and microscopic lesions. *Vet Pathol.* 1979;16(1):60-73.

Chapman RW. Canine models of asthma and COPD. *Pulm Pharmacol Ther.* 2008;21(5):731-742.

Clercx C, Peeters D. Canine eosinophilic bronchopneumopathy. *Vet Clin North Am Small Anim Pract.* 2007;37(5):917-935.

Davis KU, Sheats MK. Bronchoalveolar lavage cytology characteristics and seasonal changes in a herd of pastured teaching horses. *Front Vet Sci.* 2019;6:74. doi:10.3389/fvets.2019.00074.

Drake LY, Kita H. IL-33: biological properties, functions, and roles in airway disease. *Immunol Res.* 2017;278(1):173-184.

Hansen S, Otten ND, Birch K, Skovgaard K, Hopster-Iversen C, Fjeldborg J. Bronchoalveolar lavage fluid cytokine, cytology, and IgE allergen in horses with equine asthma. *Vet Immunol Immunopathol.* 2020;220:109976, doi:10.1016/j.vetimm.2019.109976.

Herszberg B, Ramos-Barbon D, Tamaoka M, Martin JG, Lavoie JP. Heaves, an asthma-like equine disease, involves airway smooth muscle remodeling. *J Allergy Clin Immunol.* 2006;118(2):382-388.

Hirshman CA, Malley A, Downes H. Basenji-Greyhound model of asthma reactivity to Ascaris suum, citric acid and methacholine. *J Appl Physiol.* 1980;49(6):953-957.

Johnson LR, Johnson EG, Huiseboch SE, Dear JD, Vernau W. Eosinophilic bronchitis, eosinophilic granuloma, and eosinophilic bronchopneumopathy in 75 dogs (2006-2016). *J Vet Intern Med.* 2019;33(5):2217-2226.

Kuruvilla ME, Lee FE, Lee GB. Understanding asthma phenotypes, endotypes, and mechanisms of disease. *Clin Rev Allergy Immunol.* 2019;56(2):219-233.

Lambrecht BN, Hammad H. The immunology of asthma. *Nat Immunol.* 2015;16(1):45-56.

Lambrecht BN, Hammad H, Fahy JV. The cytokines of asthma. *Immunity.* 2019;50(4):975-991.

Lange-Consiglio A, Stucchi L, Zucca E, Lavoie JP, Cremonesi F, Ferrucci F. Insights into animal models for cell-based therapies in translational studies of lung diseases: is the horse with naturally occurring asthma the right choice? *Cytotherapy.* 2019;21(5):525-534.

Gy C, Leclere M, Vargas A, Grimes C, Lavoie JP. Investigation of blood biomarkers for the diagnosis of mild to moderate asthma in horses. *J Vet Intern Med.* 2019;33(4):1789-1795.

Leguillette R. Recurrent airway obstruction – heaves. *Vet Clin North Am Equine Pract.* 2003;19(1):63-86.

Li W, Gao P, Zhi Y, et al. Periostin: its role in asthma and its potential as a diagnostic or therapeutic target. *Respir Res.* 2015;16:57.

Redman TK, Rudolph K, Barr EB, Bowen LE, Muggenburg BA, Bice DE. Pulmonary immunology to ragweed in a beagle dog model of allergic asthma. *Exp Lung Res.* 2001;27(5):433-451.

Sheats MK, Davis KU, Poole JA. Comparative review of asthma in farmers and horses. *Curr Allergy Asthma Rep*. 2019;19(11):50. doi:10.1007/s11882-019-0882-2.

Uberti B, Moran G. Role of neutrophils in equine asthma. *Anim Health Res Rev*. 2018;19(1):65-73.

White SJ, Moore-Colyer M, Marti E, et al. Antigen array for serological diagnosis and novel allergen identification in severe equine asthma [Sci Rep.:2019];9(1):15170. doi:10.1038/s41598-019-51820-7.

Wypych TP, Wickransinghe LC, Marsland BJ. The influence of the microbiome on respiratory health. *Nat Immunol*. 2019;20(10):1279-1290.

CHAPTER 14

Drug Allergies

Under certain circumstances, many drugs can initiate an allergic response. Because of their chemical diversity, allergic responses to drugs will be equally diverse, and there are many different mechanisms involved in drug hypersensitivities. Although some drugs directly or indirectly trigger type 2 helper (Th2) or Th17 cells and thus cause an immediate hypersensitivity, it is important to note that all four types of hypersensitivity responses may also be triggered in response to drugs.

In humans, it is estimated that 15%–25% of patients suffer from harmful or unintended drug reactions. Adverse drug reactions are classified into types A and B (Fig. 14.1). Type A reactions are toxic effects due directly to the known pharmacological actions of the drug. They may result from overdosing or due to the drug binding to "off-target" receptors. They are somewhat predictable and could affect anyone. Good examples of type A reactions include the drowsiness caused by certain antihistamines and the anemia caused by high doses of sulfonamides. The characteristic feature of type A reactions is that the clinical signs and severity of the reaction are directly related to the dose of drug administered. Higher doses mean greater toxicity. More than 80% of adverse drug reactions are classified as type A.

Type B reactions only occur in susceptible animals and are idiosyncratic, uncommon, and unpredictable. They are generally lumped under the term hypersensitivity. In humans, type B reactions account for 5%–10% of adverse drug reactions. These hypersensitivities include IgE-mediated allergic reactions and drug interactions with cells of the innate and adaptive immune systems that do not involve antigen-binding receptors—these are considered pseudoallergic responses. Therefore, they are drug-dependent but not necessarily antigen-dependent responses. For example, some drugs may bind directly to receptors on lymphocytes and stimulate them to respond. There are many examples of drug hypersensitivities where the pharmacological agent binds to an immune receptor to provoke an adverse response. In addition, some drugs may bind inadvertently to receptors or enzymes and induce a clinical syndrome that closely resembles an allergic response. A probability assessment should be conducted to determine the probability that an adverse reaction is mediated by a drug (Table 14.1). Type B reactions can be subdivided into three types: allergic responses, immune receptor responses, and pseudoallergic responses.

Allergic Responses

Drug-mediated allergic reactions are most conveniently classified into four main hypersensitivity types based on the system devised by Robin Coombs and Philip Gell.

TYPE I HYPERSENSITIVITY

The most significant drug hypersensitivities are type I hypersensitivity reactions resulting from type 2 immune responses and mediated by IgE and mast cells. These occur in response to many drugs, especially antibiotics and hormones. They are commonly encountered in domestic animals. They are not restricted to active drugs. Even chemicals contained in leather preservatives used in harnesses, catgut sutures, or compounds such as methylcellulose or carboxymethylcellulose used as stabilizers in vaccines may provoke IgE-mediated allergic responses.

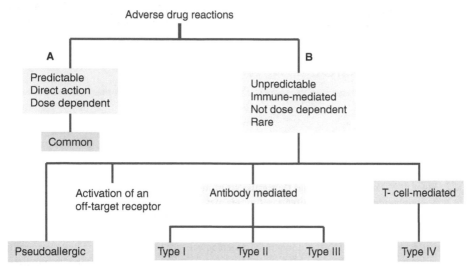

Fig. 14.1 **Classification of adverse drug reactions.** Type A reactions are a direct result of the toxic side-effects of the drug and largely predictable. Type B reactions, while less common than type A, are immunologically-mediated hypersensitivity responses and unpredictable.

TABLE 14.1 ■ **The Adverse Drug Reaction Probability Scale**

Question	Yes	No	Don't know
Are there previous conclusive reports of this adverse event?	1	0	0
Did this adverse event appear after the suspect drug was administered?	2	−1	0
Did the adverse event improve when the drug was discontinued or antagonist administered?	1	0	0
Did the adverse event reappear when the drug was readministered?	2	−1	0
Are there alternative causes that may have caused this?	−1	2	0
Did the adverse event reappear when a placebo was given?	−1	1	0
Was the drug detected in blood or tissues at a known toxic concentration?	1	0	0
Was the severity of the response affected by the dose administered?	1	0	0
Did the patient have a similar response to this drug when previously administered?	1	0	0
Was the adverse event confirmed by objective evidence?	1	0	0

The scores for all 10 questions are added together. A score of <1 is doubtful; a score of 1–4 is possible; a score of 5–8 is probable; a score of >9 is definitive.
(Naranjo CA, Busto O, Sellers EM, et al. A method of estimating the probability of adverse drug reactions. *Clin Pharmacol Ther.* 1981;30:239–245.)

Many of these drugs and their metabolites are too small to generate an immune response on their own. They must first bind covalently to proteins to generate an antigenic molecule. Thus, these drugs serve as haptens (Fig. 14.2). (Haptens are small molecules that by themselves are not antigenic; however, they can act as antigenic determinants when bound to a large carrier protein.) If these drug-protein complexes can be processed by antigen-presenting cells, they

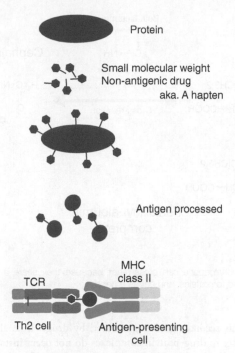

Fig. 14.2 Many low-molecular-weight drugs are only immunogenic because they can bind to proteins to form large, stable hapten-protein conjugates.

will be able to trigger immune responses. The complexes may, in theory, trigger any sort of immune response, including B cell- and T cell-mediated responses.

Examples of drugs that can bind stably and covalently to proteins and trigger immune responses include beta-lactam antibiotics such as penicillins, sulfanilamides, metamizole, some radiocontrast media, and muscle relaxants such as rocuronium.

The binding of drug molecules can change a normal protein such as serum albumin or transferrin, or even a cell surface protein such as an integrin or selectin, into a novel structure to which the immune system is no longer tolerant. Therefore, it can act as a foreign antigen. Some drugs act as pro-haptens and only gain the ability to bind to proteins after being metabolically activated.

Drug binding initially involves rapid non-covalent binding to a protein; however, covalent binding may follow. For example, the beta-lactam antibiotics react with lysine residues on proteins. There are eight exposed lysine residues on serum albumin that are accessible to beta-lactams. To be antigenic, these covalent bonds must be stable because proteins have to undergo processing by dendritic cells. This processing involves the fragmentation of antigens and their subsequent presentation on major histocompatibility complex (MHC) molecules. If the drug were to simply fall off the protein, it would no longer function as an antigen. Once processed, the drug-linked peptides can bind to MHC antigen-binding sites and induce a polyclonal immune response.

The recognition of drug-peptide complexes as foreign does not ensure that they will always trigger an immune response. Stimulation of innate immunity is also required to ensure an effective adaptive response. This innate stimulation usually occurs because the drug binds to pattern recognition receptors. This, in turn, may cause antigen-presenting cells such as dendritic cells to produce the necessary cytokines such as gamma interferon (IFN-γ) or interleukin (IL)-4. It is

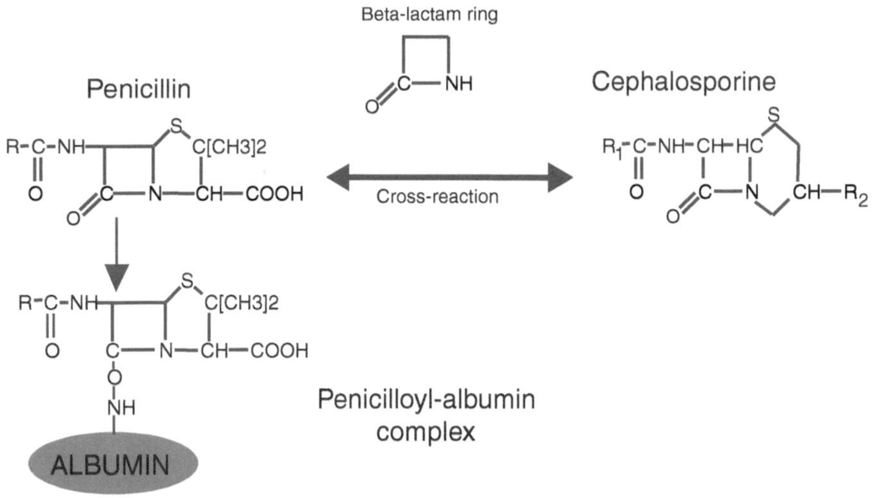

Fig. 14.3 Penicillin and cephalosporin can cross-react because they share a beta-lactam ring. This is chemically reactive, can bind to proteins, and act as a hapten.

not always clear how this second signal is generated by drugs. Like all adaptive immune responses, primary responses to drug-protein complexes do not occur instantly. It takes 7–14 days for antibodies to a drug to be produced by B cells and reach significant levels.

For example, penicillin allergy may be triggered either by therapeutic exposure or ingestion of penicillin-contaminated milk. The penicillin molecule is degraded in vivo to several compounds; the most important contains a reactive penicilloyl group. This penicilloyl group can bind to proteins, act as a hapten, and provoke an immune response (Fig. 14.3). It is not clear why some individuals develop a Th2 reaction to the drug while others develop a Th1 response. This may relate to the dose and type of drug-protein complex formed. It is probable that drugs binding to soluble proteins will be endocytosed and processed as exogenous antigens and trigger Th2 responses. On the other hand, drugs that bind to cell surface proteins will be recognized as endogenous antigens and trigger a Th1 response. Once an animal is sensitized, penicillin injection may cause acute systemic anaphylaxis or milder forms of allergy. Feeding penicillin-contaminated milk to these animals can also lead to allergic responses involving the skin or intestine. These reactions will not develop on first exposure to a drug; however, once the animal is sensitized, reactions will increase in severity with each subsequent exposure.

Mast cell degranulation requires antigen cross-linking between two IgE molecules attached to FcεRI. A single drug molecule linked to a protein will be unable to do this. Thus, two or more drug molecules must bind to a protein carrier to generate the cross-linking.

Experimental studies have generally used drug-protein complexes to both sensitize and then trigger an allergic reaction; this is not a requirement for drug-induced allergic reactions in animals. The eliciting drug-protein complex does not need to be completely identical to the sensitizing complex. Likewise, while covalent bonding is required for sensitization, rapid non-covalent bonding may be sufficient for elicitation. The complexes just need to be sufficiently stable to cross-link FcεRI on mast cells. This may explain the very rapid onset of drug-induced anaphylaxis, long before covalent bonds have had time to form.

The skin is the organ most often and obviously affected by drug-induced allergic reactions. Thus, a generalized exanthema with a red rash may develop within days following drug exposure. IgE- mediated drug responses will show typical signs of immediate hypersensitivity such as pruritic urticaria, where the edema is confined to the dermis (hives), or angioedema, where the edema spreads through the subcutis to cause an ill-defined swelling. Angioedema is often observed on the head or face. This is difficult to see in cats since their skin is elastic and wheals are indistinct. A rash with eosinophilia may also develop. The severity of the pruritus is variable. However, these reactions can also result in respiratory allergies with dyspnea and, if severe, anaphylaxis. The most dangerous forms of cutaneous drug reactions are Stevens-Johnson syndrome (SJS) and toxic epidermal necrolysis (TEN) (page 206). Both immediate and late-phase responses can occur in response to drugs. Immediate reactions occur within 1 h but occasionally up to 6 h later. Late-phase reactions mainly occur between 3 and 12 days later. Severe cutaneous adverse reactions (SCAR) may appear as late as 12–50 days post exposure.

Topical, intramuscular, and intravenous drug administration are more likely to result in allergic drug reactions than oral administration. Allergic reactions are more severe when a drug is administered rapidly, such as intravenously. Likewise, large macromolecules such as equine immune globulin and drugs that haptenate are more likely to elicit allergic reactions. In humans, atopic patients are more likely to develop type I reactions, presumably because of their predisposition to Th2 responses. Skin prick testing is used to a limited extent in humans to confirm a diagnosis of an IgE-mediated reaction. Other drug-induced skin reactions may resemble the autoimmune vesicular skin disease pemphigus foliaceus.

TYPE II HYPERSENSITIVITY

In type II hypersensitivity reactions, antibodies directed against antigens on cell surfaces acting in conjunction with complement result in target cell destruction. This is classified as cytotoxic hypersensitivity. If these antibodies are directed against drugs bound to erythrocytes or platelets, it will result in drug-induced hemolytic anemia or thrombocytopenia.

Red cells may be destroyed in drug hypersensitivity responses by three mechanisms. First, the drug and antibody may combine directly and activate the classical complement pathway, thereby destroying nearby red cells in a bystander effect.

Second, some drugs may bind to cell surface proteins. For example, penicillin, quinine, L-dopa, aminosalicylic acid, and phenacetin can bind to red cell glycoproteins. These chemically modified cells may then be recognized as foreign, trigger an immune response, and then be eliminated by antibodies, resulting in the development of hemolytic anemia. One such example, penicillin-induced hemolytic anemia, is not uncommon in horses. These conditions can be suspected based on recent treatment with penicillin and improvement in anemia when its use is discontinued. It may also be possible to detect antibodies against penicillin or penicillin-coated red cells in these animals. Sulfonamides, phenylbutazone, aminopyrine, phenothiazine, and possibly chloramphenicol may also cause agranulocytosis by binding to granulocytes. Phenylbutazone, quinine, chloramphenicol, and sulfonamides may trigger thrombocytopenia as they bind to platelets. Phenylbutazone has been implicated in the development of pancytopenia, including anemia and thrombocytopenia in dogs. If the cells of these affected animals are examined using a direct antiglobulin test, antibodies may be found bound to their surfaces. If these antibodies are eluted, they can be shown to be directed against the offending drug.

Third, drugs such as cephalosporins may chemically modify red cell membranes so that the cells will passively adsorb antibodies and then be removed by phagocytic cells. Cephalosporins have been reported to induce IgG-mediated hemolytic anemia, thrombocytopenia, and neutropenia in dogs.

TYPE III HYPERSENSITIVITY

Neutrophilic vasculitis may develop should a drug induce high-titered antibodies and generate large quantities of immune complexes. These complexes are often deposited in blood vessel walls within the skin. The resulting vasculitis can range in severity from mild to life-threatening. Anti-neutrophil antibodies have been detected in dogs with a sulfonamide allergy. Meloxicam has also been reported to induce a neutrophilic vasculitis. Fixed drug eruptions are circumscribed erythematous lesions that develop into local edema, eventually developing into bullae that may then ulcerate.

Sweet's syndrome in humans is a sterile neutrophilic dermatitis. The affected individuals develop pyrexia, a neutrophilia, and painful papules or nodules with diffuse neutrophilic infiltrate within the superficial dermis. A similar syndrome has been described in dogs. The affected animals also develop vasculitis, immune-mediated hemolytic anemia, and thrombocytopenia. Some canine cases resembling Sweet's syndrome are believed to be adverse reactions to carprofen. There have been reports of dog deaths following carprofen treatment due to neutrophilic dermatosis and the development of vasculitis.

Some drug hypersensitivities result in a clinical presentation that closely resembles the lesions of systemic lupus erythematosus. These lupoid-like lesions consist of erythema, scaling, crusting, erosions, and ulceration at mucocutaneous junctions. They have been reported to be caused by sulfonamides, hydralazine, and primidone in dogs.

TYPE IV HYPERSENSITIVITY

Type IV reactions are T cell-mediated delayed responses that do not develop for several days to 2 weeks after drug exposure. There are many different examples of these T cell-mediated drug hypersensitivities. One example is allergic contact dermatitis. In this disease, the drug covalently attaches to skin epithelial cells and acts as a hapten. The altered skin cells are then recognized as foreign and are attacked and destroyed by cytotoxic T cells. Skin patch testing may be used to confirm the existence of a drug-induced delayed T cell-mediated hypersensitivity (Chapter 19).

Severe Cutaneous Adverse Reactions (SCARs)

Some drug hypersensitivities can induce T cell-mediated life-threatening SCARs. These consist of three related mucocutaneous disorders—erythema multiforme (EM), SJS, and TEN. All are well recognized in humans and have been diagnosed in dogs and cats. All three diseases are characterized by skin loss of increasing severity. However, the three diseases overlap considerably, making precise classification sometimes difficult.

Erythema Multiforme (EM). The mildest of the three, EM is an uncommon disease of dogs affecting the skin, mucous membranes, or mucocutaneous junctions. It is characterized by sudden onset, raised patchy eruptions, skin loss affecting less than 10% of the body surface, and low morbidity. Animals develop flat or raised macular or patchy eruptions, mucocutaneous vesicles, and urticarial plaques. EM may be triggered by drugs and allergies to certain foods such as beef or soy. In dogs and cats, it is caused by diverse medications, including antibiotics, sulfonamides, aurothioglucose, propylthiouracil, and griseofulvin.

EM may disappear without sequelae within a few days when the drug is discontinued. It is subclassified into two forms, EM-minor and EM-major. EM-minor cases generally involve no more than one mucosal surface. EM-major involves two or more. A definitive diagnosis is made by examining biopsy samples, showing a cytotoxic interface dermatitis with keratinocyte destruction in the basal and suprabasal layers.

Stevens-Johnson Syndrome (SJS). SJS is much less common than EM but more severe. Its lesions are widespread and develop into confluent patchy erythematous or purpuric eruptions involving more than 50% of the body surface. However, epithelial detachment involves less than

10% of the body surface. Beginning about 14 days after drug exposure, the skin begins to blister and slough. Animals develop generalized illness, including dyspnea, vomiting, fever, and weight loss. Sloughing of the epidermis occurs over the nasal planum, footpads, and oral, pharyngeal, nasal, conjunctival, and preputial mucosa. Fluid loss leads to electrolyte imbalances, and life-threatening secondary infections are common. Biopsy shows extensive epidermal cell death.

Toxic Epidermal Necrolysis (TEN). TEN is the most serious of the three SCARs, with generalized erythematous or purpuric patches. The affected animals lose more than 30% of their epidermis, which sloughs off in large sheets, and mortality is high. Histopathological findings are similar in all three diseases. TEN/SJS overlap syndrome is similar; however, skin detachment involves 10%–30% of the body surface.

All three SCARs are associated with the development of a T cell-mediated hypersensitivity response to drugs. The drugs most commonly implicated have been antibiotics such as cephalosporins and penicillins. They also include trimethoprim-potentiated sulfonamides, carbamazepine, allopurinol, dapsone, abacavir, and phenytoin.

The skin lesions are infiltrated mainly by $CD8^+$ T cells. These cytotoxic T cells infiltrate SJS/TEN lesions and release large amounts of their cytotoxic protein, granulysin. Intradermal inoculation of granulysin solutions in mice at a concentration found in blister fluid results in the development of lesions mimicking SJS.

The question arises, how are the T cells stimulated in such an intense manner? These diseases probably result from a P-I response (see below). In these cases, the drug binds with high affinity to the specific antigen receptors on T cells and forces the cells to react unusually strongly.

Treatment of SCARs involves immediate withdrawal of the offending drug followed by symptomatic treatment, including fluid replacement. Corticosteroids should be avoided because they increase the animal's susceptibility to skin infections and worsen the prognosis. Antibiotics should only be administered if skin infections occur. Intravenous administration of high doses of human immunoglobulins have been used successfully to treat these diseases in dogs. The immunoglobulins block CD95/CD95-L (an apoptosis-triggering receptor) interactions and prevent keratinocytes from receiving the apoptosis signal.

Immune Receptor Interactions

Pharmacological interaction with immune receptors is a form of drug hypersensitivity in which a drug triggers an immune response by binding covalently to T cell antigen receptors. (This is called a P-I response.) As a result, the drugs directly activate T cells. This might result in hypersensitivities or the development of an autoimmune disease. P-I reactions are slow to develop, depending on the affinity of the drug for the T cell receptor. Thus, it takes 28–35 days for sensitivity to develop to flucloxacillin. This off-target type of response is dose dependent and somewhat predictable. It may affect both $CD4^+$ and $CD8^+$ T cells and, if the interaction is sufficiently strong, no other T cell help may be required. P-I responses may result in the activation of cytotoxic T cells. The clinical consequences will depend on the nature and affinity of the drug-receptor binding.

Some drugs may also bind to MHC molecules expressed on T cells. They can bind to the antigen-binding groove or elsewhere on the molecule, which may be important for determining the nature and severity of the T cell response.

Examples of drugs that can interact directly with immune receptors include β-lactam antibiotics, sulfanilamides, chinolones, vancomycin, and some local anesthetics such as lidocaine. Some drugs may reactivate viral infections and trigger cutaneous viral rashes. Given the diversity of drugs used in animals, it is unsurprising that multiple mechanisms may be involved. Even hypersensitivities to a single drug might be mediated via many different pathways.

Pseudoallergic Reactions

These occur when a drug interacts with receptors or enzymes in inflammatory cells to trigger acute inflammation. They are often clinically indistinguishable from true allergic reactions, although they are not associated with the production of specific antibodies or T cells. Examples of drugs that induce pseudoallergic responses include non-steroidal anti-inflammatory drugs (NSAIDs) such as acetylsalicylic acid, diclofenac, chinolones such as ciprofloxacin, radiocontrast media, muscle relaxants, and vancomycin. (These are really type A reactions that elicit immune inflammation.) Many neuromuscular-blocking drugs such as tubocurarine and fluoroquinolone antibiotics such as ciprofloxacin can trigger the MRGPRs on mast cells and provoke degranulation and histamine release. They may block enzymes such as cyclooxygenases and result in elevated leukotrienes on NSAID therapy. They may interfere with protease activity, thus resulting in persistently high bradykinin levels. Therefore, these drugs may trigger the development of acute urticaria or even non-IgE-mediated anaphylaxis. They may directly stimulate the release of mediators such as histamine, prostaglandins, leukotrienes, or kinins. NSAIDs and angiotensin-converting enzyme inhibitors are common causes of pseudoallergic reactions. Opioids such as morphine may trigger an intensely pruritic inflammatory response in the skin by directly triggering histamine release from mast cells.

Some Specific Drugs

ANTIBIOTICS

β-lactam antibiotics, which include penicillins, cephalosporins, carbapenems, and monobactams, are the drugs most associated with antibiotic allergies and delayed reactions in humans and dogs. The β-lactam ring is unstable under physiological conditions and generates bonds that bind covalently to lysine residues on host serum proteins. In general, penicillins are more reactive than cephalosporins and are significantly more allergenic. Other antibiotics reported to cause allergic responses include fluoroquinolones, macrolides, tetracyclines, and glycopeptides, especially vancomycin. Penicillin is the most frequent drug allergy in humans. In seeking substitutes, it is important to use antibiotics that do not contain the reactive penicilloyl group. Carbapenems and second-generation cephalosporins are satisfactory, but monobactams and first-generation cephalosporins may cross-react and result in multiple drug hypersensitivities.

Hypersensitivities to penicillin were first reported in the 1940s, not long after the drug was first used in humans. These included injection site reactions, serum-sickness type reactions, and delayed T cell-mediated responses. Between 5% and 15% of patients in developed countries may be allergic to penicillin. In the United States, approximately 1%–2% of patients are allergic to cephalosporins. In the case of equine responses to procaine penicillin, the procaine is rapidly dissociated from the penicillin in the bloodstream. Therefore, the adverse events may simply be due to the toxic effects of the procaine on the brain and central nervous system and may not be immune-mediated. However, horses may also develop urticaria and anaphylaxis in response to the water-soluble sodium or potassium salts of penicillin.

Surveys have shown that severe anaphylactic reactions have occurred in cats in response to the use of antibiotic ophthalmic preparations. These often contain a mixture of antibacterial molecules, including bacitracin, neomycin, oxytetracycline, and polymyxin B, and it is often difficult to determine which of these is responsible for the allergic response. However, polymyxin B is used experimentally as a mast cell degranulating agent. The most severe anaphylactic reactions occurred within 10 minutes of drug application. Rashes and "drug fever" can develop in response to cephalosporins; however, anaphylaxis is uncommon.

SULFONAMIDES

Sulfonamides and trimethoprim-sulfonamide combinations may trigger dose-dependent type A adverse reactions, such as anemia, hematuria, and thyroid hormone synthesis inhibition. However, they also trigger type B idiosyncratic allergic reactions. These generally occur several days after treatment initiation and most cases, present as T cell-mediated delayed hypersensitivity responses. In dogs, they occur on average between 5 and 36 days after treatment initiation. Thus, they may develop several days after a 7–10-day course of treatment is completed. Clinical signs include fever, polyarthritis, skin lesions such as facial swelling, hepatotoxicity, blood dyscrasias, uveitis, keratoconjunctivitis, lymphadenopathy, and proteinuria. Less common manifestations include pancreatitis, meningitis, facial palsy, polymyositis, and TEN or a lupus-like syndrome. Fever develops in about half of the affected dogs. The prevalence of these reactions is approximately 0.25% of cases in dogs and cats. Other surveys indicate a higher prevalence and suggest that sulfonamide hypersensitivity could account for about 80% of reactions to antimicrobials in dogs. It is much less common in cats.

Sulfonamide-induced polyarthritis is commonly documented, especially in large-breed dogs such as Doberman Pinschers. A single nucleotide polymorphism in the canine cytochrome-b_5 reductase gene is associated with sulfonamide hypersensitivity in Dobermans. Thus, they have a limited ability to detoxify the hydroxylamine metabolites of these drugs. Synovial fluid analysis shows high neutrophil numbers, suggesting a Th17-mediated response. Blood dyscrasias have also been reported in dogs receiving potentiated sulfonamides, including thrombocytopenia, neutropenia, and antiglobulin-positive hemolytic anemia. Acute hepatopathy also occurs as a result of severe hepatic necrosis and carries a poor prognosis. The most favored hypothesis regarding the pathogenesis of sulfonamide hypersensitivity is that they act as prohaptens. Thus, during the initial step, the parent drug is metabolized to reactive metabolites. These, in turn, haptenate tissue proteins. The adducts are then processed, leading to T cell activation. Of the three possible T cell responses, it appears that Th2-mediated antibody production by B cells is not triggered in many patients. Immediate IgE-mediated responses to sulfonamides are uncommon. Nevertheless, some affected dogs do possess anti-sulfonamide IgE. On the other hand, evidence suggests that the response is primarily mediated by T cells, most notably Th1 cells. Studies on humans and laboratory animals have detected T cells that are responsive to sulfonamides and their metabolites.

The structure of non-antibiotic sulfonamides such as the thiazide diuretics and some NSAIDs is very different from that of the antibiotic ones. They lack the arylamine portion of the molecule, which is responsible for the hypersensitivity responses. (Therefore, they cannot acetylate aromatic amines.) These can therefore be used with little risk. One exception is sulfasalazine, which is metabolized to a structure similar to sulfamethoxazole.

NSAIDS

Acetylsalicylic acid and other NSAIDs may cause allergic and pseudoallergic hypersensitivity reactions due to direct mast cell activation. These include mild reactions such as local skin rashes and gastrointestinal irritation. More severe reactions include aspirin-exacerbated respiratory disease, urticaria, angioedema, and anaphylaxis, or even SCARs such as TEN and SJS. NSAID-induced allergic reactions account for up to a third of drug-related reactions in humans. Most reactions to NSAIDs do not involve immunological responses but are related to the inhibition of cyclooxygenase (COX)-1. COX-1 inhibition shifts the arachidonic acid metabolic pathway from the production of anti-inflammatory prostaglandins such as prostaglandin E_2 (PGE_2) toward the production of pro-inflammatory leukotrienes. PGE_2 normally suppresses the sensitivity of mast cells. If PGE_2 is suppressed, the dysregulated mast cells are easily activated. IgE plays

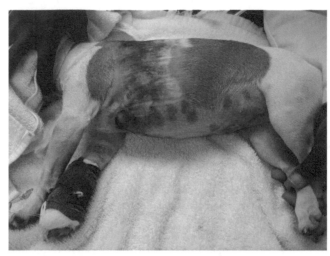

Fig. 14.4 An adverse reaction to sedation with phenobarbital. (Courtesy Dr. Robert Kennis.)

no role in the process. These non-allergic responses can be triggered by many different NSAIDs; therefore, an animal experiencing one may also react to any COX-1 inhibitor. Some of the manifestations of NSAID hypersensitivity include the exacerbation of respiratory or cutaneous diseases. Some NSAIDs induce urticaria, angioedema, or even laryngeal edema and anaphylaxis. In the case of skin disease, symptoms appear within 30 min to 4 h after ingesting the NSAID. The animal will either develop urticaria or exacerbate existing urticaria. Respiratory reactions include dyspnea, bronchospasm, eosinophilic rhinitis, and nasal congestion. T cell-mediated delayed hypersensitivity responses to NSAIDs have also been reported in humans. They occur within 24–48 h of exposure and the common symptoms are maculopapular eruptions, contact dermatitis, and photosensitivity.

ANTICONVULSIVE DRUGS

The use of anticonvulsive agents in dogs and humans is often associated with adverse reactions and is of significant concern to owners. These reactions include blood cell dyscrasias, hepatopathy, or, most commonly, skin disorders. Superficial necrolytic dermatitis or metabolic dermal necrosis has occurred after many years of therapy with drugs such as phenobarbital, primidone, and potassium bromide (Fig 14.4). These drugs produce erythematous macules that can progress to EM, and hypercutaneous crusts with fissures. In prospective studies, more than 10% of dogs receiving these drugs, especially phenobarbital, exhibited cutaneous signs. These ranged from urticaria and angioedema to severe generalized syndromes such as lupoid or pemphigoid lesions to SJS. There may be common immunological mechanisms linking skin disease and epilepsy.

LOCAL ANESTHETICS

In many cases, the allergic reactions associated with the administration of local anesthetics may be related to excipients, including preservatives and epinephrine. Anaphylaxis has been associated with the use of the local anesthetic proparacaine in eye drops. The general anesthetic alphaxalone has also been reported to cause anaphylaxis in dogs.

PROPYLTHIOURACIL

Propylthiouracil is a cytotoxic drug used for the treatment of hyperthyroidism in cats. However, its use can result in the development of a lupus-like syndrome. Thus, cats lose weight, become lethargic, and develop a fever. They eventually develop antiglobulin-positive hemolytic anemia, antinuclear antibodies, and antibodies to the enzyme myeloperoxidase. Myeloperoxidase oxidizes propylthiouracil to an active ingredient, and this is a common feature of drugs that induce lupus-like disease. It is not known how it induces autoimmunity.

Management

The most effective management strategy for drug allergies is avoidance. When available, alternative drugs with unrelated chemical structures should be substituted. Remember that drugs with similar structures may cross-react. Obviously, should the animal suffer an anaphylactic attack, immediate treatment is imperative.

Suggested Readings

Blumenthal KG, Peter JG, Trubiano JA, Phillips EJ. Antibiotic allergy. *Lancet.* 2019;393(10167):183-198.

Castells M, Khan DA, Phillips EJ. Penicillin allergy. *N Engl J Med.* 2019;381(24):2338-2351. doi:10.1056/ NEJMra1807761.

Hinn AC, Olivry T, Luther PB, Cannon AG, Yager JA. Erythema multiforme, Stevens-Johnson syndrome, and toxic epidermal necrolysis in the dog: clinical classification, drug exposure and histopathological correlations. *J Vet Allergy Clin Immunol.* 1998;6:13-20.

Hume-Smith KM, Groth AD, Rishniw M, Walter-Grimm LA, Plunkett SJ, Maggs DJ. Anaphylactic events observed within 4 h of ocular application of an antibiotic-containing ophthalmic preparation: 61 cats (1993-2010). *J Feline Med Surg.* 2011;13(10):774-751.

Kahn DA, Knowles SR, Shear NH. Sulfonamide hypersensitivity: fact and fiction. *J Allergy Clin Immunol Pract.* 2019;7(7):2116-2123.

Koch T, Mueller RS, Dobenecker B, Fischer A. Cutaneous adverse drug reactions in dogs treated with antiepileptic drugs. *Front Vet Sci.* 2016;3:27. doi:10.3389/fvets.2016.00027.

Lavergne SN, Danhof RS, Volkman EM, Trepanier LA. Association of drug-serum protein adducts and anti-drug antibodies in dogs with sulfonamide hypersensitivity: a naturally occurring model of idiosyncratic drug toxicity. *Clin Exp Allergy.* 2006;36(7):907-915.

Mellor PJ, Roulois JA, Day MJ, Blacklaws BA, Knivett SJ, Herrtage ME. Neutrophilic dermatitis and immune-mediated haematological disorders in a dog: suspected adverse reaction to carprofen. *J Small Anim Pract.* 2005;46(5):237-242.

Naranjo CA, Busto U, Sellers EM, et al. A method for estimating the probability of adverse drug reactions. *Clin Pharmacol Ther.* 1981;30(2):239-245.

Niza MM, Felix N, Vilela CL, Peleteiro MC, Ferreira AJ. Cutaneous and ocular adverse reactions in a dog following meloxicam administration. *Vet Dermatol.* 2007;18(1):45-49. doi:10.1111/j.1365-3164.2007. 00556.x.

Noli C, Koeman JP, Willemse T. A retrospective evaluation of adverse reactions to trimethoprim-sulphonamide combinations in dogs and cats. *Vet Q.* 1995;17(4):123-128.

Olsén L, Ingvast-Larsson C, Broström H, Larsson P, Tjälve H. Clinical signs and etiology of adverse reactions to procaine benzylpenicillin and sodium/potassium benzylpenicillin in horses. *J Vet Pharmacol Ther.* 2007;30(3):201-207.

Pichler W. Immune pathomechanism and classification of drug hypersensitivity. *Allergy.* 2019;74(8): 1457-1471.

Reinhart JM, Ekena J, Cioffi AC, Trepanier LA. A single-nucleotide polymorphism in the canine cytochrome b5 reductase (CYB5R3) gene is associated with sulfonamide hypersensitivity and is overrepresented in Doberman Pinschers. *J Vet Pharmacol Ther.* 2018;41(3):402-408.

Trepanier LA. Idiosyncratic toxicity associated with potentiated sulfonamides in the dog. *J Vet Pharmacol Ther.* 2004;27(3):129-138.

Uetrecht J. Role of animal models in the study of drug-induced hypersensitivity reactions. *AAPS J.* 2006;7(4):E914-E921.

Voie KL, Campbell KL, Lavergne SN. Drug hypersensitivity reactions targeting the skin in dogs and cats. *J Vet Intern Med.* 2012;26(4):863-874.

Warrington R, Silviu-Dan F. Drug allergy. *Allergy Asthma Clin Immunol.* 2011;7(suppl):S10.

CHAPTER 15

Allergies to Vaccines

Routine immunization is the most effective method of preventing death and morbidity from infectious diseases in both humans and animals; however, rare allergic reactions may occur and some may be life-threatening. Estimates of the prevalence of allergic reactions to vaccines in humans range from 1 in 100,000 to 1 in 1,000,000 doses administered.

The deliberate injection of a foreign antigen into an animal to elicit a protective response carries the risk of triggering a type 2 immune response. Therefore, vaccines have the potential to cause rare but serious allergic reactions. Allergic responses may occur when an animal produces IgE in response to the immunizing antigen and other components (excipients) present in vaccines. For example, reactions may occur after the injection of vaccines that contain trace amounts of fetal calf serum (FCS), bovine serum albumin (BSA), egg proteins (ovalbumin), or gelatin. Gelatin and serum albumin are added to vaccines as stabilizers to protect the vaccine antigens from degradation during the freeze-drying process. Some vaccines may also contain antibiotics such as neomycin to which an animal may be sensitive. All forms of hypersensitivity are more commonly associated with repeated injections of antigens and, therefore, tend to be associated with the use of killed vaccines.

A type I hypersensitivity reaction is an immediate response to an antigen and occurs within a few minutes after exposure. Reactions occurring more than 4 h after administering a vaccine reflect late-phase responses and are not consistent with acute anaphylaxis. Allergic reactions also need to be distinguished from other clinical responses often associated with vaccination. These include anxiety and local injection site reactions such as erythema and itching that may be immediate or delayed, and mild "sickness," including fever and vomiting.

Type I Hypersensitivities

THE EXCIPIENT PROBLEM

Excipients can be major contributors to vaccine-initiated immediate reactions. These are often the result of a preexisting allergy to milk, eggs, or gelatin. In human vaccines, strenuous efforts have been made to reduce the concentrations of these vaccine excipients. In veterinary vaccines, especially livestock vaccines where price is an issue, excipient reduction may not be cost-effective. Vaccines are complex mixtures with many added components designed to ensure reasonable shelf life and the proteins needed to produce sufficient quantities of viral antigens. One of the most common excipients found in vaccines is fetal calf serum. This is a complex mixture of proteins, many of which are potential allergens (Fig. 15.1). In one study that investigated the antibody profile of dogs that had developed immediate reactions following rabies vaccination, it was found that seven out of eight dogs mounted an IgE response directed against antigens in fetal bovine serum. There were large amounts of BSA and bovine IgG in these vaccines. (In theory, serum taken from a bovine fetus should lack IgG because this cannot cross the bovine placenta. In practice, however, it is inconvenient to obtain blood from a fetus at slaughter. Therefore, the serum may be taken from presuckling calves. If they had managed to suckle, however,

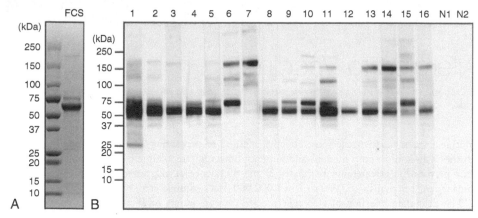

Fig. 15.1   Importance of fetal calf serum (FCS) as a vaccine allergen. (A) SDS-PAGE analysis of FCS. An FCS sample (2 mg/lane) was subjected to SDS-PAGE through a 5%–20% gradient polyacrylamide gel under reducing conditions, and the gel was stained with Coomassie brilliant blue. Molecular weight size markers are indicated along the left side. The 70 kDa band is serum albumin. (B) Immunoblot analysis of serum samples from dogs that developed post-vaccination allergic reactions to detect IgE directed against FCS components. Numbers 1–16 indicate the numbers of the dogs that exhibited allergic reactions to vaccination. N1 and N2 indicate the negative control dogs. (From Ohmori K, et al. Immunoblot analysis for IgE-reactive components of fetal calf serum in dogs that developed allergic reactions after non-rabies vaccination. *Vet Immunol Immunopathol*, 115:166-171, 2007.)

the product will contain some IgG.) Other potential allergens in FCS may include fibrinogen, fibronectin, lipoproteins, macroglobulins, and transferrin.

The eighth dog in the above study had IgE antibodies directed against gelatin and casein. These had also been added to the vaccine to serve as stabilizers. A similar phenomenon was seen in a group of children who developed anaphylaxis after exposure to the measles-mumps-rubella vaccine. Most reacted to the gelatin that had been added to the vaccine as a stabilizer. Gelatin of bovine or porcine origin is commonly added to many human vaccines and it is a known allergen. One type of allergy that is unique to gelatin-containing vaccines is galactose-alpha-1,3 galactose (alpha-gal) hypersensitivity. As described in Chapter 11, this is a tick-induced disease where bites from ticks that have fed on cattle stimulate IgE antibodies against the cross-reactive carbohydrate epitope, galactose-alpha-1,3 galactose. Therefore, sensitized individuals can develop a type I hypersensitivity response after exposure to beef- or pork-derived gelatin. This includes gelatin-containing vaccines. Casein is also recognized as a major allergen in milk-sensitive humans and dogs (and cows).

While the World Health Organization recommends that BSA in vaccines should not exceed 50 ng/dose, some animal vaccines may exceed this. One such problem occurs with Leptospira vaccines, where high levels of BSA are required to grow these organisms successfully in culture. In addition, there are more adverse events associated with a quadrivalent leptospirosis vaccine than a bivalent one. However, these are exceedingly rare. Thus, for the bivalent Leptospira vaccine the reported adverse event rate is 0.015%, or 2 adverse events reported for every 10,000 doses sold. For the quadrivalent vaccine, the rate is 0.069%, or fewer than 7 events reported for every 10,000 doses sold.

Antibiotics such as gentamycin or neomycin may be used during vaccine production to prevent bacterial growth. Most are removed during the purification process and rarely cause hypersensitivity. Similarly, preservatives such as thiomerosal and 2-phenoxyethanol are used in multidose vials of vaccine to prevent bacterial growth. Thiomerosal has been associated with the development of an allergic contact dermatitis but rarely systemic allergic responses. Contact dermatitis has also been associated with the presence of 2-phenoxyethanol in human influenza vaccines. Latex hypersensitivity is common in humans and latex may be a constituent of the rubber stoppers used in some vaccine vials. It rarely causes problems in humans and has not yet been reported in animals. Some batches of older foot-and-mouth disease vaccines induced anaphylactic reactions in cattle directed against the antifoaming agent hydroxypropylmethylcellulose.

PREVALENCE OF ALLERGIC REACTIONS

By examining the electronic records of a very large, small-animal general practice, it has been possible to determine the prevalence of vaccine-associated adverse events in over a million dogs. The use of a standardized reporting system within a very large population has permitted objective analysis of the prevalence of adverse events occurring within 3 days of vaccine administration. Out of 1,226,159 dogs receiving 3,439,576 vaccine doses, 4678 adverse events were recorded (38.2/10,000 dogs); 72.8% of these events occurred on the same day the vaccine was administered, 31.7% were considered to be allergic reactions, 1.7% were classified as anaphylaxis, and 65.8% were considered "vaccine reactions" and were likely due to innate immune responses. Three dogs died. The lowest rate of such events was associated with *Bordetella bronchiseptica* vaccination and the highest rate with *Borrelia burgdorferi* vaccination. Additional analysis indicated that the risk of adverse events was significantly greater for small dogs than for large dogs, for neutered than for sexually intact dogs, and for dogs that received multiple vaccines on a single occasion.

Each additional vaccine dose administered increased the risk of an adverse event occurring by 27% in dogs under 10 kg and 12% in dogs heavier than 12 kg (Fig. 15.2). High-risk breeds included Dachshunds, Pugs, Boston Terriers, Miniature Pinschers, and Chihuahuas. Overall, the increased prevalence of adverse events in young adult, small-breed, neutered dogs and their relationship to multiple dosing suggests that veterinarians should look carefully at the practice of giving the same vaccine dose to all dogs irrespective of their size.

In another study, 351 dogs out of 57,300 vaccinated showed an adverse event (62.7/10,000 doses). (Vaccines used included canine parvovirus, canine distemper, canine adenovirus 2, canine coronavirus, and leptospirosis.) Of these 351 dogs, 1 died, 41 had anaphylaxis, 244 developed dermatological signs, and 160 showed gastrointestinal signs. Approximately half of the anaphylaxis events occurred within 5 minutes of vaccination (Fig. 15.3). Additional analysis of these anaphylaxis cases reported 87% collapse, 77% cyanosis, and both collapse and cyanosis in 71% of affected dogs. Breeds affected included Miniature Dachshunds (50%) (these accounted for about 30% of all anaphylaxis cases), Chihuahuas (10%), mixed breeds (5%), and Toy Poodles (5%). Miniature Schnauzers were unusually prone to anaphylaxis. The highest frequency of adverse reactions occurred in dogs under 5 kg. Most adverse events were observed within 12 h after vaccination.

In a study of 27 dogs in Japan that had developed adverse reactions to rabies vaccination and were reported to the authorities, 26% developed gastrointestinal symptoms such as vomiting or diarrhea; 22% developed respiratory symptoms, including dyspnea, tachypnea, bradycardia, hypotension, or hypothermia; and 11% developed skin reactions such as urticaria, facial edema, and pruritus. In 284 cases of allergic reactions to non-rabies vaccines, 53% developed dermatologic signs, 16% developed gastrointestinal symptoms, and 14% developed respiratory/cardiovascular symptoms. The adverse event rate in Japan as reported in these studies (62.7/10,000 doses) was much higher than in the United Kingdom (0.093/10,000 doses) or in the United States (38.2/10,000 doses). Similar results have been reported in cats (Fig. 15.4).

Few studies have investigated the prevalence of adverse allergic events in livestock species. These only come to our attention if they happen in unusually large numbers. For example, multiple severe allergic responses have been reported after using some specific killed foot-and-mouth disease, rabies,

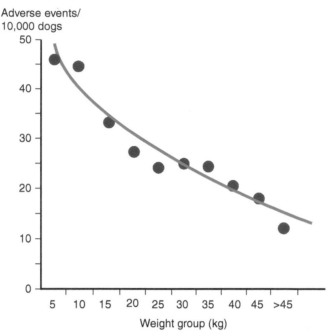

Fig. 15.2 **Prevalence of adverse events to vaccines decreases as the animal's weight increases.** It may be necessary to take this into account when vaccinating very small dogs. (Data from Moore GE, et al. *J Am Vet Med Assn* 2005;227:1102.)

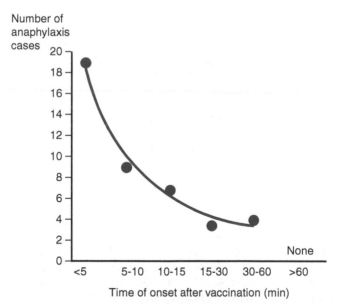

Fig. 15.3 **Timing of adverse events.** Because most adverse events are mediated by direct toxicity or type I hypersensitivity reactions, most reactions will occur within 5 minutes after vaccination. (Data from Miyaji K, Suzuki A, Shimakura H, et al. *Vet Immunol Immunopathol* 2012;145:447-452.)

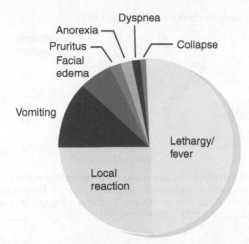

Fig. 15.4 Nature of vaccine-associated adverse events in cats occurring within 3 days post-vaccination. (Data from Moore GE, DeSantis-Kerr AC, Guptill LF, Glickman NW, Lewis HB, Glickman LT. *J Am Vet Med Assn* 2007;231:94-100.)

and contagious bovine pleuropneumonia vaccines in cattle. Signs included angioedema affecting mainly the head and ears, urticaria, pruritus, acute-onset diarrhea, vomiting, dyspnea, and collapse. Such vaccines are rapidly withdrawn from the market when problems are identified.

TREATMENT

Unlike drugs, the risks of an allergic response to vaccines is well recognized and may be anticipated. Therefore, vaccine packages invariably carry a warning regarding the risks of such occurrences. This should not be disregarded. It is good practice to keep an animal under observation for 15–25 minutes after vaccination to ensure that any immediate problems can be promptly recognized and treated. Additionally, epinephrine should always be readily available in case it is needed. Anaphylaxis is a syndrome with specific clinical features and, even if the underlying causal allergens cannot be immediately ascertained, it is important to treat all such episodes as medical emergencies.

Type II Hypersensitivities

In type II hypersensitivity reactions, antibodies directed against an animal's own cells act together with complement to bind to target cells and cause cell lysis. These antibodies can be induced by the presence of animal cells in a vaccine.

HEMOLYTIC DISEASE OF THE NEWBORN

Natural hemolytic disease in newborn calves is very rare but may result from prior vaccination against anaplasmosis or babesiosis (Fig. 15.5). These vaccines contain pooled red cells from multiple infected calves. In the case of Anaplasma vaccines, for example, the blood from infected donor animals is pooled, freeze-dried, and mixed with adjuvant before being administered to cattle. The vaccine against babesiosis consists of fresh, infected calf blood. Both vaccines result in infection and, consequently, the development of immunity in recipients. They may also stimulate

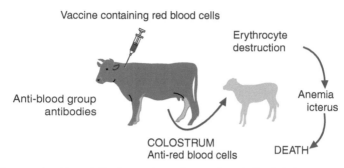

Fig. 15.5 Pathogenesis of hemolytic disease in newborn calves. In the first stage, a vaccine containing bovine erythrocytes is administered to the cow and sensitizes her. In the second stage, these antibodies are concentrated in the colostrum. When they are ingested by the suckling calf, they enter the calf's circulation and cause red cell destruction, leading to splenomegaly and anemia.

the production of antibodies against blood group antigens on the injected red cells, like an incompatible transfusion. If cows sensitized to foreign blood group antigens by these vaccines are then mated with bulls carrying the same blood groups, they can transmit these antibodies to their calves through their colostrum. The calves that drink this colostrum may then absorb the antibodies and develop hemolytic disease as the antibodies and complement destroy their incompatible erythrocytes.

In 1936, a vaccine was developed against hog cholera by adding the dye crystal violet to pooled blood from viremic pigs. The vaccine worked well and protected pigs against hog cholera. However, because it contained pig blood, it sensitized recipients to the foreign blood group antigens in the vaccine. As a result, vaccinated sows produced antibodies against these foreign blood groups. Piglets suckling colostrum ingested these antibodies in a concentrated form. If these antibodies were directed against the piglet's blood groups, their red cells were destroyed. As a result, piglets developed progressive weakness and severe anemia and many died. Those animals that survived longest developed hemoglobinuria and jaundice. The disease ceased to be a problem once the crystal violet vaccine was withdrawn.

BOVINE NEONATAL PANCYTOPENIA

Beginning in 2007, outbreaks of a hemorrhagic disease in newborn calves were reported from many countries in western Europe. It is now called bovine neonatal pancytopenia (Fig. 15.6). Affected calves showed sudden onset bleeding, including nasal hemorrhage, petechiation on mucous membranes, internal bleeding, and excessive bleeding from minor wounds such as injection or ear-tag sites. The disease developed 7–28 days after birth and the affected calves could die within 48 h of disease onset. Hematology of these calves showed that an early drop in platelets, monocytes, and neutrophils was followed by major drops in erythrocyte and lymphocyte numbers. The net result was profound pancytopenia, including thrombocytopenia, anemia, and leucopenia. The bone marrow of affected calves became completely aplastic. Mortality was as high as 90% in clinically affected calves, but there were many subclinical cases. Because the disease only occurred in suckled calves and developed within days of first suckling, it appeared to result from the consumption of colostrum. Further investigations showed that the serum and colostrum from cows known to produce affected calves contained high levels of antibodies directed against their major histocompatibility complex (MHC) class I molecules. These molecules are expressed on the surface of neonatal leukocytes and their bone marrow stem cell precursors. They are found

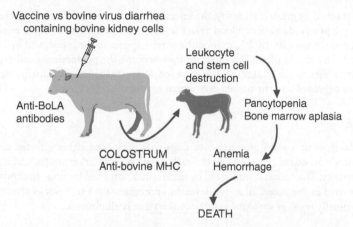

Fig. 15.6 Pathogenesis of bovine neonatal pancytopenia. This was a unique response caused by a single vaccine containing bovine kidney cells. MHC = Major histocompatibility complex, BoLA = Bovine leukocyte antigen.

on the stem cells of all major leukocyte lineages and the precursors of thrombocytes and erythrocytes. These antibodies also mediated phagocytosis of blood cells. They bound to both the α- and β-chain of MHC class I antigens. These antibodies were not present in the serum or colostrum of cows that delivered healthy calves.

It was eventually found that these antibodies were induced by administering a specific vaccine against bovine virus diarrhea. This vaccine, Pregshure, contained the virus grown in a bovine kidney cell line and then inactivated. A potent oil-in-water adjuvant was then added to the vaccine. Immunization of cattle with this vaccine induced high levels of antibodies, against the virus and the MHC antigens expressed on the bovine kidney cells. When transferred from cows to suckling calves via colostrum, these antibodies bound to their leukocytes and bone marrow stem cells, and induced bone marrow destruction, resulting in pancytopenia. Not all the calves born from mothers that received this specific vaccine developed clinical disease. The reasons for this are unknown but most likely depend on their MHC haplotype. Antibody levels remained high in cows for many years and could be boosted by each pregnancy. Therefore, bovine neonatal pancytopenia cases occurred for many years after the offending vaccine was removed from the market.

Type III Hypersensitivities

When a vaccine is administered to an animal that already possesses a high level of antibodies to the agent, immune-complexes form. If excessive immune-complex formation occurs at the injection site, an Arthus reaction may develop. This is a rare response to vaccine administration because it can only develop in animals that have high preexisting levels of antibodies (Chapter 18). The reaction is characterized by pain, swelling, tissue firmness, edema, and hemorrhage, perhaps accompanied by necrosis or ulceration at the injection site. Most cases are mild and resolve without treatment in a few days. Because of the need for high antibody levels, it rarely occurs after an animal has received its first dose of vaccine. However, the risk of excessive immune-complex formation increases progressively with each succeeding booster shot.

Immediately following antigen injection and the local formation of immune-complexes, neutrophils adhere to vascular endothelium and then emigrate into the tissues. By 6 to 8 h, when the reaction has reached its greatest intensity, the injection site is densely infiltrated by these cells. As the reaction progresses, damage to blood vessel walls results in hemorrhage and edema, platelet aggregation, and thrombosis. By 8 h, mononuclear cells appear in the lesion, and by 24 h or later, depending on the amount of antigen injected, they become the predominant cell type. Eosinophils are not a significant feature of this type of hypersensitivity. Eventually, the immune-complexes are degraded and the tissues may return to normal.

BLUE EYE

"Blue eye" develops in a small proportion of dogs that have been either infected or vaccinated with live canine adenovirus type 1. These animals develop an anterior uveitis leading to corneal edema and opacity. The cornea is infiltrated by neutrophils, attracted by virus-antibody complexes that are deposited in the tissue. Blue eye develops approximately 1 to 3 weeks after the onset of infection. It usually resolves spontaneously once the virus is eliminated.

VACCINE-INDUCED VASCULOPATHY

It is not uncommon for a local vasculitis to develop at the injection site following rabies vaccination in dogs and cats. The presence of rabies viral antigen can be demonstrated in the walls of cutaneous blood vessels, resulting in vasculitis and ischemic dermatitis. It can also be found in the epithelium of hair follicles.

This response is most frequently diagnosed in small-breed dogs such as Toy or Miniature Poodles, Shih Tzu, Shetland Sheepdogs, Lhasa Apsos, Bichons Frises, and Yorkshire and Silky Terriers. It is rarely reported in large-breed dogs. There are no apparent age or sex predilections. The lesion develops between 1 and 4 months after vaccination. However, it may take much longer to develop. It develops slowly as an area of alopecia with irregular margins. The site eventually becomes scaly, indurated, and pigmented, but visible inflammation is minimal. Smaller satellite lesions may develop nearby. Erosion and ulceration of the skin may occur in severe cases. A subgroup of these dogs may develop a generalized vaccine-induced ischemic dermatopathy. However, these dogs will usually have a focal lesion at the subcutaneous vaccine site. Local muscle atrophy may be significant. Dogs may also show systemic signs such as lethargy, depression, and fever.

The lesion should be biopsied. Histopathology reveals evidence of long-term deoxygenation, including dermal pallor, smudging, and prominent follicular atrophy in the superficial dermis, with perivascular accumulations of lymphocytes, monocytes, and occasional plasma cells in the deep dermis and panniculus (Fig. 15.7). There may be evidence of vasculitis/vasculopathy and some hemorrhage. Secondary dermal and epidermal vesiculation may also develop. There are few eosinophils in these reactions. Hair regrowth may eventually occur, but it may take up to a year and may be associated with changes in skin pigmentation. Similar reactions have been observed in response to leptospirosis vaccination.

Treatment consists of appropriate anti-inflammatory and immunosuppressive therapy. Administering prednisolone supplemented by pentoxifylline is effective. Topical glucocorticoids may also be useful. Animals should not be revaccinated.

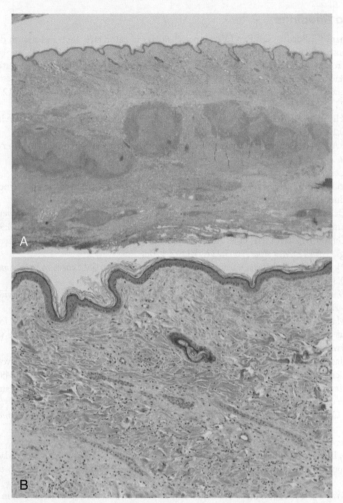

Fig. 15.7   Lesion of a vaccine-induced vasculopathy in a dog. (A) The vasculitis lesion (×40). (B) Showing follicular atrophy, lymphocytic infiltration, and edema (×10). (Courtesy Dr. Dominique Wiener.)

Type IV Reactions

Delayed inflammatory reactions to vaccines may result from type IV hypersensitivities or less well defined T cell responses. They are rare and primarily directed against the vaccine adjuvants such as aluminum salts. They are not considered a contraindication for subsequent revaccination.

Suggested Readings

Black L, Menard FJ, Beadle GG, Pay TW. Hypersensitivity in cattle after foot-and-mouth disease vaccination: response to hydroxpropylmethylcellulose. *J Hyg (Lond)*. 1975;75(1):79-86.

Bonetto C, Trotta F, Felicetti P, et al. Vasculitis as an adverse event following immunization-Systematic literature review. *Vaccine*. 2016;34(51):6641-6651.

Davis G, Rooney A, Cooles S, Evan GS. Pharmacovigilance: suspected adverse events, 2012. *Vet Rec*. 2013; 173(23):573-576.

Fritsche PJ, Helbling A, Ballmer-Weber BK. Vaccine hypersensitivity—update and overview. *Swiss Med Wkly*. 2010;140(17-18):238-246.

Gershwin LJ. Adverse reactions to vaccination: from anaphylaxis to autoimmunity. *Vet Clin North Am Small Anim Pract*. 2018;48(2):279-290.

Meyer EK. Vaccine-associated adverse events. *Vet Clin North Am*. 2001;31(3):493-515.

Miyaji K, Suzuki A, Shimakura H, et al. Large-scale survey of adverse reactions to canine non-rabies combined vaccines in Japan. *Vet Immunol Immunopathol*. 2012;145(1-2):447-452.

Moore GE, DeSantis-Kerr AC, Guptill LF, Glickman NW, Lewis HB, Glickman LT. Adverse events after vaccine administration in cats: 2,560 cases (2002-2005). *J Am Vet Med Assoc*. 2007;231(1):94-100.

Moore GE, Guptill LF, Ward MP, et al. Adverse events diagnosed within three days of vaccine administration in dogs. *J Am Vet Med Assoc*. 2005;227(7):1102-1108.

Moore GE, Hogenesch H. Adverse vaccinal events in dogs and cats. *Vet Clin North Am Small Anim Pract*. 2010;40(3):393-407.

Moore GE, Ward MP, Kulldorff M, et al. A space-time cluster of adverse events associated with canine rabies vaccine. *Vaccine*. 2005;23(48-49):5557-5562.

Ohmori K, Masuda K, DeBoer DJ, Sakaguichi M, Tsugimoto H. Immunoblot analysis for IgE-reactive components of fetal calf serum in dogs that developed allergic reactions after non-rabies vaccination. *Vet Immunol Immunopathol*. 2007;115(1-2):166-171.

Ohmori K, Masuda K, Maeda S, et al. IgE reactivity to vaccine components in dogs that developed immediate-type allergic reactions after vaccination. *Vet Immunol Immunopathol*. 2005;104(3-4):249-256.

Ohmori K, Masuda K, Sakaguchi M, Kaburagi Y, Ohno K, Thujimoto H. A retrospective study on adverse reactions to canine vaccines in Japan. *J Vet Med Sci*. 2002;64(9):851-853.

Shmuel DL, Cortes Y. Anaphylaxis in dogs and cats. *J Vet Emerg Crit Care (San Antonio)*. 2013;23(4): 377-394.

Tizard IR. *Vaccines for Veterinarians*. 1st ed. Elsevier; 2020.

Turnquist SE, Bouchard G, Fisher JR. Naturally occurring systemic anaphylactic or anaphylactoid reactions in four groups of pigs injected with commercially available bacterins. *J Vet Diagn Invest*. 1993;5(1): 103-105.

Willcock BP, Yager JA. Focal cutaneous vasculitis and alopecia at sites of rabies vaccination in dogs. *J Am Vet Med Assoc*. 1986;188(10):1174-1177.

Treatments

CHAPTER 16

Allergen-specific Immunotherapy

While drug treatments, such as systemic glucocorticosteroid therapy, may provide immediate relief, they are not a long-term solution to the problem of atopic disease. This is especially true in cases of atopic dermatitis involving large areas of the skin. The only proven effective, sustained treatment for such cases is allergen-specific immunotherapy (ASIT). ASIT is a procedure that, in effect, forces the immune system to change direction and move from an excessive type 2 immune response to a more balanced situation. ASIT is considered the only satisfactory long-term treatment for allergies caused by environmental allergens. Ideally, ASIT reduces the clinical signs associated with allergic diseases, with minimal adverse events and long-lasting effectiveness.

The Science of Immunotherapy

The first successful immunotherapy for seasonal allergic rhinoconjunctivitis (hay fever) in humans was reported in 1911. At that time, it was believed that hay fever was caused by a toxin in pollen grains, and that it made sense to make a vaccine against it! The administration of the offending allergen in the form of a vaccine seemed to be effective. Since then, it has been realized that the reasons for its effectiveness are much more complex. Nevertheless, it is useful to consider immunotherapy as a form of vaccination designed to induce diverse protective immune responses and minimize the relative dominance of type 2 immune responses in the process.

Allergic diseases occur as a result of the dominance of Th2 cells in the immune response to a foreign allergen and the subsequent production of allergen-specific IgE. Immunotherapy injections were originally believed to counteract this effect by promoting IgG rather than IgE production. IgG antibodies were believed to compete with IgE for circulating allergens, neutralize them, and prevent them from reaching the IgE molecules present on mast cell surfaces. This is now considered unlikely for several reasons. For example, many IgE-coated mast cells are located on mucosal surfaces and encounter allergens before IgG can block their response. It is also apparent that the rise in IgG in response to immunotherapy follows, rather than precedes, any clinical benefit. There is also a poor correlation between IgG levels and protection. The magnitude of the IgG response is unrelated to the clinical benefit.

By injecting allergens subcutaneously, it is possible to bypass the type 2 environment in the epidermis: epithelial alarmins are not released, epidermal dendritic cells are not converted to DC2 cells, and as a result, Th2 and ILC2 cells are not stimulated to respond. Thus, immunotherapy changes the balance between Treg cells, Th1 cells, and Th2 cells (Fig. 16.1). In acute atopic dermatitis, Treg cells are reduced in both number and activity, while Th2 responses predominate. Subcutaneous immunotherapy (SCIT) reverses this and causes a shift in the dominant helper cell response from Th2 to Treg cells.

Immunotherapy thus generates allergen-specific Treg cells and their accompanying suppressive cytokines, IL-10 and TGF-β. During ASIT, IL-10 production increases within two to four weeks. IL-10 inhibits the expression of many inflammatory cytokines, chemokines, and their receptors. IL-10 also inhibits Th2 cell activation. Treg cells also produce TGF-β, a cytokine that is both immunosuppressive and anti-inflammatory. As a result, Treg-derived cytokines effectively increase the threshold stimuli required for mast cell and basophil histamine release.

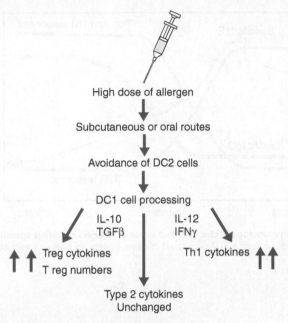

Fig. 16.1 The principle of allergen-specific immunotherapy. Increasing doses of allergen administered by routes that avoid the epidermis (and epidermal dendritic cells) promote both a Th1 and a Treg response, while at the same time reducing the relative contribution of Th2 responses.

Immunotherapy also selectively promotes Th1 responses. The ratio of IFN-γ to IL-4 is low in atopic dogs, indicating a dominant Th2 cytokine profile. After immunotherapy, this ratio shifts. IFN-γ levels increase, and the cytokine balance therefore shifts away from the Th2 response. IFN-γ reduces the effects of Th2 cells on IgE antibody synthesis and, ideally, switches allergen-specific immunoglobulin production from IgE to IgG. Immunotherapy does not appear to directly suppress Th2 responses. Rather, it suppresses them indirectly by inducing DC1 cell-mediated production of IL-12 and IL-18 and, consequently, upregulating Th1 responses.

As a result of immunotherapy, several other changes occur in cell behavior. For example, there is an eventual decrease in the number of IgE-producing B cells. (Prior to that time, there may be a transient increase in IgE levels) (Fig. 16.2). Internalization of mast cell FcεRI together with its bound IgE occurs, thereby reducing the availability of cell-surface IgE. An increase in IgG and IgA levels may also occur, but this takes several weeks to develop. Immunotherapy in asthmatic humans has been shown to reduce mast cell and eosinophil numbers in the lungs, as well as the infiltration of CD4$^+$ T cells and eosinophils into the skin. In some cases, blood eosinophil counts may also decline to normal levels. With sublingual immunotherapy (SLIT), it is possible that oral tolerance mediated through oromucosal dendritic cells may also serve to reduce Th2 responses.

BASIC PRINCIPLES

The key features of ASIT are as follows: first, the administration of allergens by a route that does not involve skin contact, usually through the subcutaneous or sublingual routes. During this induction phase, the dominant helper T cell response switches from Th2 to Th1 and/or Treg cells. This is followed by a maintenance phase, which can last for several years in an effort to make these changes permanent. These are accompanied by appropriate dose adjustments for

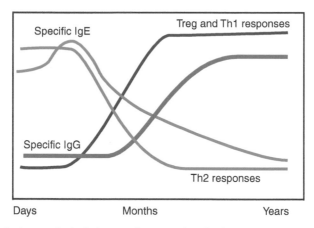

Fig. 16.2 **The major immunological changes that occur in animals receiving specific immunotherapy.** The net effect is a change from a Th2-dominated immune system to a more balanced Treg and Th1 response.

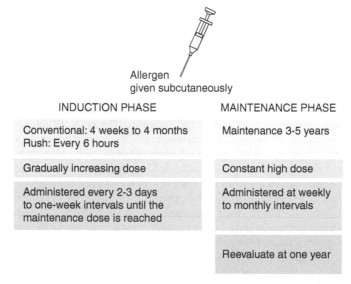

Fig. 16.3 **The time course of allergen-specific immunotherapy.** The procedure is conveniently divided into two phases: an induction phase, wherein the balance of the animal's immune responses is converted, and a maintenance phase that effectively seeks to make this a permanent state.

each individual patient, management of any adverse reactions, and continuous assessment of clinical responses.

ASIT therefore involves giving patients a course of specific allergen injections, starting with a very low dose and building up gradually until a maintenance dose is reached and the severity of subsequent allergic disease is minimized (Fig. 16.3). Once the desired dose of allergen is reached, maintenance therapy involves injection of the same dose every few weeks or monthly for up to several years. Unfortunately, this takes a long time and clinical improvement may not be observed until 6–9 months after the therapy is initiated. In practice, ASIT should be pursued for at least one year before discontinuation. It is possible to time immunotherapy for seasonal allergens to ensure maximal effectiveness during the peak pollen season. In dogs, the subcutaneous route is primarily used for allergen administration, although sublingual administration has advantages and is gaining popularity. There is limited data on subcutaneous administration in cats where ASIT was used to treat cutaneous hypersensitivity dermatoses. In horses, ASIT has been studied primarily for the treatment of Culicoides hypersensitivity.

As a result of the need for a prolonged course of treatment and the delay in generating clinical improvement, numerous attempts have been made to speed the process. Some rapid therapies (rush protocols) or the use of specific adjuvants designed to switch the type of immune response have been investigated with mixed results.

IMMUNOTHERAPY IN HUMANS

The effectiveness of subcutaneous immunotherapy in inducing "sustained unresponsiveness" has been confirmed by multiple controlled studies in human patients. It appears to be the most effective treatment for allergic rhinitis (hay fever), asthma, and allergies to insect stings. Its effectiveness is less clear in the treatment of allergic dermatitis. Patients with moderate asthma appear to benefit most from ASIT, largely because of the decreased need to use inhaled glucocorticosteroids. Rush schedules are also efficient; however, because of the accelerated induction phase, adverse local reactions may occur in as many as 40% of patients. There is also limited evidence that ASIT may prevent new allergen sensitization in some patients.

In humans, allergens used for immunotherapy have been administered via various routes, including subcutaneous, epicutaneous, intralymphatic, and oral routes, to improve results. Oral therapy has been studied intensively. Like other immunotherapies, it begins by administering a very low dose of allergen that is then progressively increased over a period of months until it eventually reaches a maintenance level. The allergen is usually delivered in the form of drops or lozenges to the sublingual mucosa. The lozenge is held there for several minutes while the allergen is slowly released. It may take several years for this type of immunotherapy to achieve sustained unresponsiveness. In general, oral immunotherapy in humans has focused on asthma and allergic rhinitis, rather than eczema. It has also been effective in desensitizing many allergic subjects to eggs, milk, and peanuts. Remission occurs in approximately 50% of cases. Adverse reactions are common in food-allergic individuals. Approximately 15–20% of patients may be unable to tolerate the therapy because of persistent gastrointestinal symptoms.

IMMUNOTHERAPY IN DOGS

The predominant allergic syndrome in dogs is atopic dermatitis. Once diagnosed, it is essential to identify the allergens responsible. This can be done by either intradermal skin testing or by measurement of allergen-specific IgE. Both tests have advantages, and a combination of both may yield the best results (Chapter 20). The success rate of ASIT is similar irrespective of the diagnostic test used. As pointed out elsewhere, there is a high prevalence of false-positive results in these tests. Thus, in interpreting positive skin test results, it is important to ensure that these are plausible and compatible with the animal's clinical history. Once identified, a decision must be made as to which allergens should be incorporated into the injectable and what the optimal desensitization schedule will be. Important and relevant allergens include dust mites, molds, and a variety of pollens. ASIT is best used in dogs with perennial severe allergic disease or in animals with severe and unresponsive seasonal allergies. It should also be considered for dogs whose lesions are so extensive that they cannot be easily managed by topical therapy. Animals that have had the disease for a prolonged period may not respond well. This is an important consideration, since ASIT is often not considered until other treatments have been attempted and failed. Patients that are the best candidates for ASIT are young animals with generalized progressive or widespread lesions that have been present for six or more months per year. Animals with short-duration seasonal allergies may be better managed using topical glucocorticoids to control itching.

Allergen Selection

Immunotherapy is designed to trigger a specific adaptive immune response. Thus, allergens are administered to generate a Th1 or Treg response to a specific allergen. Therefore, allergen selection is critical. Elicitation of a Treg response to allergen A will have absolutely no benefit if the animal is in fact hypersensitive to allergen B. In practice, the best results have been obtained in animals with known hypersensitivity to a specific allergen accompanied by specific immunotherapy against the same allergen.

In humans, ASIT is conducted using either single-allergen preparations or mixtures of related allergens. However, because dogs are often sensitized to multiple allergens, allergen mixtures are commonly used for immunotherapy. Conventionally, it is recommended that allergen mixtures containing more than 10–12 allergens should not be used. By convention, solutions containing 10,000–20,000 protein nitrogen units/mL of allergen are used as maintenance doses, but there is also minimal data to support this or determine whether this dose is optimal. Open studies suggest that higher doses may yield better results.

Only allergens with known positive skin responses by intradermal testing or antigen-specific serology should be used for immunotherapy. The greater the severity of the response or the antibody titer, the more likely that the allergen is important and therefore should be included in the immunotherapy solution. Allergenic preparations that contain ill-defined mixtures of allergens may work on occasion, but the results are unpredictable and often unrepeatable. A limited number of well-defined allergens have been identified for house dust mites, Culicoides midges, and some foods and pollens, but these are relatively few when compared to the diversity of allergens implicated in atopic diseases. Likewise, there have been very few studies determining the optimal dose and dosing intervals in animals. The optimal number of allergens in a mixture and their ratios have not been determined. Most allergen extracts are water-soluble preparations. Many of these are complex mixtures, where the specific responsible allergen may be at subthreshold concentrations. Key allergenic components, such as lipids, may be missing entirely. They are rarely standardized completely. Their potency may also be affected by the source of the allergen, extraction procedures, and conditions used, including filtration and storage. In addition, the presence of preservatives such as glycerol or phenol may affect the results. In humans, the FDA has established standards for some allergens based on bioequivalent allergy units (BAU)/mL and establishing identical potencies. This is not the case with allergens used in animals. These are usually standardized based only on their protein content.

Technique

In classical immunotherapy, small amounts of dilute aqueous solutions or alum-precipitated suspensions of mixed allergen extracts are injected subcutaneously. In North America, aqueous extracts with phenol preservatives are used almost exclusively, whereas aluminum hydroxide-precipitated allergens tend to be preferred in Europe. The aluminum hydroxide is believed to provide a slower release and thus requires fewer injections. Allergens may be administered singly or as a mixture containing not more than 12 allergens. Typically, allergen manufacturers provide two- or three vial sets of each allergen solution at different concentrations. The first injections contain very little allergen (either low volume or very dilute). Over four weeks to four months during the induction phase, the dose is gradually increased until the allergen concentration reaches the maintenance level. The allergen is usually administered subcutaneously using a sterile 1-mL syringe. The first doses usually start at 0.1 mL of a 1:100–1:10 dilution of the allergen concentrate. Lower doses may be used at the veterinarian's discretion if there is a concern regarding extreme sensitivity. The volume injected may be increased by approximately 0.2 mL every other day until the syringe reaches capacity. Then, a switch can be made to a higher concentration of the allergen solution. It is important to follow the recommendations provided by the allergen manufacturers.

Once the maintenance dose has been reached, it is customary to administer this dose every three to four weeks. The doses may be adjusted to ensure the best possible control of pruritus. The optimal interval between injections, whether for the initial loading or maintenance dose, has not been evaluated in dogs. By convention, loading protocols are generally administered at intervals ranging from to two to three days to one week. Maintenance protocols generally use intervals between five days and one month. Epinephrine and a fast-acting corticosteroid injectable should be readily available in cases of unexpectedly severe reactions. Animals may potentially develop hives, dyspnea, vomiting, diarrhea, or acute anaphylaxis with collapse.

Immunotherapy should be continued for at least 12 months before the procedure is re-evaluated. Some animals may require prolonged life-long therapy. Other dogs may remain symptom-free for months or even years after discontinuation of therapy. If an animal's allergy is seasonal, the course of injections should be timed to reach completion just before the anticipated allergen exposure.

Results

Positive responses include objective clinical improvement and a reduction in the amount of medication required to maintain health and comfort.

With the growing impetus of evidence-based medicine, it has been a challenge to provide data that supports the use of immunotherapy. ASIT protocols in domestic animals are not standardized and as a result, it is difficult to objectively compare treatments. Animals tend to be treated with bespoke combinations of allergens following the identification of those to which they are sensitized. Its true efficacy and optimal clinical protocols remain unclear because few randomized controlled trials have been published. Nevertheless, multiple clinical reports have suggested that this therapy is effective in the treatment of atopic dermatitis in many but not all animals. Retrospective studies evaluating allergen doses or allergen mixtures have shown similar levels of positive results. However, many of these trials have used small numbers of dogs over a relatively short time period, and there have been few well-controlled, long-term, double-blind studies. Collectively, open studies report that at least half of atopic dogs show a clinical improvement, although 60–70% is a widely quoted figure and some investigators have reported a 100% success rate. Many such trial results are based on owner opinions and are thus very subjective. After all, the owners themselves may be affected by the placebo effect. A recent Australian study of the outcome of 9 months of immunotherapy in 37 dogs indicated that it had excellent results in 20%, good results in 15%, modest results in 18%, and failure in 47%.

The key advantage of immunotherapy is its potential to modify the course of the disease over the long term and its relative safety. On the other hand, it is slow and may be costly compared to symptomatic treatment. However, it should be considered as a component of an integrated approach for the control of atopic dermatitis. It is especially important if the animal has severe disease mediated by environmental allergens that cannot readily be avoided or in cases where symptomatic therapy is not working.

It is essential to determine as objectively as possible whether the patient is improving. One way to do this is to establish a consistent pruritus scoring system. This commonly requires owners to score their animal responses on a scale from 1 to 10, with 1 representing no itch and 10 reflecting constant scratching, chewing, licking, and rubbing (see Fig. 6.9). A much more complex scoring system, the CADESI-03 system, was specifically developed for use in clinical trials. It is a thorough but very complex system, and as a result is not routinely used in practice. However, recent modifications and simplification have helped considerably (see Chapter 9). Another problem associated with ASIT is determining what constitutes a successful response. Dermatologists may regard a >50% reduction in pruritus scores as a success. Owners may think differently. The key feature in measuring success is the quality of life of the animal and the owner.

Adverse events tend to occur more commonly with the subcutaneous method than with the sublingual approach. They are also provoked more readily by native allergens than by allergoids. The most common adverse event associated with SCIT is an increase in pruritus. This may be alleviated by administering antihistamines prior to injection or by reducing the dose of the allergen injected. Systemic reactions occur in approximately 1% of dogs and may include gastro-intestinal signs such as diarrhea and vomiting, as well as evidence of histamine toxicity, urticaria, angioedema, and anaphylaxis. Other systemic responses that have been observed include mood changes, such as sleepiness or hyperactivity.

Client Education

Immunotherapy requires that dogs receive frequent subcutaneous injections of allergens over a very long period of time. Therefore, it requires a long-term commitment on the part of both veterinarians and owners, and it is well recognized that owner compliance may be low. It is common to request clients to inject their animals at home rather than requiring them to travel frequently to their veterinarians. If the client elects to perform SCIT at home and can follow the schedule, they must be provided with needles and syringes with a sharps container, appropriate vials of allergen, and careful and detailed instructions and training on how to inject their animals. Owners should receive an instruction sheet and contact information for the attending veterinarian. They should also be provided with a printed list of potential side effects to look out for, and these should also be discussed with the owner.

Informed consent is always paramount. The advantages and disadvantages of ASIT must be explained and discussed with the owners before a final decision is taken to initiate this procedure. Owners must be made aware that it may take a year for improvement to develop and given realistic expectations of what results to expect. Expectations should not be unjustifiably raised. Unrealistic expectations are an important reason why clients discontinue immunotherapy.

Compliance with these instructions can become a significant issue, especially if the client fails to see any apparent improvement in their pet's condition. Much depends on the frequency of the injections. Better compliance is seen with weekly to monthly administration compared to required daily injections. Certainly, many owners (and their animals) eventually become accustomed to the procedure. Generally, if the patient becomes clinically normal and remains so for at least a year, then ASIT may be discontinued. Even then, almost half of patients may relapse to some degree, and the therapy may have to be restarted. It is important to provide appropriate counseling and follow-up visits to assess results and maximize compliance. Clients should be encouraged to contact their veterinarians regarding any questions or concerns. Veterinarians should also contact owners regularly to ensure that the therapy is proceeding in an appropriate fashion, that no problems have arisen, and eventually, to discuss discontinuation of the therapy at an appropriate time.

SUBLINGUAL IMMUNOTHERAPY

SLIT using "allergy drops" is an effective treatment modality in atopic dogs and is widely used in humans (where allergen tablets are preferred). In humans, it is considered safe and effective in treating allergic rhinitis caused by pollen or house dust mites. Oral immunotherapy against food allergens is also used in humans but carries a higher risk of adverse events. It appears to be moderately effective in inducing desensitization to food allergens, such as peanuts, where SCIT is unsafe. The adverse reaction rate of SLIT is considerably lower than that of SCIT.

SLIT is based on the concept that allergen administered into the oral cavity, specifically to the sublingual mucosa, reaches mucosal dendritic cells efficiently, activates Treg cells, triggers IL-10 release, and thus induces oral tolerance (Fig. 16.4). Published data suggest that its efficacy in dogs is similar to that of SCIT, although its mechanism of action is somewhat different.

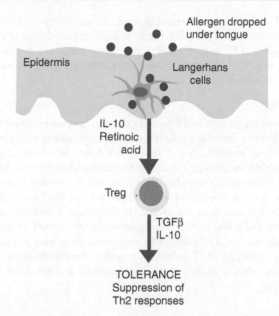

Fig. 16.4 Possible mechanisms of action of sublingual immunotherapy. It is designed to generate oral tolerance by restoring a generalized Treg cell predominance.

Technique

The great advantage of SLIT is its ease of administration, which is an important consideration for owners who dislike administering injections. In SLIT, gradually increasing doses of an allergen solution are applied by drops between the tongue and gums once or twice daily. Allergen solutions may contain glycerin. This not only tastes sweet and improves palatability, but also increases the persistence of the allergen on the oral mucosa. Ideally, the allergen solution should remain for as long as possible in contact with the mucosa in order to maximize absorption.

As with SCIT, SLIT begins with the administration of a low dose of allergen, which then gradually increases. For example, owners may be provided with three pump bottles containing progressively increasing concentrations of allergens. The process starts with the administration of a standard dose (two pumps) of the allergen solution to the underside of the tongue. The bottle with the lowest concentration is used first, twice daily, every day. Once the first bottle is emptied, the second bottle is used, and finally, the third bottle, which contains the highest maintenance dose. The allergen must be squirted into the empty oral cavity, and the dog should not be fed or allowed to drink for ten minutes after dosing.

Results

As with many areas of canine allergy, assessment of results has proven difficult as a result of differences in treatment schedules, doses, and allergen formulations. SLIT has been used in dogs with mixed results. Thus, in experimental Beagles sensitized to house dust mites, feeding the allergen had no apparent effect. Conversely, in a pilot study in naturally mite-sensitive dogs, SLIT induced clinical improvement, as determined by decreased pruritus and medication scores in 80% of animals. In a larger, uncontrolled, open clinical study involving over 200 dogs, improvements were seen by 6 months in 60% of dogs suffering from atopic dermatitis that had not previously received immunotherapy. It also appeared to be effective in approximately half of dogs that had previously failed SCIT. SLIT appears to work well against food allergies in dogs. A more recent study on SLIT in dogs with non-seasonal atopic dermatitis reported that only 14% of dogs returned to normal. Other studies have demonstrated a significant change in some T cell populations in dogs undergoing SLIT, suggesting that they play a role in the desensitization process. It has also been shown that SLIT directed against food allergens induces the secretion of IL-10 by canine blood mononuclear cells.

Client Education

SLIT has practical advantages over SCIT because many clients are reluctant to inject their pets. They prefer giving drops to their dogs and, as a result, compliance tends to be better. Dogs may also respond positively to sweet fluids and view it as a treat. As a result, it may be difficult to prevent them from rapidly swallowing the allergen solution. One problem, however, is the need to administer drops twice daily every day. This may not be possible if the owners are busy. Adverse reactions tend to be rare (about 4%), although a few dogs may rub their mouths for several minutes in an apparent response to oral itching, while others may develop a transient worsening of pruritus and a few may develop gastrointestinal upsets. It remains unclear how long the treatment should last, but it should be continued for at least 10 months. Dogs appear to respond relatively rapidly to SLIT (within 6 months). Premature discontinuation of SLIT is a common problem when animals improve and pruritus declines. Unfortunately, this may lead to a relapse.

IMMUNOTHERAPY IN CATS

The diagnosis of allergic reactions in cats is not as sophisticated as in dogs, and the diagnostic criteria are not as well defined. A variety of clinical presentations are diagnosed as allergies, often with very little proof. Feline atopic skin syndrome is largely diagnosed by excluding other causes, such as flea or food allergies. However, cats can develop an allergic respiratory syndrome, feline asthma (Chapter 13), eosinophilic granuloma complex, and miliary dermatitis. The role of environmental allergens in cats is unclear. Intradermal skin testing of cats is sometimes difficult to interpret because of their failure to develop distinct wheals. Immunotherapy studies have generally been limited to experimental studies involving small numbers of cats. The results suggest that cats may respond to ASIT even better than dogs, with success rates ranging from 60–78%. The reported incidence of adverse effects is low and mainly consists of increased pruritus. The use of SLIT has been investigated in cats with encouraging results and appears to be well tolerated.

IMMUNOTHERAPY IN HORSES

Most immunotherapy studies in horses have been designed to treat allergic dermatitis resulting from Culicoides hypersensitivity. As in many other species, experimental studies have generally employed a small number of horses and have delivered contradictory results. Thus, in one study, Culicoides immunotherapy failed to affect the course of the disease, whereas in another study, 8 of 10 horses improved clinically. These studies had different designs and used different allergen preparations, so they are difficult to interpret.

Stepnik et al. reported the use of ASIT in 54 horses over a 17-year period, with results determined via a telephone survey of the owners. The presenting signs included pruritus and/or urticaria. Twenty-eight of the horses presented with non-pruritic urticaria alone. Of the owners, 84% reported that their horses' clinical condition had improved to the extent that 59% of them were able to manage by receiving ASIT alone. Others required the use of corticosteroids or sedatives. The only adverse events noted were swelling at the injection site in 5 horses. Twenty-four owners discontinued ASIT on average after 2 years; of these, 10 reported no recurrence, while 5 had a recurrence within 2 years of discontinuing the therapy. There is evidence to suggest that IgE levels drop while IgG levels rise in horses undergoing ASIT.

OTHER IMMUNOTHERAPY TECHNIQUES

ASIT essentially involves administering an allergen to an animal to elicit a specific type of immune response. Thus, in many ways, it resembles vaccination. In recent years, many new and innovative techniques have been developed to increase vaccine efficacy while at the same time improving safety. Similar novel approaches to allergen administration for ASIT are currently being investigated to determine whether they may be safer and more effective. These include the use of allergoids, peptide therapy, recombinant allergens, and the use of new adjuvants as well as new routes of allergen administration.

Intralymphatic Immunotherapy

In an effort to bypass conventional allergen processing by Langerhans cells and skin DC2 cells, ultrasound-guided intralymphatic therapy is a novel approach. In humans, this involves administering three injections of the allergen solution directly into the popliteal or submandibular lymph nodes. Thus, a low dose of allergen is delivered to a very large number of lymphocytes. Ideally this increases the chance of inducing tolerance while, at the same time, minimizing the risks of adverse events. Its first use in humans involved the administration of the cat allergen Fel d 1. While adverse events still occurred, they appeared to work better than subcutaneous administration. Intralymphatic immunotherapy has been studied in dogs using aluminum hydroxide-precipitated allergens injected into the popliteal lymph nodes once a week for four weeks. This was followed by SCIT. It appeared to work as well or better than conventional subcutaneous therapy.

Epicutaneous Immunotherapy

Another method currently being investigated as a means of delivering immunotherapy is epicutaneous therapy. The allergen was simply deposited onto the intact healthy skin. This activates dermal dendritic cells and induces an effective and well-regulated immune response (this method also acts well for vaccination). It is also effective in inducing long-lived Treg populations. The method involves applying an allergen patch to the arm or back and changing it daily. Other methods involve applying a chamber to the skin into which allergens can be sprayed, or alternatively, the use of a microneedle array that deposits the allergen directly into the epidermis. Epicutaneous therapy using a skin patch appears to increase the tolerated threshold dose of food allergens.

Rush Protocols

One important factor reducing owner compliance with SCIT is the length of time needed to obtain positive results. Attempts to accelerate the desensitization process, including reduced doses, rushed schedules, or simply omitting the induction phase have been investigated, but there is little evidence that they improve on the conventional procedure.

For example, the multiweek induction period may be shortened to 6-8 hours. Allergens are injected hourly to reach a maintenance dose of 20,000 PNU/mL. In humans, this method is used in patients who are highly sensitive to insect venom, and anaphylactic responses are common. It is reported to be effective in 77–84% of patients with honeybee venom allergy.

In dogs, rush procedures have been well tolerated, and severe adverse events have been rare, although pruritus may be an issue. Thus, it is recommended that an antihistamine be administered 1-2 hours before initiating the procedure. Adverse reactions, such as wheal formation or generalized pruritus, may require steroid treatment. In this procedure, the dogs received allergen injections every few minutes for six hours while being closely monitored. In a double-blind randomized study, subcutaneous rush therapy was compared with the conventional technique. Both worked, and reduced lesion, pruritus, and medication scores, but there was no significant difference in the results between the two methodologies. Similar studies have been performed with alum-adjuvanted allergens, and they appear to produce satisfactory results. However, as with all canine immunotherapy studies, there is a lack of double-blind, high-powered randomized studies. In one notable blind, placebo-controlled trial that involved 51 dogs, 59% of the dogs receiving allergen responded positively, while 21% in the placebo-treated group showed improvement. In a double-blinded study using the rush procedure, the benefits were apparent 2-3 months before those in dogs receiving conventional ASIT. It appeared to have a safety and effectiveness profile similar to that of conventional subcutaneous therapy.

Vaccine Technologies

The addition of adjuvants to allergen solutions to promote a Th1 response makes sense. There have been major improvements in adjuvant technology in recent years, which can be used to improve the process of immunotherapy. After all, ASIT is nothing more than a form of vaccination. Newer vaccine technologies such as those involving the use of allergens displayed on viruslike particles can induce maximal IgG responses while simultaneously avoiding IgE responses.

Native allergens may be chemically polymerized. The resulting large molecules will be more readily captured and processed by dendritic cells, while at the same time may be less likely to trigger Th2 responses or mast cell degranulation. Thus, the safety and potency may be improved. Hypoallergenic, glutaraldehyde-modified allergens (polymerized allergoids) have an improved safety profile, permitting accelerated immunotherapy. For example, polymerized allergoids derived from grass pollens and coupled to non-oxidized mannans are effectively delivered to dendritic cells in such a way that IL-10 and TGF-β are increased and IL-4 production is reduced, thus promoting the generation of Tregs. A similar polymerized allergoid from *Dermatophagoides farinae* attached to oxidized mannan has also been developed. It has a reduced reactivity with canine IgE and increases IL-10 while suppressing IL-4. A DNA-plasmid vaccine for peanut allergy has been tested in humans.

Another method of improving the allergens used in ASIT employs low-molecular-weight recombinant dust mite allergens Der f 2 and Der p2 conjugated with the large fungal carbohydrate maltotriose pullulan. Administration of this compound resulted in clearance of cutaneous lesions in five of six dogs and their reduction in the remaining animal. Its use in dogs reduces both clinical severity and glucocorticoid use in mite-allergic dogs. This product is commercially available in Japan.

Suggested Readings

Bachmann MF, Mohsen MO, Kramer MF, Heath MD. Vaccination against allergy: a paradigm shift? *Trends Mol Med.* 2020;26(4):357-368. doi: 10.1016/j.molmed.2020.01.007

DeBoer DJ. The future of immunotherapy for canine atopic dermatitis: a review. *Vet Dermatol.* 2017;28(1): 25-e6. doi: 10.1111/vde.12416

DeBoer DJ, Verbrugge M, Morris M. Clinical and immunological responses of dust mite sensitive, atopic dogs to treatment with sublingual immunotherapy (SLIT). *Vet Dermatol.* 2016;27(2):82-7e23. doi: 10.1111/vde.12284

Fischer NM, Rostaher A, Favrot C. A comparative study of subcutaneous, intralymphatic and sublingual immunotherapy for the long-term control of dogs with nonseasonal atopic dermatitis. *Vet Dermatol.* 2020;31(5):365-e96. doi: 10.1111/vde.12860

Foj R, Carrasco I, Clemente F, et al. Clinical efficacy of sublingual allergen-specific immunotherapy in 22 cats with atopic dermatitis. *Vet Dermatol.* 2021;32(1):67-e12. doi: 10.1111/vde.12926

Gunawardana NC, Durham SR. New approaches to allergen immunotherapy. *Ann Allergy Asthma Immunol.* 2018;121(3):293-305. doi: 10.1016/j.anai.2018.07.014

Han C, Chan WY, Hill PB. Prevalence of positive reactions in intradermal and IgE serological allergy tests in dogs from South Australia, and the subsequent outcome of allergen-specific immunotherapy. *Aust Vet J.* 2020;98(1-2):17-25. doi: 10.1111/avj.12892

Kawano K, Mizuno T. A pilot study of the effect of pullulan-conjugated Der f 2 allergen-specific immunotherapy on canine atopic dermatitis. *Vet Dermatol.* 2017;28(6):583-e141. doi: 10.1111/vde.12470

Maina E, Devriendt B, Cox E. Food allergen-specific sublingual immunotherapy modulates peripheral T cell responses of dogs with adverse food reactions. *Vet Immunol Immunopathol.* 2019;212(6):38-42. doi: 10.1016/j.vetimm.2019.05.003

Mueller RS. Update on allergen immunotherapy. *Vet Clin North Am Small Anim Pract.* 2019;49(1):1-7. doi: 10.1016/j.cvsm.2018.08.001

Mueller RS, Jensen-Jarolim E, Roth-Walter F, et al. Allergen immunotherapy in people, dogs, cats and horses – differences, similarities and research needs. *Allergy.* 2018;73(10):1989-1999. doi: 10.1111/all.13464

Olivry T, Paps JS, Dunston SM. Proof of concept of the preventative efficacy of high-dose recombinant mono-allergen immunotherapy in atopic dogs sensitized to the *Dermatophagoides farinae* allergen Der f 2. *Vet Dermatol.* 2017;28(2):183-e40. doi: 10.1111/vde.12395

Radwanski NE, Morris DO, Boston RC, Cerundolo R, Lee KW. Longitudinal evaluation of immunological responses to allergen-specific immunotherapy in horses with IgE associated dermatological disease, a pilot study. *Vet Dermatol.* 2019;30(3):255-e78. doi: 10.1111/vde.12732

Soria I, Alvarez J, Manzano AI, et al. Mite allergoids coupled to nonoxidized mannan from Saccharomyces cerevisiae efficiently target canine dendritic cells for novel allergy immunotherapy in veterinary medicine. *Vet Immunol Immunopathol.* 2017;190:65-72. doi: 10.1016/j.vetimm.2017.07.004

Stepnik CT, Outerbridge CA, White SD, Kass PH. Equine atopic skin disease and response to allergen-specific immunotherapy: a retrospective study at the University of California-Davis (1991-2008). *Vet Dermatol.* 2012;23(1):29-35, e7. doi: 10.1111/j.1365-3164.2011.01001.x.

Tordesillas L, Berin MC, Sampson HA. Immunology of food allergy. *Immunity.* 2017;47(1):32-50. doi: 10.1016/j.immuni.2017.07.004

Trimmer AM, Griffin CE, Rosenkrantz WS. Feline immunotherapy. *Clin Tech Small Anim Pract.* 2006;21(3):157-161. doi: 10.1053/j.ctsap.2006.05.009

Yu Y, Kumar MN, Wu MX. Delivery of an allergen powder for safe and effective epicutaneous immunotherapy. *J Allergy Clin Immunol.* 2020;145(2):597-609. doi: 10.1016/j.jaci.2019.11.022

CHAPTER 17

Drug Therapy

Allergic diseases, whether affecting the skin or elsewhere in the body, are commonly treated with a diverse array of pharmaceuticals and other agents. The diversity of available treatments testifies to the generally unsatisfactory results obtained. Nevertheless, as science progresses, the effectiveness of treatments also improves. Natural selection ensures that only the most effective treatments persist.

To date, the most satisfactory treatment for extrinsic allergic disease is the avoidance of exposure to the offending allergens. Allergen-specific immunotherapy provides a good response in many cases. It has the potential to induce stable, long-term remissions, but is not appropriate in all situations and is not a substitute for allergen avoidance.

The majority of the drugs used to treat allergic diseases are not designed for prevention, but are used specifically for symptomatic relief. Indications for drug therapy thus include short-term temporary relief, either while waiting to begin immunotherapy or while waiting for it to take effect. Drugs or shampoos may also be useful for the relief of transient recurrences or in animals in which immunotherapy is not possible.

As pointed out earlier, atopic diseases encompass diverse syndromes with a multitude of clinical presentations and multiple endotypes within each syndrome. There is no clear evidence that different therapies have different efficacies in different endotypes.

The major factors that influence treatment selection are whether the disease is chronic or acute, the lesions local or generalized, and is the animal suffering from severe pruritus that requires immediate attention. They are also determined by the severity of the lesion and the presence of secondary bacterial or fungal infections. Additionally, in complex disease syndromes such as atopic dermatitis (AD), there are factors other than simple mast cell degranulation that contribute to the disease pathogenesis, such as skin barrier defects, that need to be addressed.

Inhibition of Mast Cell Products

ANTIHISTAMINES

Histamine exerts its effects through four different receptors, numbered in the order of their discovery. The term "antihistamine" applies to drugs that specifically interfere with histamine receptor signaling. These antihistamines are inverse agonists, not competitive receptor antagonists. Histamine 1 receptors (H1R) exist in both active and inactive forms. Antihistamines preferentially bind to and stabilize the inactive form of H1R. As a result, they prevent receptor activation (Fig. 17.1). H1Rs are principally associated with signals that transmit pruritus, pain, and increased vascular permeability. H1 antihistamines act quickly, are relatively inexpensive, and are generally safe. Unfortunately, their efficacy in many allergic diseases is limited or unclear. More than 40 H1 antihistamines are available worldwide and are among the most widely used medications for the control of animal allergies. There are two functional classes of H1 antihistamines. First-generation antihistamines include diphenhydramine, chlorpheniramine, cyproheptadine, and hydroxyzine. These have some unfavorable side effects because they are lipid soluble and can cross the blood–brain barrier to induce somnolence and possibly tremors. They may also cause gastrointestinal problems, such as vomiting and diarrhea. Second-generation H1 antihistamines,

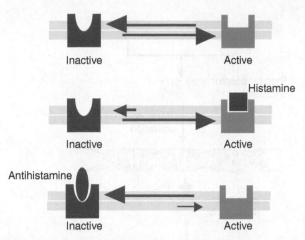

Fig. 17.1 The mode of action of antihistamines. Instead of simply blocking receptors as was once believed, they act as inverse activators. They effectively stabilize histamine receptors in their inactive state and hence prevent their activation.

such as loratadine, fexofenadine, and cetirizine, lack these adverse effects and are relatively safe but not necessarily more effective.

H1 antihistamines have several different pharmacological effects in addition to preventing histamine activity. For example, they can prevent the release of mediators from mast cells and basophils by inhibiting the formation of calcium ion channels. They can also inhibit eosinophil migration. Thus, H1 antihistamines, such as diphenhydramine, can effectively inhibit many histamine activities. However, since histamine is one of the large number of mast cell-derived mediators and its levels do not correlate well with skin disease severity, antihistamines are not effective in controlling acute canine pruritus. Likewise, they cannot replace epinephrine in the treatment of anaphylaxis. If antihistamines are to be effective, they must bind to the inactive histamine receptors. Once histamine binds to its activated receptors, antihistamines are ineffective. As a result, antihistamines cannot markedly reduce the severity of skin reactions that have already developed.

H2 antihistamine drugs also act as inverse agonists. They are used to treat peptic ulcers and gastrointestinal reflux diseases. These H2R inhibitors also appear to be of limited usefulness in the treatment of cutaneous allergic diseases or anaphylaxis. They include famotidine, ranitidine, and cimetidine.

For all the above reasons, antihistamines are not recommended as the first-line treatment for acute allergic diseases such as anaphylaxis, AD, or asthma. However, they may be used to supplement long-term therapy and help reduce the required dose of other more toxic drugs such as glucocorticoids.

GLUCOCORTICOIDS

Until recently, glucocorticosteroids were the only medications proven to ameliorate AD. Corticosteroids are lipid-soluble and can be absorbed directly into cells, where they bind to receptors in the cytosol (Fig. 17.2). These corticosteroid-receptor complexes are then translocated to the nucleus, where they bind to DNA sequences called glucocorticoid response elements and regulate gene transcription. As a result, they stimulate the synthesis of a family of proteins called IκBs.

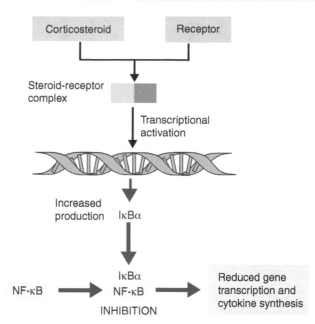

Fig. 17.2   The mode of action of corticosteroids. Normally, signal transduction and cytokine synthesis occur when the transcription factor NF-κB dissociates from its inhibitor IκBα. The released IκBα is rapidly degraded. Corticosteroids stimulate the synthesis of excessive amounts of IκBα, which binds to NF-κB. It thus persists and continues to prevent NF-κB activation.

These act as inhibitors of the key regulator of gene transcription, NF-κB. In resting cells, NF-κB remains inactive since its nuclear binding site is masked by an IκB. When a lymphocyte is stimulated by antigens or cytokines, the two molecules dissociate, the IκB is degraded, and the released NF-κB is free to move into the nucleus, where it activates the genes involved in inflammation and immunity. Corticosteroids, however, stimulate the production of IκBs and as a result, they persist and continue to block NF-κB-mediated processes. These include cytokine synthesis and T cell responses to allergens. Therefore, corticosteroids are able to suppress both immunological and inflammatory responses.

Corticosteroids influence four aspects of the immune system: they affect leukocyte production and circulation and thus reduce innate immunity; they influence the effector mechanisms of lymphocytes and suppress adaptive immunity; they modulate the activities of inflammatory mediators; and they modify protein, carbohydrate, and fat metabolism.

Effects on Lymphocytes

By blocking NF-κB signaling, corticosteroids inhibit the ability of T cells to produce IL-1, IL-6, IL-8, IL-12, IFN-γ and TNF-α. These are the major cytokines that promote type 1 immune responses and inflammation. However, paradoxically, glucocorticoids can upregulate the production of IL-4, IL-10, and IL-13 by Th2 cells. As a result, they cause a change in the Th1/Th2 balance rather than non-specific immunosuppression. The suppression of type 1-mediated inflammation is the most obvious therapeutic benefit. Corticosteroids also upregulate the expression of the IL-1 receptor, CD121b. This is a decoy receptor that can bind active IL-1 but will not generate a signal, thus blocking IL-1 function. In addition to suppressing Th1 responses, glucocorticoids increase Treg numbers and stimulate their activity. They do this in part by upregulating the expression of their transcription factor, FoxP3, in addition to modulating the cytokine mixture within the T cell environment. Experimental studies have shown that glucocorticoids lose their therapeutic effect in the absence of FoxP3 Treg cells.

The effects of corticosteroids on antibody responses are variable and depend on timing and dose. In general, B cells tend to be resistant to corticosteroids, and enormous doses may be required to suppress antibody synthesis.

Glucocorticoid treatment of patients with asthma reduces the number and activity of ILC2 cells. They act through JAK-STAT signaling pathways to reduce ILC2 production by IL-5, IL-9, and IL-13. They enhance the production of lipocortin, which inhibits phospholipase A_2 and interrupts arachidonic acid metabolism. This, in turn, inhibits leukotriene synthesis. They also inhibit cyclooxygenase (COX-2) gene transcription, thus blocking prostaglandin production.

Effects on Leukocytes

The effects of corticosteroids on leukocytes vary among species. In horses and cattle, the number of circulating eosinophils, basophils, and lymphocytes declines within a few hours of corticosteroid administration as a result of sequestration in the bone marrow. On the other hand, the number of neutrophils increases as a result of decreased adherence to the vascular endothelium and reduced migration into inflamed tissues. Corticosteroids suppress neutrophil, monocyte, and eosinophil chemotaxis. Corticosteroids suppress the cytotoxic and phagocytic abilities of neutrophils in some species, but in other species, such as horses and goats, they have no effect on phagocytosis. They also block nitric oxide synthase and prevent the production of nitric oxide. Macrophage production of prostaglandins and cytokines, such as IL-1, as well as antigen processing, is reduced in some species.

In humans, glucocorticoids inhibit eosinophil production of IL-1, TNF-α, IL-4, IL-3, IL-5, and GM-CSF. As a result, they also inhibit eosinophil migration. They reduce eosinophil life-span by enhancing apoptosis. They cause a rapid and profound decrease in the number of circulating eosinophils and, as a result, decrease the recruitment of eosinophils to sites of allergic inflammation.

Synthetic corticosteroids suppress acute inflammation by preventing increased vascular permeability and vasodilation, thus preventing edema formation and fibrin deposition. In the later stages of inflammation, they inhibit capillary and fibroblast proliferation and enhance collagen breakdown. As a result, corticosteroids delay wound healing and fracture healing.

Glucocorticoids can be classified based on their biological half-lives. Hydrocortisone is a short-acting molecule with a half-life of 8–12 hours. Prednisone, prednisolone, and methylprednisolone have intermediate half-lives of 12–36 hours and have less sodium retention activity than hydrocortisone. Long-acting corticosteroids, such as dexamethasone and triamcinolone, have half-lives of 24–54 hours.

Topical, intralesional, or oral treatment with glucocorticosteroids is the standard of care for humans with AD. It is also clear that they work in dogs. Oral and low-dose glucocorticoids effectively treat skin lesions in atopic dogs. Systemic glucocorticoid treatment of canine AD reduces the number of inflammatory cells within these lesions, effectively suppresses local inflammatory responses, and reduces pruritus. Glucocorticoids act rapidly and are relatively inexpensive. They have no apparent effect on skin microbiota.

Adverse Effects

Although highly effective, glucocorticoid treatment is not without significant risks. Most importantly, it has the potential to supply the body's corticosteroid needs, suppress the pituitary-adrenal axis, and induce Cushing's syndrome—iatrogenic hyperadrenocorticism. Side effects include polyuria and increased thirst and appetite, leading to obesity. They also cause skin and muscle atrophy. In addition, corticosteroids can render animals susceptible to infection by effectively suppressing inflammation and phagocytosis. For example, they predispose dogs to bacterial urinary tract infections, fungal infections, and demodicosis.

Because these adverse events are generally a result of prolonged high doses, oral glucocorticoids are best used for short-term palliative treatments such as the suppression of acute disease or pruritus as well as occasional flares. They may also serve as a first response while alternatives such as immunotherapy are being initiated. Once a satisfactory clinical response has been induced, the dose of corticosteroids should be gradually reduced to enable the adrenal cortex to resume its normal functions. This is generally achieved by lengthening the dose interval and decreasing the amount given.

When systemic corticosteroid therapy is initiated, medium-acting oral prednisolone (0.5–1 mg/kg orally) or methylprednisolone (0.4–0.8 mg/kg orally) are usually the agents selected for companion animal treatment. They can be administered once daily or divided and administered twice in the first week. Thereafter, the dose and frequency should be reduced in accordance with the patient's clinical state. If improvement is not noted by two weeks, consideration should be given to alternative diagnoses such as skin infections or food allergies. If long-term treatment is necessary, the dose should be gradually reduced by first administering the second daily dose on alternate days and continuing to reduce it to the minimal dose that controls the disease. Animals receiving long-term treatment should be regularly examined to monitor for adverse effects. Cats may require higher doses than dogs to achieve a significant clinical response, although an initial dose of 1–2 mg/kg daily of prednisolone is usually effective. As in other species, the dose should be tapered as soon as possible to the lowest dose that controls pruritus.

Given the severity of the potential side effects of systemic glucocorticoid therapy, there is a trend toward increased use of topical glucocorticoids. Topical corticosteroid treatments may be a satisfactory solution if the skin lesions are small and localized. They are safer for animals, and the owner can readily observe any changes. Triamcinolone acetonide spray (0.015%) is effective in controlling pruritus when applied to allergic dogs for 4 weeks. However, it may still cause skin thinning and some systemic effects such as polyuria. Thus, the lowest effective dose should be employed. The effective dose of prednisolone may also be significantly reduced with the use of oral essential fatty acid supplements.

Efforts have been made to improve the efficacy and safety of glucocorticoids. Diester topical glucocorticoid sprays such as hydrocortisone aceponate appear to be effective, especially in mild cases of AD. They are highly active but are metabolized in situ to inactive molecules and are thus much less likely to cause systemic adverse effects. They can be used for prevention or treatment. Studies on the efficacy of hydrocortisone aceponate sprays (Cortavance) have shown significant effectiveness against experimental IgE-mediated inflammatory lesions. Systemic glucocorticoid treatment may be used to induce remission, followed by topical treatment of small lesions to prevent disease recurrence.

CALCINEURIN INHIBITORS

Perhaps the single most important recent advance in the treatment of allergic skin diseases has been the application of very potent but selective immunosuppressive agents. Of these, cyclosporine is by far the most successful (Fig. 17.3). Cyclosporine (also called ciclosporin) is a cyclic polypeptide derived from the soil fungus *Tolypocladium inflatum*. This fungus yields several natural forms of cyclosporine, of which the most important is cyclosporin A, a circular peptide of 11 amino acids. Cyclosporine has two distinct surfaces that allow it to bind to two proteins simultaneously. When it enters the T cell cytosol, one surface binds to cyclophilin, an intracellular receptor, whereas the other binds to calcineurin, an intracellular transmitter (Fig. 17.4). Therefore, cyclosporine prevents cyclophilin-calcineurin interactions and blocks many T cell functions, such as production of IL-2, IL-3, IL-4, GM-CSF, TNF-α, and IFN-γ. The primary effect of cyclosporine treatment is, therefore, blocking helper T cell responses.

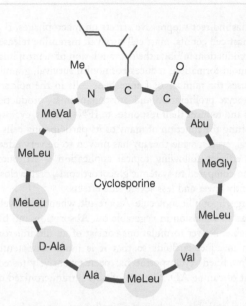

Fig. 17.3 The structure of the immunosuppressive cyclic peptide cyclosporine.

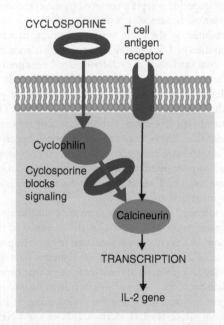

Fig. 17.4 The mode of action of cyclosporine. It prevents activation of the signaling molecule calcineurin by blocking its binding to cyclophilin. As a result, the transcription factor NF-AT is inhibited, and activation of genes such as those encoding IL-2 are prevented.

Cyclosporine also has indirect suppressive effects on macrophages, B cells, and natural killer cells. It reduces skin mast cell counts, mast cell survival, histamine release, and mast cell prostaglandin and cytokine production; inhibits the degranulation of neutrophils, eosinophils, and mast cells; suppresses eicosanoid formation; reduces eosinophil survival, granule release, and cytokine production; and decreases the number of Langerhans cells in the epidermis. Cyclosporine also inhibits canine keratinocyte proliferation and prostaglandin E_2 production. It inhibits the production of chemokines and reduces their responses to IFN-γ. Thus, cyclosporine prevents allergic inflammation by inhibiting the function of many of its participating cells.

Oral, but not topical, cyclosporine therapy has proven to be very effective in treating AD in humans. The lack of efficacy following topical application is attributed to poor absorption through the skin. When compared to systemic glucocorticoids, oral cyclosporine is equally effective, but with significantly fewer and less severe side effects.

Cyclosporine is a large, lipophilic molecule. As a result, when first developed, oral cyclosporine had to be formulated as a suspension in vegetable oil. Absorption and blood levels were highly variable and unpredictable. Newer formulations consist of an ultramicronized product that can form a microemulsion in aqueous fluids so that it is more consistently absorbed across the small intestine. This "modified" cyclosporine has been extensively tested and approved by the FDA for the treatment of canine AD. The use of non-ultramicronized oral cyclosporine is not recommended.

An appropriate initial oral dose in dogs is 5 mg/kg twice daily, but this should be adjusted according to disease severity and clinical response. Oral modified cyclosporine in liquid or capsules develops peak blood levels approximately two hours after dosing (the molecule has a high affinity for red cells and plasma lipoproteins). It accumulates in the skin, liver, kidneys, and adipose tissues. In the liver, cyclosporine is rapidly removed by the cytochrome P450 enzyme system. This actively transports it across hepatocytes to the bile, where it is excreted into the intestine. This P450 pathway is inhibited by the azole antifungal drugs, ketoconazole and fluconazole. Thus, concurrent administration of 2.5–5 mg/kg of ketoconazole once daily reduces cyclosporine secretion and permits the dose (and cost) of cyclosporine to be reduced by 30–50%.

Cyclosporin is a satisfactory alternative to glucocorticoid therapy. It has a wide safety margin in dogs. However, it is slower to act, taking at least a week to show evidence of effectiveness. Therefore, it is not suitable for the treatment of acute AD flares. The major adverse effects reported in dogs are gastroenteritis (vomiting, and diarrhea) but these tend to resolve spontaneously. Other less common side effects may include gingival hyperplasia, lymphadenopathy, persistent otitis externa, footpad hyperkeratosis, and coat shedding. Opportunistic infections are rare, and cyclosporine has no apparent effect on the skin microbiota. Once cyclosporine therapy is established, usually by around 4 to 6 weeks, the daily dose may be gradually reduced to a level that maintains the disease in remission.

Cyclosporine is a well-tolerated alternative to glucocorticoid therapy in cats. As in dogs, improvements are not usually seen until 2–3 weeks after the initiation of therapy. As in dogs, vomiting and diarrhea may occur. In a small prospective open trial, cyclosporine administered subcutaneously at an initial dose of 2 mg/kg once daily on alternate days appears to be effective in treating feline AD. This may be a practical alternative for cats that cannot be treated orally.

Tacrolimus is a macrolide antibiotic produced by the fungus *Streptomyces tsukubaensis*. It acts as a calcineurin-blocking agent in a manner similar to cyclosporine. It inhibits the production of several key cytokines, including IL-2, IL-3, IL-4, IL-5, IFN-γ, and TNF-α. Tacrolimus is a much more potent immunosuppressant than cyclosporine. It downregulates cytokine production by mast cells, basophils, eosinophils, keratinocytes, and Langerhans cells. Oral administration causes severe intestinal toxicity in dogs, resulting in ulceration, vasculitis, anorexia, and vomiting. Unlike cyclosporine, however, it is topically effective. Topical tacrolimus has been successfully used to treat AD in dogs. It reduces erythema, pruritus, and subsequent excoriation. It may be used as a 0.1% ointment to treat local lesions and pruritus. However, it may also cause skin irritation.

OCLACITINIB (APOQUEL)

Many cytokines signal to cells through surface receptors that consist of paired identical transmembrane proteins (homodimers). When a cytokine binds to these receptors, the two proteins come together. This dimerization results in the phosphorylation and activation of two tightly associated JAK proteins (Fig. 17.5). These activated JAK molecules then phosphorylate STAT proteins. Phosphorylated STAT proteins dissociate from JAK and move to the cell nucleus, where they act as transcription factors and induce the expression of target genes. There are four JAK and seven STAT family members currently recognized. For example, hematopoietic growth factor receptors usually use JAK2, IFN-γ receptors use JAK1 and JAK2, and IL-4 receptors use JAK1 and JAK3. Presumably, the genes turned on by this signaling depend on these specific combinations of JAK and STAT proteins as well as the cell type involved.

The synthetic JAK inhibitor, oclacitinib maleate (Apoquel), blocks signal transduction by the cell receptor kinases, JAK1 and JAK3. These are components of the receptors for IL-31, IL-2, IL-4, IL-6, and IL-13. IL-31R is expressed on NP3 prurinergic neurons, where it triggers an itch sensation. IL-4R and IL-13R are found in other NP neurons, where they enhance neuronal responsiveness to multiple other pruritogens. As a result, oclacitinib can inhibit not only Th2 responses but, more importantly, severe chronic pruritus associated with AD. It has been approved for use in dogs over 12 months of age for the control of IL-31-mediated pruritus associated with allergic skin diseases. It is effective and fast acting, has a good safety profile, and improves the quality of life of many animals. It is given orally in tablet form at 0.4 to 0.6 mg/kg twice daily for up to 14 days and once daily thereafter. Oclacitinib appears to be as effective as prednisolone or cyclosporine in controlling pruritus. It is ideal for short-term treatment of dogs while animals are being initiated for immunotherapy. Excessive blocking of IL-31 function may be undesirable since IL-31-regulated genes are also involved in forming an intact skin barrier, and IL-31 stimulates the production of antimicrobial peptides. Adverse events may include anorexia, vomiting, and diarrhea. As an immunomodulating drug, it may increase the susceptibility to neoplasia or infections. Therefore, it should not be used in dogs less than 12 months of age or in those with serious infections.

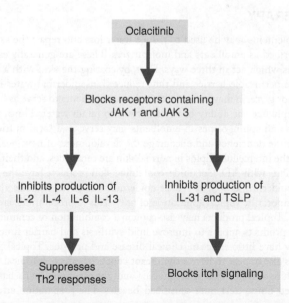

Fig. 17.5 The consequences of oclacitinib blocking signal transmission through JAK receptors.

PENTOXIFYLLINE

Phosphodiesterases are enzymes with multiple functions. Most importantly, they stimulate cell signaling. Allergic humans and dogs exhibit increased phosphodiesterase activity. This leads to excessive cytokine production and exaggerated immune responses. Pentoxifylline is a widely employed competitive phosphodiesterase inhibitor that can reverse this effect. By decreasing the production of inflammatory cytokines and leukotrienes, it can act as an anti-inflammatory agent. It is safe and moderately effective in reducing the severity of some hypersensitivity diseases, especially those mediated by T cells. Therefore, it may be used in the treatment of allergic contact dermatitis. It should be administered orally twice or three times daily at 10–20 mg/kg since it has a very short half-life. It may take 1–2 months of treatment before the benefits are observed.

OTHER DRUGS

Disodium cromoglycate (cromolyn sodium) stabilizes mast cells and thus can reduce mast cell-mediated allergic reactions. It is not widely employed in animals except in the case of eye drops used to treat allergic conjunctivitis in dogs.

Misoprostol is a synthetic prostaglandin E_1 analog that has been shown to elevate intracellular levels of cyclic AMP. This, in turn, reduces the production of the inflammatory cytokines IL-1, TNF-α and leukotriene B_4. It also reduces lymphocyte proliferation and granulocyte activation. In humans, misoprostol selectively inhibits late-phase allergic responses and eosinophil chemotaxis. It significantly improves the clinical score and reduces pruritus in dogs with AD. Misoprostol is inexpensive and may be administered "off-label" at 3–6 µg/kg three times daily to reduce the effective dose of glucocorticoids.

Epidermal Barrier Dysfunction

Transepidermal water loss as a result of defective skin barrier function is a major contributor to the pathogenesis of AD. As pointed out earlier, the restoration of the barrier is an essential step in treating AD.

TOPICAL THERAPY

Topical lipid supplements may be used to reduce water loss and repair the skin barrier in atopic dogs and are described as emollients and moisturizers. These are generally emulsions consisting of water and lipids which act in three ways. First, by coating the skin with a layer of lipids, they provide a water-impermeable barrier and thus reduce transepidermal water loss. Second, molecules such as urea or glycerin may be incorporated into emollients to serve as humectants (hydrating agents) that enhance the ability of keratinocytes to retain water. Third, physiological lipids such as ceramides and sphingosines in emollients may serve as a local nutrient source that can help replace ceramide deficiency and encourage the development of new, healthy keratinocytes.

Nearly half of the intercellular lipids in normal skin are ceramides, and their levels are decreased in the skin of patients with AD. Ceramide-containing skin products have the potential to protect and hydrate the epidermis as well as reduce epidermal water loss and effectively repair the skin barrier, at least temporarily. Topical application of fatty acids or proceramide cream appears to have moderate benefits. Topical products may also contain a combination of ceramides, cholesterol, and fatty acids. These products appear to improve lipid synthesis and barrier function in the stratum corneum, but may have little effect on clinical disease and pruritus. Topical products containing phytosphingosines also appear to have a significant beneficial effect. A topical formulation using a preparation of sphingomyelin-rich sphingolipids and glycosaminoglycans has been tested in repeatedly challenged house dust mite-sensitized Beagles. The preparation attenuated the clinical

> ### BOX 17.1 ■ The Use of Colloidal Oatmeal
>
> Oats (*Avena sativa*) have traditionally been used in colloidal form as a topical treatment for irritating and itchy skin reactions, including rashes and eczema. They are currently widely marketed in both human and canine shampoos and promoted for their soothing effects in atopic dermatitis. Such oatmeal preparations contain numerous potentially bioactive agents. It is believed that the principal active constituents in oatmeal are polyphenolic alkaloids, called avenanthramides. These have been shown to suppress inflammation in mouse models of allergic contact dermatitis. Oatmeal extracts have been reported to decrease arachidonic acid, phospholipase A2, and TNF-α production in keratinocytes. They appear to act by inhibiting NF-κB activation. They also have potent antioxidant activity. Colloidal oatmeal also inhibits keratinocyte release of IL-8 and histamine. They have been demonstrated to reduce scratching in a murine itch model. Oatmeal-based preparations are widely used in skin, hair, and sun-care products. Colloidal oatmeal is incorporated in numerous shampoos used for bathing pets.
>
> Fowler JF. Colloidal oatmeal formulations and treatment of atopic dermatitis. *J Drugs Dermatol* 2014;13(10):1180-1183

worsening of AD and reduced pruritus visual scores. While this treatment also increased the subcutaneous polyunsaturated fatty acid content, it had no significant effect on skin barrier function (Box 17.1).

NUTRITIONAL THERAPY

While it is generally agreed that the current allergy pandemic is largely a result of changes in the commensal microbiota, a case can be made for a linkage to alterations in Western diets, especially in fatty acid intake. As a result, one common approach to improving skin barrier function and reducing allergic inflammation involves supplementation of an animal's diet with essential fatty acids. These long-chain polyunsaturated fatty acids (PUFAs) are considered essential because they cannot be synthesized by mammals. The most important fatty acids include alpha-linolenic (omega-3 or n-3) and linoleic (omega-6 or n-6) fatty acids.

Omega-3 Fatty Acids

Upon ingestion, the n-3 fatty acid alpha-linolenic acid is elongated and desaturated to form eicosapentaenoic and docosahexaenoic acids. All three n-3 PUFAs are also found naturally in fish oils. When ingested, they are incorporated into anti-inflammatory eicosanoids. These anti-inflammatory mediators are classified as resolvins, protectins, or maresins. Produced by endothelial cells, resolvins and protectins reduce neutrophil and eosinophil migration from the bloodstream and enhance macrophage ingestion of apoptotic neutrophils. Maresins are produced by macrophages and enhance tissue repair while acting on nerves to reduce pain. Thus, n-3 PUFAs compete with arachidonic acid to neutralize pro-inflammatory n-6 eicosanoid production. As a result, they have moderate anti-inflammatory effects. n-3 PUFAs may also be incorporated into phospholipids in keratinocyte cell membranes. As a result, feeding fish oil to experimental rats reduced transepidermal water loss, increased skin hydration, and reduced itch-related scratching. Oral administration or feeding diets enriched in n-3 PUFAs may therefore be beneficial when fed to dogs with chronic AD. Unfortunately, there have been relatively few controlled canine studies on the subject, and optimal timing, duration, and dose have yet to be established.

Omega-6 Fatty Acids

Defective fatty acid metabolism in atopic skin can lead to reduced lipid levels in the stratum corneum and decreased barrier function. Upon ingestion, linoleic acid (an n-6 fatty acid) is elongated to form arachidonic acid. This is then incorporated into the plasma membrane phospholipids of keratinocytes in the stratum corneum. n-6 PUFAs are also components of the lipid barrier ceramides. Dietary supplementation may therefore help restore skin barrier function and reduce transepidermal water loss. Oral administration or feeding diets enriched in these PUFAs (usually in the form of vegetable oils such as evening primrose or sunflower seed oils) may therefore be beneficial.

Balanced diets supplemented with n-3 and n-6 essential fatty acids fed to dogs with AD increased their skin lipid content and have been reported to decrease pruritus and clinical severity scores in the short term, but there is not much data on their long-term use. Essential PUFA supplementation is considered safe, but its benefits may be slow to appear.

It is interesting to note that in human studies, the greatest protective effects of PUFA supplementation were observed in individuals with the lowest pre-existing fatty acid levels. Likewise, children with the highest levels of PUFAs in their bloodstream have a significantly reduced risk of developing asthma or allergic rhinitis. Measurement of PUFA levels in animals may therefore identify those most likely to benefit from fatty acid supplementation. It is important to note that unsaturated oils, especially omega-3 fatty acids, readily oxidize, generate peroxides, turn rancid, and lose efficacy. They must be stored correctly.

In a study designed to screen other nutritional components for their ability to upregulate canine epidermal lipid synthesis, seven components were identified as having a positive effect. These included pantothenate, choline, nicotinamide, histidine, proline, pyridoxine, and inositol. The five best performing nutrients were fed to dogs in a 12-week study, while barrier function was measured by determining transepidermal water loss. It was found that a combination of pantothenate, choline, nicotinamide, histidine, and inositol reduced epidermal water loss after 9 weeks of feeding.

Other Treatments

ANTIDEPRESSANT DRUGS

It is widely believed that stresses of many types exacerbate allergic dermatitis in dogs, cats, and horses, while persistent pruritus is very stressful in itself. As a result, many veterinarians prescribe antidepressants to these animals. These drugs increase serotonin and noradrenalin levels in the brain, but they may also act as H1R blockers and analgesics. Thus, tricyclic antidepressants (TCAs), specific serotonin reuptake inhibitors, and N-methyl-D-aspartate (NMDA) receptor antagonists may help animals. TCAs such as doxepin (1–2 mg/kg orally twice daily) and amitriptyline (1–2 mg/kg orally twice daily) have been used. It is possible that any benefit obtained may result from H1R-blocking activity. Dextromethorphan is an NMDA receptor antagonist that has also been used in dogs (2 mg/kg orally twice daily). It may benefit dogs when major behavioral issues develop as a result of chronic pruritus. Likewise, fluoexetine (Prozac) has been used successfully in some dogs for the treatment of compulsive disorders such as acral lick dermatitis.

INHALATION THERAPY

In humans with respiratory allergies, the recommended treatment commonly involves the administration of bronchodilators or anti-inflammatory drugs via the respiratory route through the use of nebulizers and inhalers. In this way, high drug doses can be delivered directly to lesions in the respiratory tract. While humans can control the depth and duration of inhalation, this is not possible in animals. Thus, dry powder inhalers are not suitable for use in animals. Nevertheless, there are methods available for administering controlled doses of drugs to animals via inhalation. One method is to use spacers between the drug inhaler and the animal's face. These spacers serve to decrease the amount of drug that reaches the oropharynx. Spacers are available specifically for use in cats and horses.

Short-acting β2-agonists such as albuterol (salbutamol) reduce bronchoconstriction in acute airway obstruction by relaxing smooth muscle. They appear to be safe when used appropriately in animals. Their effects are seen within minutes and persist for 3–6 hours.

Inhaled glucocorticoid formulations are also available. These include fluticasone, beclomethasone, flunisolide, and triamcinolone. Fluticasone is the most potent, with the longest duration of action. Other drugs that may be used for inhalation therapy include ipratropium (an atropine-like bronchodilator) used in cases of severe asthma in horses.

Biological Therapy

The development of allergic diseases involves communication between many different cell types through a network involving many different cytokines. In seeking to prevent or control these diseases, it makes sense to try to block intercellular communication. One way to achieve this is through the use of highly specific monoclonal antibodies (mAbs). These mAbs may be directed against cytokines themselves or against their receptors. Either way, by interfering with the interaction between the cytokine and its receptor, signals are effectively blocked (Fig. 17.6). Monoclonal antibodies were first produced in the 1970s in mouse cells. If these are administered to humans or other animals, they generate anti-mouse antibodies. Over time, however, it has been proven possible to modify these mAbs by replacing their constant regions with human amino acid sequences. In effect, the mouse antibodies were humanized, and they were no longer antigenic in humans. The first of these humanized monoclonal antibodies to be employed was omalizumab, sold under the name Xolair. This monoclonal antibody is directed against the constant domains of IgE. When it binds to IgE, it effectively blocks IgE from binding to its high-affinity receptor on mast cells and basophils. It downregulates IgE production by B cells. As a result, allergic responses are blocked, and mast cells and basophils do not degranulate. It is widely used to treat severe, persistent allergic asthma and chronic urticaria.

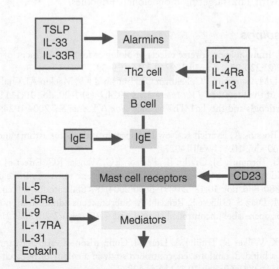

Fig. 17.6 Current and proposed monoclonal antibody therapy is primarily directed against certain key cytokines or their receptors that participate in the Th2 response pathway (red rectangles). While few are currently available for use in domestic species, the remarkable successes of many of these treatments in humans ensures that this is changing rapidly.

Omalizumab was just the beginning. Several new humanized monoclonal antibodies have been produced and marketed or are undergoing clinical trials. Some have been used to suppress inflammation by blocking TNF-α or its receptor. In the search for allergy treatments, monoclonal antibodies are being developed against all major cytokines and/or their receptors. However, monoclonal antibodies are expensive to produce, and the process of humanization is also expensive. If resources are available to produce successful mAbs, the profits would be enormous; however, this is not the case in veterinary medicine. The costs of development and production will almost inevitably mean that mAbs will only be available for companion animal species in the foreseeable future.

Monoclonal anti-IL-31 is marketed for the relief of itching in canine AD. IL-31 is the major cause of severe itching observed in AD in dogs. The production of IL-31 in the affected skin can be inhibited by oclacitinib, a JAK inhibitor. It can also be neutralized by administration of a caninized monoclonal antibody, lokivetmab (Cytopoint), directed specifically against canine IL-31 (90% of this monoclonal antibody is "caninized" and hence identical to dog immunoglobulins). Lokivetmab is injected subcutaneously. It binds to circulating IL-31, thus preventing its binding to the IL-31 receptor. In double-blind, placebo-controlled trials, a single dose has provided relief from itching, prevention of flares, and a reduction in disease severity in dogs with chronic AD. It has a prolonged duration of action and is administered subcutaneously every 4–8 weeks as needed. Thus, it appears to be safe and effective. It is approved for use in dogs under one year of age and is well tolerated. Reported adverse events include vomiting, diarrhea, lethargy, incontinence, and pain. Anaphylaxis and other allergic reactions have also been reported.

Monoclonal antibody therapy is increasingly being employed in human medicine and will eventually be used in domestic animal species. For example, monoclonal antibodies used successfully in human AD include those directed against mediators of innate immunity, including IL-1 and IL-6, and those directed against type 2 immunity, including IL-4R, IL-5, IgE, CD20, IL-13, TSLP, IL-33, and IL-33R. Other monoclonal antibodies directed against cytokines participating in Th1 and Th17 responses, such as TNF-α, while effective, may effectively immunosuppress recipients and unacceptably increase their susceptibility to secondary infections. This appears to be less of an issue with Th2-targeting monoclonal antibodies.

Suggested Readings

Aranez V, Ambrus J. Immunologic adverse effects of biologics for the treatment of atopy. *Clin Rev Allergy Immunol.* 2020;59(2):220-230. doi: 10.1007/s12016-019-08739-8

Archer TM, Boothe DM, Langston VC, Fellman CL, Lunsford KV, Mackin AJ. Oral cyclosporine treatment in dogs: A review of the literature. *J Vet Intern Med.* 2014;28(1):1-20. doi: 10.1111/jvim.12265

Elenkov IJ. Glucocorticoids and the Th1/Th2 balance. *Ann N Y Acad Sci.* 2004;1024:138-146. doi: 10.1196/annals.1321.010

Eyerich S, Metz M, Bossios A, Eyerich K. New biological treatments for asthma and skin allergies. *Allergy.* 2020;75(3):546-560. doi: 10.1111/all.14027

Hall JA, Van Saun RJ, Tornquist SJ, Gradin JL, Pearson EG, Wander RC. Effect of type of dietary polyunsaturated fatty acid supplement (corn oil or fish oil) on immune responses in healthy horses. *J Vet Intern Med.* 2004;18(6):880-886. doi: 10.1892/0891-6640(2004)18<880:eotodp>2.0.co;2

Koch SN, Torres SM, Diaz S, Gilbert S, Rendahl A. Subcutaneous administration of ciclosporin in 11 allergic cats – a pilot open-label uncontrolled clinical trial. *Vet Dermatol.* 2018;29(2):107-e43. doi: 10.1111/vde.12505

Marsella R, Ahrens K, Wilkes R, Trujillo A, Dorr M. Comparison of various treatment options for canine atopic dermatitis: a blinded, randomized, controlled study in a colony of research atopic beagle dogs. *Vet Dermatol.* 2020;31(4):284-e69. doi: 10.1111/vde.12849

Marsella R, Segarra S, Ahrens K, Alonso C, Ferrer L. Topical treatment with sphingolipids and glycosaminoglycans for canine atopic dermatitis. *BMC Vet Res.* 2020;16(1):92. doi: 10.1186/s12917-020-02306-6

Michels GM, Ramsey DS, Walsh KF, et al. A blinded randomized, placebo controlled, dose determination trial of lokivetmab (ZTS-00103289), a caninized, anti-canine IL-31 monoclonal antibody in client owned dogs with atopic dermatitis. *Vet Dermatol.* 2016;27(6):478-e129. doi: 10.1111/vde.12376

Miyata J, Arita M. Role of omega-3 fatty acids and their metabolites in asthma and allergic diseases. *Allergol Int.* 2015;64(1):27-34. doi: 10.1016/j.alit.2014.08.003

Mueller RS, Nuttall T, Prost C, Schulz B, Bizikova P. Treatment of the feline atopic syndrome – a systematic review. *Vet Dermatol.* 2021;32(1):43-e8. doi: 10.1111/vde.12933

Olivry T, DeBoer DJ, Favrot C, et al. Treatment of canine atopic dermatitis: 2015 updated guidelines from the International Committee on Allergic Diseases of Animals (ICADA). *BMC Vet Res.* 2015;11:210. doi: 10.1186/s12917-015-0514-6

Olivry T, Banovic F. Treatment of canine atopic dermatitis: time to revise our strategy? *Vet Dermatol.* 2019;30(2):87-90. doi: 10.1111/vde.12740

Ozdemir C. Monoclonal antibodies in allergy: updated applications and promising trials. *Recent Pat Inflamm Allergy Drug Disc.* 2015;9(1):54-65. doi: 10.2174/1872213x09666150223115303

Palmeiro BS. Cyclosporine in veterinary dermatology. *Vet Clin North Am Small Anim Pract.* 2013;43(1):153-171. doi: 10.1016/j.cvsm.2012.09.007

Peters LJ, Kovacic JP. Histamine: metabolism, physiology, and pathophysiology with applications in veterinary medicine. *J Vet Emerg Crit Care (San Antonio).* 2009;19(4):311-328. doi: 10.1111/j.1476-4431.2009.00434.x

Santoro D. Therapies in canine atopic dermatitis: an update. *Vet Clin North Am Small Anim Pract.* 2019;49(1):9-26. doi: 10.1016/j.cvsm.2018.08.002

Saridomichelakis MN, Olivry T. An update on the treatment of canine atopic dermatitis. *Vet J.* 2016;207: 29-37. doi: 10.1016/j.tvjl.2015.09.016

Simons FER. Advances in H1-antihistamines. *N Engl J Med.* 2004;351(21):2203-2217. doi: 10.1056/NEJMra033121

Tater KC, Gwaltney-Brant S, Wismer T. Dermatological topical products used in the US population and their toxicity to dogs and cats. *Vet Dermatol.* 2019;30(6):474-e140. doi: 10.1111/vde.12796

Venter C, Meyer RW, Nwaru BI, et al. EAACI position paper: Influence of dietary fatty acids on asthma, food allergy, and atopic dermatitis. *Allergy.* 2019;74(8):1429-1444. doi: 10.1111/all.13764

Watson AL, Fray TR, Bailey J, Baker CB, Beyer SA, Markwell PJ. Dietary constituents are able to play a beneficial role in canine epidermal barrier function. *Exp Dermatol.* 2006;15(1):74-81. doi: 10.1111/j.0906-6705.2005.00385.x

White AG, Santoro D, Ahrens K, Marsella R. Single blinded, randomized, placebo-controlled study on the effects of ciclosporin on cutaneous barrier function and immunological response in atopic beagles. *Vet Immunol Immunopathol.* 2018;197(1):93-101. doi: 10.1016/j.vetimm.2018.02.001

Yosipovitch G, Misery L, Proksch E, Metz M, Ständer S, Schmelz M. Skin barrier damage and itch: Review of mechanisms, topical management and future directions. *Acta Derm Venereol.* 2019;99(13):1201-1209. doi: 10.23540/00015555-3296

Other Hypersensitivities

CHAPTER 18

Type III Hypersensitivity Diseases

Immune complexes formed by the combination of bivalent antibodies and polyvalent antigens can form large molecular aggregates. Under normal conditions, circulating immune complexes are rapidly and completely removed from the bloodstream by macrophages in the liver and spleen, without any pathological consequences. When, however, large amounts of immune complexes form within tissues, they trigger inflammation. Complement is activated and generates C3a and C5a anaphylatoxins, that degranulate mast cells and attract neutrophils. The accumulated neutrophils and their granules then release oxidants and enzymes, causing inflammation and tissue destruction. Inflammation generated in this way is classified as a type III or immune complex-mediated hypersensitivity reaction. It should be noted, however that the combination of an antigen with an antibody always produces some immune complexes. However, the occurrence of clinically significant type III hypersensitivity reactions results from the deposition of excessive amounts of these complexes in the wrong places. Minor immune complex-mediated lesions probably develop relatively frequently following an antibody response without causing clinically significant disease or tissue damage.

Pathogenesis

The severity and significance of type III hypersensitivity reactions depend, as might be expected, on the amount and site of deposition of the immune complexes. One form of reaction occurs locally when immune complexes are generated within tissues. Another type results when large quantities of immune complexes form within the bloodstream. This can occur, for example, when an antigen is administered intravenously to an immune recipient. Immune complexes that form within the bloodstream are deposited in glomeruli in the kidneys, and the development of glomerulonephritis is characteristic of this type of hypersensitivity. If the complexes bind to blood cells, anemia, leukopenia, or thrombocytopenia may also result. Immune complexes may also be deposited in blood vessel walls to cause vasculitis or in joints to cause arthritis.

LOCAL REACTIONS

Immune complexes that form in tissues first bind to Fc and complement receptors on cells, especially neutrophils. When the immune complexes bind to these receptors, they activate the neutrophils and stimulate their release of oxidants, leukotrienes, prostaglandins, cytokines, and chemokines, as well as extracellular traps (NETs). Immune complexes can also bind to mast cells through their IgG receptors (FcγRIII), causing them to degranulate. Among the molecules released by mast cells are proteases that activate complement and kinins. All these mediators promote inflammation by binding to vascular endothelium and stimulating neutrophil adherence and immigration (Fig. 18.1).

Immune complexes activate the complement system, resulting in the production of two small chemotactic peptides: C3a and C5a. Neutrophils, attracted by these peptides as well as by mast cell–derived chemokines, emigrate from the bloodstream, bind to the complexes, and promptly phagocytose them. Eventually, the complexes are digested and destroyed. During this process,

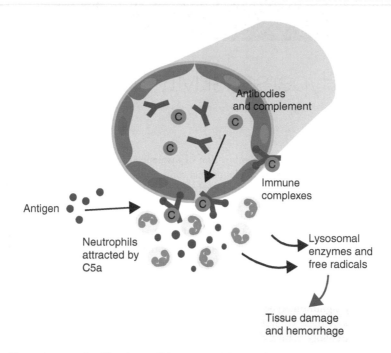

Fig. 18.1 The pathogenesis of local type III hypersensitivity reactions such as the Arthus reaction as well as immune-mediated vasculitis. The deposition of immune complexes in blood vessel walls results in an influx of neutrophils, local inflammation, and tissue damage.

however, more proteases and oxidants are released into tissues. For example, if neutrophils attempt to ingest immune complexes attached to large structures such as basement membranes, they simply release their granule contents directly into the surrounding tissues. As a result, neutrophil proteases disrupt collagen fibers and destroy ground substances, basement membranes, and elastic tissues. The released NETs also contribute to inflammation. Normal tissues contain proteases that inhibit neutrophil enzymes. However, these inhibitors can be overwhelmed by oxidants such as hypochlorite (OCl^-). OCl^- destroys the inhibitors and allows tissue destruction to proceed. Neutrophil proteases can also act on complement to generate more C3a and C5a, which then promote further neutrophil accumulation and degranulation. Other enzymes released by neutrophils may cause mast cells to degranulate and generate kinins. As a result of all this, inflammation and destruction of blood vessel walls result in edema, vasculitis, and hemorrhage.

Arthus Reaction

If an antigen is injected subcutaneously into an animal that already has a high level of antibodies in its bloodstream, inflammation develops at the injection site within 4 to 8 hours. This is called an Arthus reaction, after the French scientist who first described it. The reaction starts as a red, edematous swelling; eventually, hemorrhage and thrombosis occur, and if severe, it culminates in local tissue destruction.

Immediately following antigen injection, neutrophils adhere to vascular endothelium and migrate into the tissues. By 6 to 8 hours, when the reaction reaches its greatest intensity, the injection site is densely infiltrated by these cells. As the reaction progresses, neutrophil-mediated damage to blood vessel walls results in vasculitis, hemorrhage, edema, platelet aggregation, and thrombosis. By 8 hours, macrophages begin to appear in the lesion, and by 24 hours or later, depending on the amount of antigen injected, they become the dominant cell type. Eosinophils are not a significant feature of type III hypersensitivity reactions.

The injected antigen diffuses from the injection site through tissue fluid. When it encounters small blood vessels, the antigen diffuses into the vessel walls, where it meets the circulating antibodies. Immune complexes form and are deposited between and beneath vascular endothelial cells.

Although the classical Arthus reaction is produced by local injection of an antigen into hyperimmunized animals, any technique that generates large quantities of immune complexes in tissues will provoke a similar inflammatory response. It should be noted that is unusual for pure hypersensitivity reactions of only a single type to occur under natural conditions; however, there are diseases in domestic animals in which type III reactions play a predominant role.

For example, several different local type III hypersensitivity reactions may be triggered by vaccination (Chapter 15).

Staphylococcal Hypersensitivity

Staphylococcal hypersensitivity is a pruritic pustular dermatitis in dogs, described in Chapter 10. Skin testing with staphylococcal antigens suggests that types I, III, and IV hypersensitivity responses may be involved. Histological findings of a neutrophilic dermal vasculitis suggest that a type III reaction may predominate in some cases.

Hypersensitivity Pneumonitis

Immune complexes may form in the lungs when sensitized animals inhale foreign antigens. For example, cattle housed in winter are exposed to dust from hay. Normally, these dust particles are relatively large and are deposited in the upper respiratory tract, trapped in nasal mucus, and eliminated. However, if the hay is stored when damp, bacterial growth and metabolism will result in heating. As a result of this warmth, thermophilic actinomycetes grow well. One of the most important of these thermophilic actinomycetes is *Saccharopolyspora rectivirgula*, an organism that produces large numbers of very small spores (~1 μm diameter). When inhaled, these spores can penetrate deep into the alveoli. If cattle are fed moldy hay for long periods, such as over winter, constant inhalation of *S. rectivirgula* spores will result in the development of high-titered precipitating IgG antibodies to *S. rectivirgula* antigens in serum. These antibodies are produced in sufficient amounts to form large, insoluble immune complexes when they bind to their antigens. As a result, when inhaled spore antigens encounter antibodies within the alveolar walls, the resulting immune-complex formation and complement activation result in neutrophil immigration, NET release, and the development of alveolar inflammation.

Hypersensitivity pneumonitis consists of an acute alveolitis, vasculitis, and exudation of fluid into the alveolar spaces. The alveolar septa become thickened, and the entire lesion is infiltrated by inflammatory cells (Fig. 18.2). Since many of these infiltrating cells are eosinophils and lymphocytes, it is obvious that the reaction is not a pure type III reaction. It also involves the activation of antigen-specific T cells and high concentrations of proinflammatory cytokines. Respiratory challenge with the antigen also triggers both immediate and delayed dyspneic responses. Examination of the affected lungs by immunofluorescence demonstrates immune complexes and complement deposited in the alveolar walls. Bronchoalveolar lavage fluid from affected animals characteristically contains high numbers (60–80%) of CD8+ T cells. In cattle that inhale smaller amounts of an antigen over a long period, proliferative bronchiolitis and fibrosis may be observed. Clinically, hypersensitivity pneumonitis presents as pneumonia occurring between 5 and 10 hours after acute exposure to grossly moldy hay. The animal may have difficulty breathing and develop a severe cough. In chronically affected animals, dyspnea may be continuous. The most effective

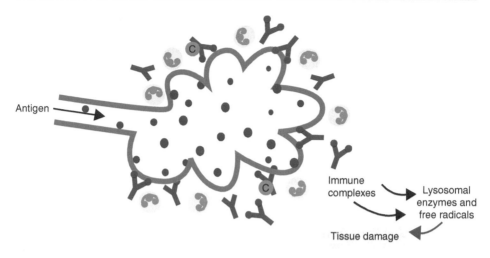

Fig. 18.2   The pathogenesis of the alveolitis that gives rise to hypersensitivity pneumonitis. It too is an immune complex-mediated lesion that forms in the alveolar walls following inhalation of large quantities of foreign antigens.

method for managing this condition is to remove the source of the antigen. Administration of systemic glucocorticoids may be beneficial.

A similar hypersensitivity pneumonitis also occurs in farmers chronically exposed to *S. rectivirgula* spores from moldy hay and is called "farmer's lung." This is also caused by the prolonged inhalation of large quantities of spores from thermophilic actinomycetes growing in damp hay. It has been estimated that between 1% and 19% of farmers exposed to moldy hay develop the disease. Many other syndromes in humans have identical pathogeneses. Collectively, these diseases are classified as extrinsic allergic alveolitis. However, different syndromes are usually named after the source of the offending antigen. For example, "bird fancier's lung" is another form of hypersensitivity pneumonitis. This develops in about 6% to 20% of individuals following prolonged exposure to proteins in the dust from avian feces and feathers. This is a significant cause of morbidity in bird fanciers. It has been reported that pigeon fancier's lung affects approximately 10% of pigeon breeders in the UK. The disease presents with fever, sweats, headaches, coughing, and severe dyspnea. It usually develops 4–8 hours after exposure (often wakening the victim in the middle of the night) and resolves within 24 hours after leaving the dusty environment. If the exposure is prolonged, chronic disease may develop, resulting in pulmonary fibrosis.

GENERALIZED REACTIONS

If large quantities of an antigen are administered intravenously to animals with circulating antibodies, immune complexes form in the bloodstream. These immune complexes are removed by binding to either erythrocytes or platelets, or if very large, by mononuclear phagocytes. However, if excessive amounts of complexes are produced, they may be deposited in blood vessel walls, especially medium-sized arteries, and in vessels where there is a physiological outflow of fluid such as glomeruli and joint synovia. An example of this type of generalized hypersensitivity is serum sickness.

Serum Sickness

During the First World War, when the use of antisera for passive immunization was in its infancy, it was observed that wounded soldiers who had received a very large dose of equine anti-tetanus serum developed a characteristic illness about 10 days later. This "serum sickness" consisted of a generalized vasculitis with skin erythema, edema, and urticaria, and neutropenia, lymph node enlargement, joint swelling, and proteinuria. The sickness was usually of short duration and subsided within a few days. A similar response can be produced experimentally in rabbits by administering a single large intravenous dose of antigen. The development of serum sickness coincides with the formation of large amounts of immune complexes in the circulation. The experimental disease may be acute if it is caused by a single, large injection of an antigen, or chronic if caused by multiple small injections. In either case, animals develop glomerulonephritis and vasculitis.

Serum sickness has been described in dogs that had received equine polyvalent antivenin for the treatment of a suspected rattlesnake bite. One week after receiving antivenin, the dogs develop signs of hypersensitivity, including generalized swelling, mild facial edema, urticaria, gastrointestinal signs, and vasculitis. These episodes may be successfully treated with glucocorticoids and antihistamines. In one case, there was a recurrence of the reaction a week later with vomiting, diarrhea, urticaria, and facial swelling. The treatment was repeated, and recovery was rapid. Biopsies demonstrated that the skin lesions consisted of vasculitis with mild to moderate neutrophil infiltration as well as leukocytoclastic changes and fibrinoid necrosis in blood vessel walls.

A similar reaction has been reported in hypoalbuminemic dogs that had received human serum albumin (HSA) as a plasma expander. Vasculitis developed 8–16 days after receiving the albumin. The dogs developed epidermal pallor and generalized edema. Histopathology revealed hemorrhage, degenerative neutrophil perivascular infiltrates with "nuclear dust," and multifocal areas of neutrophilic or leukocytoclastic vasculitis. Immunohistochemistry showed the presence of HSA-antigen-antibody complexes in the dermis. The dogs were successfully treated with glucocorticoids and antihistamines.

All these cases developed vasculitis affecting arterioles, venules, and capillaries. The lesions were characterized by endothelial swelling and neutrophilic inflammatory infiltrates in the vessel walls and surrounding tissues. There was karyorrhexis of neutrophils and extravasation of erythrocytes.

Immunothrombosis

Immune complexes are highly effective in triggering the release of NETs. Trap formation is triggered when the complexes bind and activate Fc receptors on neutrophils. This not only occurs during infections but also in allergic and hypersensitivity diseases. The interaction between these netlike chromatin structures, platelets, and the coagulation pathway can result in intravascular thrombus formation, or immunothrombosis (Fig. 18.3).

NET formation can be triggered by platelet activation. Thus, when immune complexes interact with platelet Fc receptors, they cause platelet activation and aggregation. These aggregated platelets can then bind to neutrophils and form neutrophil-platelet clusters. Platelets express CD40L, which can bind to neutrophil CD40, triggering a respiratory burst that drives NET formation. These interactions, together with the release of platelet clotting factors such as von Willebrand factor (VWF), PAF, platelet factor 1, and HMGB-1, trigger NET release.

When neutrophils are activated, they release a netlike structure consisting of DNA and histones intermixed with their granules and granule contents. These NETs interact with VWF, a key component of the clotting system, and bind to endothelial surfaces. NETs also provide a scaffold to which the clotting factors, VWF, and tissue factor (TF) can bind and be activated. The histones and DNA in the nets are also proinflammatory and induce TF production. This combination of NET-bound VWF and TF is sufficient to trigger local thrombus formation.

In addition to thrombosis, these NETs also trigger inflammation. Both NETs and VWF are proinflammatory. Activated neutrophils release cytokines, proteases, peptides, and reactive oxygen species (ROS), such as H_2O_2 and OCl^-. NETs are also potent activators of the alternative

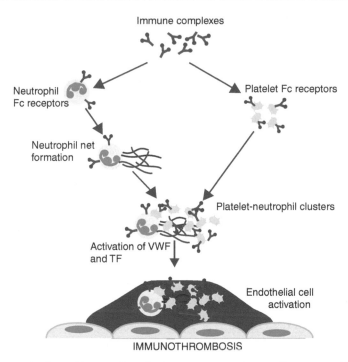

Fig. 18.3 The mechanism of immunothrombosis. Immune complexes activate neutrophils resulting in NETosis. Immune complexes also activate platelets so that they bind to NETs. The neutrophil-platelet clusters bind to vascular endothelial cells, activate von Willebrand factor (VWF) and tissue factor (TF), and a thrombus develops on the vessel wall. NET, neutrophil extracellular trap.

complement pathway. These can all cause direct damage to the vascular endothelium and further promote clotting and thrombus formation. Immunothrombosis has been implicated in many different syndromes, including IgE-independent anaphylaxis, sepsis, myocardial infarction, and some autoimmune diseases. It is probably a major contributor to the pathogenesis of systemic vasculitis in animals.

Vasculitis

On occasion, focal vascular lesions characterized by neutrophil infiltration may develop in dogs and cats. The lesions develop in the walls of small blood vessels throughout the body, especially in the skin. As a result of blood vessel leakage, they may present as hemorrhagic or purpuric lesions. Although called hypersensitivity vasculitis, a foreign antigen can be identified in only a small proportion of cases. For this reason, a better name for this condition may be leukocytoclastic vasculitis.

Pathogenesis. Leukocytoclastic vasculitis is a necrotizing inflammatory reaction involving the walls of small blood vessels. Its pathogenesis is complex, and there are likely many causative factors and endotypes. Its clinical manifestations depend on the severity of inflammatory lesions as well as their distribution. However, in this chapter, we will focus specifically on vasculitis resulting from type III hypersensitivity responses mediated by immune complexes deposited in blood vessel walls. As a result, interference with local blood flow can lead to edema, hemorrhage, immunothrombosis, and purpura. Skin necrosis and ulceration may occur. Both cutaneous and systemic forms occur as a result of impaired blood vessel function.

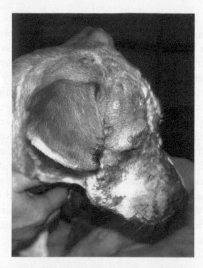

Fig. 18.4 Generalized vasculitis in an 8-month-old mixed breed dog. No triggers could be identified in this patient, but the dog was successfully managed with 5 mg/kg cyclosporine. (From Innerå M. Cutaneous vasculitis in small animals. *Vet Clin North Am Small Anim Pract.* 2013;43(1):113-134. doi: 10.1016/j. cvsm.2012.09.011)

Numerous triggers of leukocytoclastic vasculitis have been identified, and a careful history including recent drug treatments is needed if the trigger is to be identified. The most common cause of these vasculitides in small animals is a type III hypersensitivity reaction, but at least half of canine vasculitis cases are idiopathic (Fig. 18.4). Lesions can develop at any site in the body, including the oral cavity and mucus membranes. These lesions may evolve over time, and ulcers may develop several days after the first appearance of the lesions.

Clinical Disease. Dogs suffering from vasculitis present with anorexia, depression, malaise, and fever. Ulcers may form on the pinnae, oral mucosa, and lips. The affected skin may be very painful, especially during the initial phase of the disease. These dogs can develop mucocutaneous ulcers, bullae, edema, polyarthropathy, myopathy, anorexia, intermittent fever, and lethargy. If necrosis and ulcerations are extensive, secondary bacterial and fungal infections may invade the raw skin lesions. Epidermal lesions include exudation, crusting, and ulceration. Many animals develop purpuric plaques, hemorrhages, papules, and edema. Purpuric lesions darken over time.

The skin overlying the extremities, including the pinnae, feet, and over the hocks, is most commonly affected. Vasculitis is often associated with anemia, thrombocytopenia, neutropenia, protein-losing nephropathy, and musculoskeletal lesions. Vasculitis-associated immunothrombosis may cause the thrombocytopenia.

Pathology. Histological examination of the dermis and panniculus is required to identify the presence of vasculitis. It affects both small- and medium-sized blood vessels. Damage to these vessels can lead to hemorrhage and edema. The vasculitis is usually leukocytoclastic. Thus, the fragmentation of the nuclei of infiltrating pyknotic or karyorrhexic neutrophils results in the accumulation of fragments of nuclear material around blood vessels. This is called leukocytoclasia (or nuclear dust). This nuclear dust is often the only evidence of a vascular lesion. Other criteria that need to be satisfied include intramural inflammation, endothelial cell swelling, hemorrhage, and fibrinous necrosis in the blood vessel walls. In most cases, cellular infiltration is neutrophilic. Hypoxic changes will result in pale collagen and faded hair follicles.

Diagnosis and Treatment. The underlying causes of vasculitis may include drugs, insect bites, infections, food allergies, and some autoimmune diseases. In reviewing the animal's history, care should be taken to obtain a history of all drugs and vaccines administered, as well as any diet or dietary supplements. If an infectious cause is suspected, blood culture is required.

Most commonly, the disease is caused by type III hypersensitivity to a drug. A temporal relationship with drug administration can often be identified, although it may be difficult to determine which specific drug is the cause, especially in patients receiving multiple medications. Three commonly used drugs known to trigger cutaneous vasculitis in dogs and cats include itraconazole, fenbendazole, and meloxicam. The immune complexes found in vessel walls contain antigens derived from the parent drug or its metabolites coupled with host antibodies. The first step in treatment is to remove and avoid subsequent exposure to the offending drug. However, it may not be the drug itself that causes vasculitis. For example, gelatin capsules may trigger a response in beef-allergic animals. Once a diagnosis of vasculitis is confirmed by histology, treatment and follow-up should be tailored to the specific animal. In general, patients should receive glucocorticoid therapy or cyclosporine. Immunosuppressive doses are required to induce remission, and relapses are not uncommon.

Other Vasculitides. Several other forms of immune-mediated vasculitis have been described in domestic animals. Their precise relationships are unclear, and as a result, they have been given several different names, including canine juvenile polyarteritis and polyarteritis nodosa.

Canine juvenile polyarteritis primarily affects Beagles less than 2 years of age. The animals show episodes of anorexia, persistent fever over 40°C, and a hunched stance with a lowered head and a stiff gait, indicating severe neck pain. They may show cyclical remissions and relapses. These dogs have a neutrophilia, elevated acute-phase proteins, and elevated serum IgM and IgA levels, but normal IgG levels. Circulating B cells are increased, but their T cells are decreased, as is their response to mitogens. Necropsy reveals few gross lesions. There may be some hemorrhage within the lymph nodes. Histologically, there was systemic vasculitis and perivasculitis. In acute cases, there may be necrotizing vasculitis with fibrinoid necrosis and massive inflammatory cell infiltration involving small- and medium-sized arteries of the heart, mediastinum, and cervical spinal cord. Immunoglobulins are deposited on the walls of these arteries. During remissions, the vascular lesions consist of intimal and medial fibrosis and mild perivasculitis, the residue of previous acute attacks. Chronically affected dogs may develop generalized amyloidosis.

Polyarteritis nodosa occurs in humans, pigs, dogs, and cats. It is characterized by widespread focal necrosis of the media of small- and medium-sized muscular arteries. Lesions are found in many organs, especially the kidneys. The vessels in the skin are rarely involved. Polyarteritis nodosa is usually an incidental finding on necropsy, although ocular defects may present clinically if the arteries of the eye are involved.

The cause or causes of polyarteritis nodosa and canine juvenile polyarteritis are unknown. Their histopathology suggests that they are type III hypersensitivity reaction, perhaps triggered by an infectious agent. Immunosuppression with corticosteroids, together with cyclophosphamide, has given encouraging results in the treatment of canine hypersensitivity vasculitis. Pentoxifylline, a phosphodiesterase inhibitor, appears to be effective in the treatment of cutaneous vasculitis. It has anti-inflammatory effects and it reduces neutrophil adherence to the vascular endothelium. In dogs, combined treatment with glucocorticoids and pentoxifylline appears to produce the best results. However, pentoxifylline is slow to act and patience is required.

Drug Hypersensitivities

In a previous chapter, it was pointed out that if a drug attached itself to a cell such as an erythrocyte, the immune response against the drug could lead to elimination of the cell. A similar reaction may occur through type III hypersensitivity reactions if drug-antibody complexes bind to host cells. In this case, the cells are recognized as foreign, opsonized, and removed by phagocytosis. As might be predicted, if immune complexes bind to erythrocytes, anemia results, whereas if they bind to platelets, immunothrombosis, thrombocytopenia, and purpura result. Binding to granulocytes leads to granulocytopenia and, consequently, recurrent infections. However, in many cases, it is difficult to distinguish between type A responses to a drug and type III hypersensitivity unless specific antibodies can be eluted from the affected cells.

Purpura Hemorrhagica

Purpura hemorrhagica is a necrotizing vasculitis of horses that may develop following infections in which suppuration is present in some region of the body. For example, 2 to 4 weeks after an acute *Streptococcus equi* infection, horses may develop urticaria, followed by severe, well-demarcated, subcutaneous edema, especially involving the distal limbs, and the development of hemorrhages in the mucosa and subcutaneous tissues (Fig. 18.5). Other triggers of purpura hemorrhagica include *Corynebacterium pseudotuberculosis*, *Prescottella equi*, equine influenza virus, and equine herpesvirus type 1. In some cases, purpura may develop in the absence of any obvious prior bacterial or viral infections.

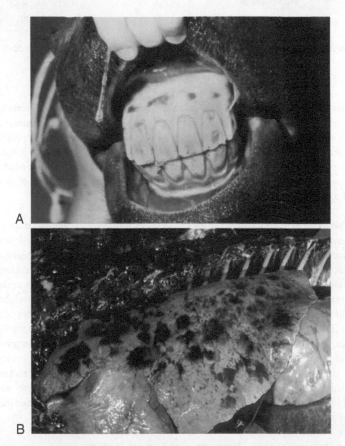

Fig. 18.5 A, Petechial hemorrhages of oral mucous membranes in a horse with purpura hemorrhagica. **B**, Hemorrhages on the surface of the lungs in a horse with purpura hemorrhagica. (From Sellon DC, Long MT. *Equine Infectious Diseases*, Saunders, 2007.)

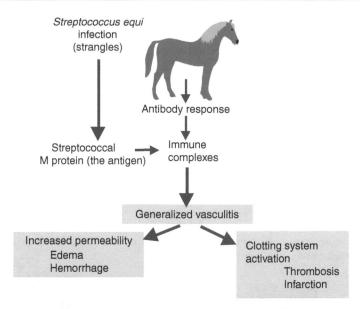

Fig. 18.6   The pathogenesis of equine purpura hemorrhagica following a *Streptococcus equi* infection.

Pathogenesis. Immune complexes are found in the serum of affected horses and consist of streptococcal M or R protein complexed with IgM or IgA (Fig. 18.6). These immune complexes are deposited in blood vessel walls and cause membranoproliferative glomerulonephritis, resulting in proteinuria and azoturia. Deposition of these complexes in blood vessel walls results in vasculitis, immunothrombosis, edema, and hemorrhage. Complement may also be deposited in association with antigen-antibody complexes. Preexisting high serum antibody levels in *S. equi* may predispose horses to this condition.

Clinical Disease. There are great variations in disease severity and clinical course, ranging from mild transient reactions to fatal disease. Clinical signs develop within 2 to 4 weeks following natural or vaccinal exposure to streptococcal antigens. The most prominent signs include severe subcutaneous edema in all four limbs and the ventral abdomen. Petechial or ecchymotic hemorrhages develop on the visible mucous membranes. Other signs may include depression and reluctance to move, fever, anorexia, tachycardia, tachypnea, colic, epistaxis, and weight loss. Edema may result in skin exudation, ulceration, crusting, and sloughing. Severe edema of the head may compromise breathing and eating. Other abnormalities include anemia, neutrophilia, hyperglobulinemia, elevated muscle enzymes (due to rhabdomyolysis), and hyperproteinemia. The vasculitis may also affect the gastrointestinal tract, lungs, and muscles. In severe cases, some horses may develop a generalized leukocytoclastic vasculitis that can lead to thrombosis and infarction. Intussusception in the small intestine may complicate the disease, as does muscle infarction. Hemorrhage and necrosis of the skeletal muscle may occur. Infarctive purpura hemorrhagica is a rare and fatal form of the disease.

Pathology. Skin biopsies show the presence of a severe leukocytoclastic vasculitis with marked neutrophilic infiltration around the affected blood vessels. This vasculitis may be associated with necrosis of the infarcted muscle. Affected horses may have unusually high blood IgA levels.

Diagnosis and Treatment. Immediate medical attention should be sought for affected horses. Any inducing infection should be treated. Inflammation should be suppressed by the use of systemic glucocorticoids (dexamethasone and/or prednisolone). Horses may also receive nonsteroidal anti-inflammatory drugs (phenylbutazone or flunixin meglumine) and antibiotics to limit secondary infections.

Pigs also suffer from sporadic cases of immune complex-mediated thrombocytopenic purpura syndrome. This has been a specific problem in Gottingen minipigs, a line of small pigs used in experimental studies. The animals develop severe thrombocytopenia, anemia, excessive bleeding, and membranoproliferative lesions in their glomeruli. Some animals have necrotizing vasculitis. The cause is unknown, although it is assumed to be due to type III hypersensitivity. The same line of pigs may also develop spontaneous polyarteritis. Its cause is unknown but is likely immune-mediated.

Suggested Reading

Asmundsson T, Gunnarsson E, Johannesson T. "Haysickness" in Icelandic horses: precipitin tests and other studies. *Equine Vet J.* 1983;15(3):229-232. doi: 10.1111/j.2042-3306.1983.tb01774.x

Carrasco L, Madsen LW, Salguero FJ, Nunez A, Sanchez-Cordon PJ, Bollen P. Immune complex-associated thrombocytopenic purpura syndrome in sexually mature Gottingen minipigs. *J Comp Pathol.* 2003;128(1):25-32. doi: 10.1053/jcpa.2002.0601

Delph KM, Beard LA, Trimble AC, Sutter ME, Timony JF, Morrow JK. Strangles, convalescent Streptococcus equi subspecies equi M antibody titers and the presence of complications. *J Vet Intern Med.* 2019;33(1):275-279. doi: 10.1111/jvim.15388

Galan JF, Timony JF. Immune complexes in purpura hemorrhagica of the horse contain IgA and M antigen of *Streptococcus equi. J Immunol.* 1985;135(5):3134-3137.

Gunson DE, Rooney JR. Anaphylactoid purpura in a horse. *Vet Pathol.* 1977;14(4):325-331. doi: 10.1177/030098587701400403

Innerå M. Cutaneous vasculitis in small animals. *Vet Clin North Am Small Anim Pract.* 2013;43(1):113-134. doi: 10.1016/j.cvsm.2012.09.011

Jasani S, Boag AK, Smith KC. Systemic vasculitis with severe cutaneous manifestation as a suspected idiosyncratic hypersensitivity reaction to fenbendazole in a cat. *J Vet Intern Med.* 2008;22(3):666-670. doi: 10.1111/j.1939-1676.2008.0092.x

Kaese HJ, Valberg SJ, Hayden DW, et al. Infarctive purpura hemorrhagica in five horses. *J Am Vet Med Assoc.* 2005;226(11):1893-1898. doi: 10.2460/javma.2005.226.1893

Lee BM, Zersen KM, Schissler JR, Sullivan LA. Antivenin-associated serum sickness in a dog. *J Vet Emerg Crit Care (San Antonio).* 2019;29(5):558-563. doi:10.1111/vec.12874

Martinod K, Deppermann C. Immunothrombosis and thromboinflammation in host defense and disease. *Platelets* 2020;32(3):314-324. doi: 10.1080/09537104.2020.1817360

Morris DD. Cutaneous vasculitis in horses: 19 cases (1978-1985). *J Am Vet Med Assoc.* 1987;191(4):460-464.

Nichols PR, Morris DO, Beale KM. A retrospective study of canine and feline cutaneous vasculitis. *Vet Dermatol.* 2001;12(5):255-264. doi: 10.1046/j.0959-4493.2001.00268.x

Powell C, Thompson L, Murtaugh RJ. Type III hypersensitivity reaction with immune complex deposition in 2 critically ill dogs administered human serum albumin. *J Vet Emerg Crit Care (San Antonio).* 2013;23(6):598-604. doi: 10.1111/vec.12085

Spagnolo P, Rossi G, Cavazza A, et al. Hypersensitivity pneumonitis: a comprehensive review. *J Investig Allergol Clin Immunol.* 2015;25(4):237-250.

CHAPTER 19

Selected Type IV Hypersensitivities

When injected into the skin of sensitized animals, some antigens provoke a slowly developing inflammatory response at the injection site after a delay of 12 to 24 hours. These delayed hypersensitivity reactions are classified as type IV hypersensitivities and result from interactions between the injected antigen and effector T cells. Delayed hypersensitivity reactions can be considered T-cell-mediated inflammatory responses directed against organisms or other foreign antigens that are resistant to elimination by conventional antibody-mediated responses.

Cutaneous Basophil Hypersensitivity

As pointed out in Chapter 12, it is common for animals to mount both type I and type IV hypersensitivity responses to arthropod allergens. In most cases, type I responses predominate. However, tick bites are different. The exposure to tick antigens is not transient. Ticks remain attached to an animal for many days; sufficient time for a delayed T cell response to have an effect. When ticks feed, their injected salivary antigens induce a complex mixture of immune responses in their host. Feeding ticks trigger a delayed cellular response in the skin in which basophils and mast cells predominate (Fig. 19.1). Basophils constitute up to 70% of the infiltrating cells in experimental tick bites in guinea pigs. This type of reaction is called cutaneous basophil hypersensitivity (CBH) (Fig. 19.2).

When a tick first inserts its mouthparts into the skin, its salivary antigens are taken up by DC2 cells and present to Th2 cells. This triggers IgE and IgG responses that recruit and activate basophils. These basophils accumulate around the tick mouthparts and contribute to the local tissue defense. On second exposure, IgE-coated basophils are recruited to tick feeding sites, where they release histamine, resulting in pruritus and epidermal hyperplasia that promotes anti-tick resistance. This basophil accumulation increases significantly in the early phase of a second tick bite as a result of IL-3 production by $CD4^+$ memory T cells. When the inflammatory reactions around tick bite lesions in cattle are examined, it is clear that these lesions are also densely infiltrated with eosinophils and basophils. Infiltration is greater in tick-resistant cattle than in tick-susceptible breeds. CBH reactions may also contribute in part to the development of flea allergy dermatitis in dogs, as well as their response to the scabies mite *Sarcoptes scabiei*.

Contact Dermatitis

It has been estimated that out of approximately 140,000 chemicals in common use worldwide, about 80,000 are potentially reactive and damaging to animals. As a result, the incidence of contact dermatitis is rising, especially in industrialized countries. Chemically induced skin diseases are now the second most common form of occupational disease. The skin is a protective barrier that excludes these chemicals from the body, and interactions between these reactive chemicals and the body's defenses often occur first in the skin. The resulting response may generate the hypersensitivity reactions, known as contact dermatitis. There are two types of contact dermatitis: irritant contact dermatitis and allergic contact dermatitis (Table 19.1).

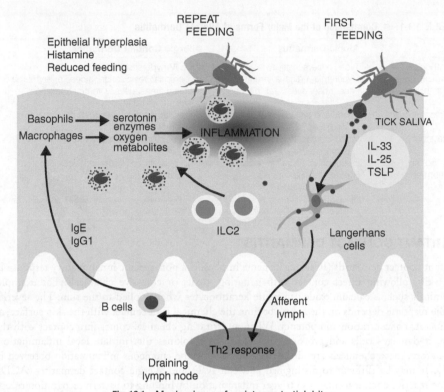

Fig. 19.1 Mechanisms of resistance to tick bites.

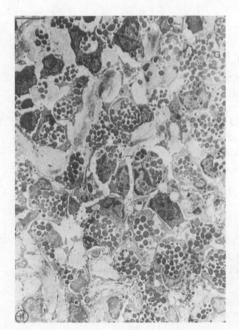

Fig. 19.2 A section of guinea pig skin 18 hours after attachment of a tick in an animal sensitized by prior infestation with tick larvae. The skin is infiltrated with large numbers of basophils. (From McLaren D, Worms MJ, Askenase PW: Cutaneous basophil-associated resistance to ectoparasites (ticks). Electron microscopy of *Rhipicephalus appendiculatus* larval feeding sites in actively sensitized guinea pigs and recipients of immune serum. *J Pathol* 1983;139(3):289).

TABLE 19.1. ■ Comparison of the Major Forms of Allergic Dermatitis

	Atopic Dermatitis	Allergic Contact Dermatitis
Pathogenesis	Type I hypersensitivity	Type IV hypersensitivity
Clinical signs	Hyperemia, urticaria, pruritus	Hyperemia, vesiculation, alopecia, erythema
Distribution	Face, nose, eyes, feet, perineum	Hairless areas, usually ventral abdomen, scrotum, and feet
Major allergens	Foods and pollens, fleas, inhaled allergens	Small but reactive chemicals coming into contact with skin
Diagnosis	Intradermal testing, immediate response	Delayed response on patch testing
Pathology	Eosinophilic infiltration, edema	Mononuclear cell infiltration, vesiculation
Treatment	Steroids, antihistamines, hyposensitization	Steroids, cyclosporine

IRRITANT CONTACT DERMATITIS

Irritant contact dermatitis (ICD), as its name implies, is a non-specific inflammatory response in the skin following direct contact with irritating, toxic, or corrosive chemicals. For example, chemicals such as calcium oxide can injure keratinocytes when applied to the skin. The severity of the response depends on the length of time the chemical is in contact with the skin surface, as well as its concentration and potency. When an irritating chemical comes into contact with the skin, it damages cells and provokes the release of cytokines that initiate local inflammation. Therefore, these chemicals are directly responsible for the cutaneous inflammation observed in ICD. It may be difficult to distinguish between ICD and allergic contact dermatitis (ACD). Some reactive chemicals may also trigger inflammation by binding to pattern recognition receptors (PRRs) and inflammasomes. For example, TLR4 is a PRR that can bind multiple contact sensitizers, including nickel and trinitrochlorobenzene. They therefore trigger dermatitis by releasing IL-1β and TNF-α.

ALLERGIC CONTACT DERMATITIS

ACD is also a chemically induced inflammatory skin response. However, the response is immunologically mediated rather than simply due to the toxic effects of the chemical (Fig. 19.3). The chemical induces a defensive immune response, which is expressed as an acute cutaneous inflammatory reaction. This antigen-specific response develops within hours or days following contact of the skin with a specific chemical sensitizer. ACD reactions are, in effect, equivalent to type B drug-mediated adverse events. As such, they are idiosyncratic and not dose dependent. Some sensitizers, such as nickel, are not only contact irritants, but are also immunogenic. Despite being considered rare in dogs, the reported prevalence of ACD has been as high as 10% in dermatological cases in one canine study.

CONTACT SENSITIZERS*

Contact sensitizers are chemically reactive compounds that covalently bind to proteins on epithelial cells. Unlike some drug responses where the chemical binds covalently to soluble proteins and thus triggers an antibody response, these chemicals bind to cell surface proteins and therefore

---

*A database of known contact-sensitizing chemicals is available at the website of the Contact Dermatitis Institute at https://www.contactdermatitisinstitute.com/database.php

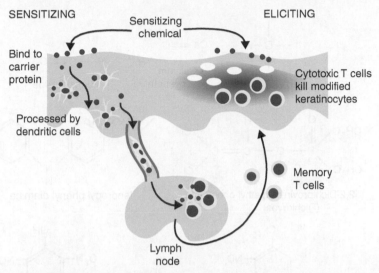

Fig. 19.3 The pathogenesis of allergic contact dermatitis. Note that this is a two-stage process with a sensitizing phase followed by an eliciting phase on subsequent exposure to the contact sensitizer.

trigger a T cell–mediated response that resembles the graft rejection process. As with many drugs, most skin-sensitizing chemicals are too small to be immunogenic on their own. Therefore, they must first covalently bind to epidermal cell proteins to create antigenic hapten-protein complexes. In fact, most known contact sensitizers are small molecules, such as cations or metals. They are delivered to the skin as drugs, oils, cosmetics, skin creams, or fragrances. Many do not bind to conventional major histocompatibility complex (MHC) antigen-binding sites. However, a nonpolymorphic MHC-related molecule, CD1a, can bind and present hydrophobic molecules, including lipids, to T cells.

Chemicals that induce ACD are usually highly reactive. They tend to be lipophilic and readily penetrate the skin. Their upper size limit is approximately 500 Da if they are to pass through the stratum corneum.

Contact sensitizers originate from a wide variety of sources. Many are natural products derived from plants; for example, the reactive oils (urushiols) of the poison ivy plant (*Rhus radicans*) are major contact allergens in humans. Some plants can also cause ACD in dogs. For example, dermal contact with *Plumbago auriculata* can cause contact dermatitis. Other plants reported to induce ACD in dogs include hippeastrum, Asian jasmine, oleander, dandelion, and plants belonging to the family *Commelinceae* (spiderworts) such as *Commelina cyanea* and *Callista fragrans* (commonly called the inch plant or basket plant).

Many contact allergens are relatively small compounds (Fig. 19.4). For example, dogs may develop contact dermatitis in response to dihydroxyacetone, an ingredient in sunless tanning solutions. ACD can occur on pathologists' fingers because of exposure to formaldehyde, on the ears of dogs treated with neomycin for otitis externa, on the foot pads and ventral abdomens of dogs exposed to carpet dyes and deodorizers, and around the necks of animals as a result of exposure to dichlorvos (2,2-dichlorovinyldimethylphosphate) in flea collars. This may also cause contact dermatitis in pet owners who handle these collars. Hardwood floor varnish has also been implicated in some canine cases.

Severe lesions have developed on the teats of dairy cattle as a result of contact dermatitis to a component of milking machine rubber (N-isopropyl-N-phenyl diamine). Powdered calcium

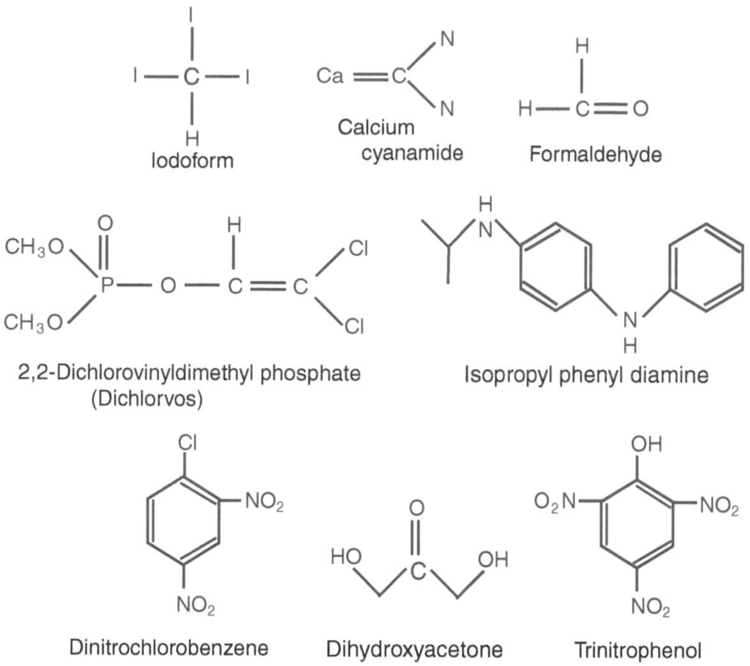

Fig. 19.4 Some of the simple chemicals that can cause allergic contact dermatitis in domestic animals.

cyanamide ($CaCN_2$) was used to reduce *Escherichia coli* levels in bedding. Dairy cattle developed severe dermatitis upon contact with calcium cyanamide spread on the floor of a cattle shed.

The list of other potential contact allergens is long and includes simple metal salts, such as potassium bichromate, cobalt chloride, and nickel sulfate; and mixtures of chemicals used in the natural and synthetic rubber industries, such as thiuram mix, black rubber mix, naphthyl mix, and carba mix. Other chemical allergens include lanolin alcohols, epoxy resins, quinoline mix (used in antibacterial creams), fragrance mix (used to mask unpleasant smells), ethylenediamine, wood tar, concrete, and dinitrochlorobenzene. Even pure metals, such as nickel and chromium, may cause ACD. For example, dogs have also developed ACD in response to the chromium in stainless steel cages.

PATHOGENESIS

ACD is a T cell-mediated delayed hypersensitivity reaction. It is therefore slow to develop, antigen-specific, and is primarily mediated by $CD8^+$ cytotoxic T cells. It can be conveniently divided into two distinct phases: sensitization and elicitation.

Sensitization Phase

The development of ACD first requires sensitization of an animal to a specific antigen. This sensitization phase develops over a period of weeks to months following chemical exposure. There are two mechanisms by which an animal may become sensitized. Compounds that covalently bind to cell proteins are treated as endogenous antigens. This means that they are processed and presented by MHC class II molecules. The second mechanism is used for lipids. Lipids are processed and then bound to a non-polymorphic antigen-presenting molecule called CD1a. CD1a is abundantly expressed in Langerhans and dermal dendritic cells. It rapidly binds to its ligands without the need for complex antigen-processing pathways. CD1a binds to small hydrophobic oily molecules. For example, it readily binds urushiol from poison ivy.

Chemically modified proteins are first taken up by epidermal Langerhans cells, which then migrate to the draining lymph nodes. Here, they mature into dendritic cells that process the hapten-carrier conjugates and then present them to T cells. They also release pro-inflammatory cytokines and chemokines that stimulate the helper cell response. They prime T cells, promoting their clonal expansion and differentiation into CD8$^+$ and CD4$^+$ cells. The migration of hapten-bearing antigen-presenting cells to the draining lymph nodes is essential for the development of memory T cells.

Elicitation Phase

Once an animal has been sensitized, it may take 6 to 12 months after priming before dermatitis develops. The memory T cells generated during the sensitization phase will mount a response when they encounter the chemically modified epidermal cells a second time. The Langerhans cells activate both Th1 and Th17 cells. These helper cells in turn produce large amounts of IFN-γ and IL-17 and promote the activity of CD8$^+$ cytotoxic T cells.

Primed cytotoxic CD8$^+$ T cells migrate from the local lymph nodes into the bloodstream and eventually reach the site of chemical exposure on the skin. These primed T cells carry a skin homing marker called cutaneous lymphocyte antigen, which is a ligand for E-selectin, an adhesive cell surface protein expressed in chronically inflamed skin. This allows T cells to specifically target the lesion site in the skin. This marker also induces the release of pro-inflammatory cytokines and the expression of adhesion molecules by keratinocytes and Langerhans cells. This attracts and activates yet more T cells.

Following exposure to the sensitizing chemical, macrophages and CD8$^+$ T cells infiltrate the dermis. They take approximately 24 hours to generate a significant response. The cytotoxic T cells target and kill skin cells that express chemically modified proteins. Cytotoxic T cells also release IFN-γ, which activates keratinocytes and enhances the expression of IL-33, IL-25, and TSLP. In addition to killing chemically modified keratinocytes, cytotoxic T cells also kill any dendritic cells carrying the chemical. Eventually, these cytotoxic T cells kill so many altered cells that gaps form and intraepithelial vesicles develop.

This destructive T cell response, together with the production of IL-33 and accompanying inflammatory products, results in an intensely pruritic inflammatory skin reaction. In addition to α/β T cells, other cell types, such as γ/δ T cells, ILC1 cells, NK cells, B cells, mast cells, and NKT cells, contribute to the reaction. Inflammation is eventually moderated by IL-10 and TGF-β production by Treg cells.

Mast cells are found in close proximity to infiltrating T cells in ACD. As a result, the two cell types signal to each other. For example, T cell-derived IL-3, MIP-1α, and MCP-1 signal from T cells to mast cells. Conversely, activated mast cells signal to T cells. They may attract T cells by releasing lymphotactin, IL-16, or leukotriene B$_4$. They may bind T cells through E-selectin, ICAM-1, or VCAM-1. Since mast cells can release both IL-4 and IL-13, they may also polarize T cells and convert them to Th2 cells. The intense pruritus associated with ACD is probably not mediated directly by T cells but by mast cells. A molecule called proadrenalomedullin produced in lesional ACD skin activates mast cells through the MRGPRX2 receptor. This results in the production of tryptase, leukotrienes, and serotonin, all of which contribute to the itch sensation.

Canine Contact Dermatitis

Because of their haired skin, dogs and other domestic animals are generally less susceptible to developing ACD than hairless species such as humans. Nevertheless, ACD can occur in these species, especially when the hairless areas come in contact with chemically treated surfaces (Fig. 19.5).

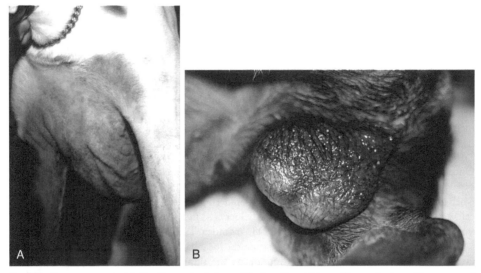

Fig. 19.5   A severe case of allergic contact dermatitis in a Great Dane. The contact sensitizer was not identified, but it appeared to originate in the concrete surrounding a newly constructed swimming pool. Chloride ions appear to release a contact sensitizer from concrete. (Courtesy Dr. R. Kennis)

A colony of Mexican hairless dogs has been established for the purpose of studying atopic dermatitis. These dogs have been used to investigate hypersensitivities to agricultural chemicals and hair dyes. They spontaneously developed contact dermatitis upon contact with chromium in stainless steel cages. The primary changes were erythema, edema, macules, and papules. Initially, pruritus developed over the thoracic and abdominal skin, and the lesions gradually progressed to cover the dorsum and extremities. The affected areas developed lichenification, hyperkeratosis, hyperpigmentation, scaling, and skin fissuring. When the dogs were patch tested, positive reactions were obtained in response to potassium dichromate 24, 48, and 72 hours after application. Histopathology of the lesional skin showed epidermal hyperplasia and intercellular edema. In the upper dermis of the involved skin, dense mononuclear cell infiltrates were observed. Lymphocytic infiltration developed around the base of the hair follicles and sebaceous glands. There was also marked mast cell infiltration. Chromium is one of the most common causes of occupational dermatitis in humans, and the histopathological changes in these dogs closely resemble those in humans. Hexavalent chromium penetrates epidermal cells and enters their organelles, where it is converted to trivalent chromium. Trivalent chromium reacts with proteins to induce T cell responses and dermatitis.

Only one study has looked for any breed predisposition to the development of canine ICD, and none has been identified. The use of Mexican hairless dogs to study ACD was based on their lack of hair and the ability of the sensitizing chemical to reach their skin surface rather than any specific genetic markers.

The development of ACD in dogs and cats is similar to that reported in humans. Affected sites usually include areas of skin that come into direct contact with the sensitizer. The lesions tend to be restricted to thinly haired areas. These include the groin, face, ears, paws, perineum, scrotum, and ventral tail. The distribution of these lesions may help identify the source of the irritant. For example, generalized lesions point to liquid shampoo components as a possible cause. If the lesions are restricted to the groove between the shoulder blades, this suggests that a drop-on product is responsible. Because ACD lesions are often generally restricted to the sites of contact with the sensitizer, the ventral abdomen is the most commonly affected site.

Acute lesions of ACD include erythema and erosions, vesicles, crusts, edema, and papule formation. However, due to intense pruritus, self-trauma, excoriation, ulceration, secondary Malassezia infections, and staphylococcal pyoderma often mask the true nature of the lesion. If exposure to the allergen persists, chronic lesions include scaling, fissuring, lichenification, hyperpigmentation, or depigmentation. Hyperkeratosis, acanthosis, and dermal fibrosis may eventually occur.

Scrotal skin is thin with few hair follicles, and as a result, it is commonly affected by contact dermatitis. Case studies in dogs have suggested that floor detergents, bleach, cement, laundry detergents, and some plastics may act as contact allergens (see Fig. 9.5). In these cases, the predominant clinical sign is severe pruritus, accompanied by licking and rubbing. It is important to note that the scrotum is not commonly involved in canine atopic dermatitis.

ACD involving the muzzles of dogs has been reported to result from sensitivity to plastics in food bowls. Some dogs, instead of developing the usual type I hypersensitivity to pollen proteins, experience ACD to pollen resins. The period required for sensitization ranges from 6 months to several years.

It is important to note that veterinarians and their assistants may also come into contact with potential contact allergens during their work. For example, ACD has been observed in veterinary assistants following exposure to carprofen, a canine nonsteroidal anti-inflammatory drug. It is interesting to note that the reaction is more severe when the lesion is exposed to light, an example of a photoallergic response.

HISTOPATHOLOGY

Histologic examination cannot always distinguish between ICD and ACD. This is especially true for chronic lesions. Therefore, it is best to sample lesions within the first 48 hours. The major feature of acute disease is intracellular vacuolation with cell necrosis (Fig. 19.6). Collagen degradation may also occur. The cellular infiltrate consists mainly of monocytes and lymphocytes infiltrating the dermis and epidermis. In chronic lesions, there may be hyperkeratosis, parakeratosis, and acanthosis. ACD lesions show varying degrees of superficial perivascular dermatitis with

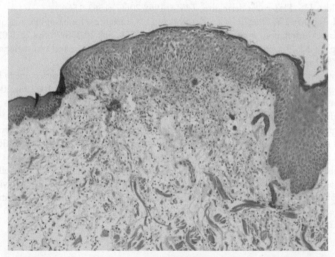

Fig. 19.6 Histopathology of allergic contact dermatitis showing the presence of spongiosis, edema, infiltration with lymphocytes, neutrophils, and eosinophils. The presence of these latter cells suggests that this is a mixed type I and type IV reaction. (Courtesy Drs. Dominique Wiener and Aline Rodrigues Hoffman).

epidermal spongiosis that may proceed to vesiculation. Some reactions show infiltration with lymphocytes, whereas others contain eosinophilic or neutrophilic epidermal pustules. Presumably, these reflect different mechanisms mediating the development of the lesion and possibly point to the existence of different endotypes.

DIAGNOSIS AND TREATMENT

ACD is diagnosed by the removal of the suspected antigen and patch testing. In "closed" patch tests, suspected sensitizers are used to impregnate gauze swabs that are then attached to the shaved skin with tape. After 48 to 72 hours of contact, the dressing is removed, and the areas in contact with the sensitizers are examined. A positive reaction is indicated by local erythema and vesiculation. Closed patch tests may be impractical for some dogs and cats. An "open" patch test may therefore be employed. In this procedure, a solution of the suspected sensitizer is applied to a small area of shaved normal skin, and the area is examined daily for up to 5 days. Identification of the offending allergen and its avoidance is the optimal therapy for ACD.

Steroids may be used to treat acute cases, with antibiotics to control secondary infections. Topical treatments may also include bathing in an effort to remove the irritant and soothe the epidermis. Topical corticosteroids can be used in the short term for the treatment of local lesions to reduce inflammation and discomfort. However, they are not appropriate for long-term treatment. Calcineurin inhibitors, such as cyclosporine, are clearly indicated for long-term treatment. They are often used in animals that do not respond well to glucocorticoid therapy. The use of pentoxifylline at a dose of 10 mg/kg has been reported to be effective in the treatment of ACD to plants of the *Commelinceae* family. Because ACD is T cell-mediated, antihistamines are of no benefit in treating it, and ACD is not responsive to allergen-specific immunotherapy.

Suggested Reading

Carvalho WA, Franzin AM, Abatepaulo ARR, et al. Modulation of cutaneous inflammation induced by ticks in contrasting phenotypes of infestation in bovines. *Vet Parasitol*. 2010;167(2-4):260-273. doi: 10.1016/j.vetpar.2009.09.028

Cronce PC, Alden HS. Flea-collar dermatitis. *JAMA*. 1968;206(7):1563-1564.

Karasuyama H, Tabakawa Y, Ohta T, Wada T, Yoshikawa S. Crucial role for basophils in acquired protective immunity to tick infestation. *Front Physiol*. 2018;9:1769-1776. doi: 10.3389/fphys.2018.01769

Ho KK, Campbell KL, Lavergne SN. Contact dermatitis: a conmparative and translational review of the literature. *Vet Dermatol*. 2015;26(5):314-e67. doi: 10.1111/vde.12229

Kimura T. Contact dermatitis caused by sunless tanning treatment with dihydroxyacetone in hairless descendants of Mexican hairless dogs. *Environ Toxicol*. 2007;22(5):176-184. doi: 10.1002/tox.20456

Kimura T. Contact hypersensitivity to stainless steel cages (chromium metal) in hairless descendants of Mexican hairless dogs. *Environ Toxicol*. 2009;24(2):506-512. doi: 10.1002/tox.20243

Nicolai S, Wegrecki M, Cheng T-Y, et al. Human T cell response to CD1a and contact dermatitis allergens in botanical extracts and commercial skin care products. *Sci Immunol*. 2020;5(43):eaax5430. doi: 10.1126/sciimmunol.aax5430

Seavers A, Robson D, Weingarth JM. A vesicular (blistering) skin condition in a dog following putative contact exposure to Plumbago auriculate. *Aust Vet J*. 2016;94(8):290-292. doi: 10.1111/avi.12461

Trenti D, Carlotti DN, Pin D, Bensignor E, Toulza O. Suspected contact scrotal dermatitis in the dog: a retrospective study of 13 cases (1987 to 2003). *J Small Anim Pract*. 2011;52(6):295-300. doi: 10.1111/j.1748-5827.2011.01069.x

CHAPTER 20

Diagnostic Assays

Throughout this book, it has been made clear that the diagnosis of allergic diseases requires demonstration that affected animals are generating an IgE response to a specific allergen or allergens. In other words, is the animal is making these antibodies and can they be detected in the bloodstream? Once specific sensitization has been confirmed, clinical judgment is required to determine if this is significant and relevant to the animal's clinical state. Subsequent treatment options include drugs or specific immunotherapy. If a decision is made to use specific immunotherapy, it is essential to determine the precise allergens to which the animal is responding. These sensitization assays are divided into two broad areas. Laboratory-based in vitro assays measure total IgE levels; additionally, they may measure, at least semi-quantitatively, the presence of allergen-specific IgE. In vivo assays performed in the clinic rely on the ability of specific allergens to react with IgE bound to skin mast cells, trigger the release of inflammatory mediators, and cause a local tissue reaction when injected into an animal's skin.

In Vitro Assays

TOTAL IgE

It is worth reiterating that the measurement of total IgE levels in the bloodstream has intrinsically limited usefulness. The IgE found in blood is in transit. It is on its way from B cells in the lymphoid organs to basophils and mast cells in the tissues where it binds to their receptors (Fig. 20.1). The quantity of IgE in the blood will therefore be determined not only by its rate of production by B cells but also by the rate of its removal by receptors on mast cells and its rate of catabolism. Serum IgE assays measure IgE that has yet to bind to mast cells. Therefore, its level depends not only on its production rate but also on the availability of unoccupied mast cell receptors. An increase in IgE levels may suggest increased IgE production in lymphoid organs. It may also reflect a reduction in mast cell uptake because there are too few available receptors. Recall that the primary storage site for IgE is the mast cell surface. As pointed out in Chapter 2, when IgE binds to a mast cell receptor, it stabilizes its expression. As IgE levels rise, so do the number of available mast cell receptors. This is not a proportional increase; a 10-fold rise in IgE levels will cause only a 2.7-fold increase in receptor expression. If the increase in IgE is due to irrelevant antibodies, then these may saturate the mast cell receptors before specific IgE can bind and thus functionally reduce a mast cell's ability to respond.

As discussed in Chapter 2, it has been demonstrated that the biological activity of IgE largely depends on its degree of glycosylation, specifically its sialylation. Thus, non-atopic humans have a much lower level of IgE sialylation than atopic individuals. This is another reason for the limited clinical usefulness of measuring total IgE. It also explains why many animals may possess allergen-specific IgE in the absence of clinical disease.

An elevated serum IgE level is suggestive of an atopic predisposition, but it provides no information on the responsible allergen or on its likelihood of developing allergic disease.

While serum IgE levels are very low compared to other immunoglobulins, they also vary over a much wider range. Non-atopic individuals do not make IgE against most antigens.

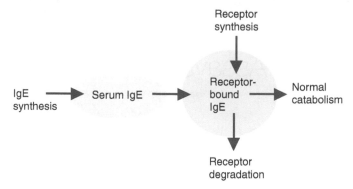

Fig. 20.1   The dynamics of total IgE levels in serum. These are influenced by not only its rate of synthesis and catabolism but also the availability of receptors on mast cells and basophils. In some situations, the rate of production of FcεR1 may not be coincident with the rate of production of IgE and, as a result, IgE levels may rise or fall. These assays do not measure either IgE specificity or its affinity for allergens.

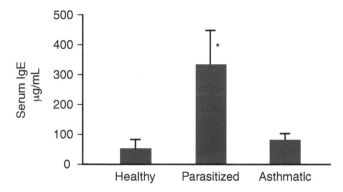

Fig 20.2   Comparison of the mean total serum IgE concentration between healthy, parasitized (obvious ecto- and endoparasites), and asthmatic cats. Healthy cats had the lowest total serum IgE concentrations. There was a significantly higher IgE concentration in parasitized cats when compared to healthy cats (* $P<0.05$ compared to the healthy group). IgE levels in asthmatic cats did not differ significantly from healthy cats. (From Delgado C, Lee-Fowler TM, DeClue AE, Reinero CR. Feline-specific serum total IgE quantitation in normal, asthmatic, and parasitized cats. *J Feline Med Surg.* 2010;12(12):991-994. doi: 10.1016/j.jfms.2010.08.006)

Despite these known issues, total IgE measurement using an enzyme-linked immunosorbent assay (ELISA) has been widely used in humans as a method of distinguishing atopic patients from "normal" individuals. However, serum IgE levels are highly variable (Table 2.1). Many factors, such as season, sex, genetics, parasites, and the occurrence of other non-allergic diseases, can influence IgE levels. Elevated IgE levels in infancy are associated with a significantly increased risk of developing asthma in later childhood. The usefulness of measuring total IgE levels declines with age. In adults, IgE levels are bimodal, but there remains a considerable overlap between atopic and non-atopic populations. Note also that quantitative IgE assays cannot distinguish between low- and high-affinity IgE, which is also reflected in the poor correlation between blood IgE levels and the severity of an allergy. This also means that, in effect, there is no "normal" IgE level.

The situation in dogs and cats is similar to that in humans: Measurement of total serum IgE is of questionable usefulness and varies according to age and breed, but most significantly with the presence of parasites (Fig. 20.2). The most common cause of elevated IgE in animals is parasite infestation. In cats, IgE levels are correlated with the absence of flea control or deworming. Thus, worms and fleas can have a potentially significant effect on serum IgE levels.

When an IgE response is mounted against a specific allergen, it frequently accounts for a large portion of the total serum IgE. In humans, the ratio of specific IgE to total IgE can be as high as 54% in patients allergic to Hymenoptera venom, 33% in peanut allergy, and 27% in milk allergy. This is very different from typical IgG responses, where each specific antibody only accounts for a small fraction of the total circulating IgG. Atopic animals may demonstrate elevated IgE levels, but as in humans, these may be limited to specific allergen responses in different individuals.

MULTIALLERGEN SCREENING ASSAYS

In contrast to the measurement of total IgE, in vitro assays that measure the presence of IgE directed against a specific allergen or set of allergens can confirm the diagnosis of a specific allergy. These tests measure the amount of IgE directed against the most important aeroallergens or foods. They also serve as diagnostic confirmatory tests, provided that their results are compatible with the clinical history and presentation. Therefore, these tests should only be used for confirmation after a clinical diagnosis has been made. One important reason for this is that many non-atopic dogs and horses may have high levels of allergen-specific IgE. For example, up to 20% of apparently healthy dogs may have high levels of IgE against house dust mites and common pollens.

Serologic assays for IgE all work in the same basic manner. The allergens are first covalently bound to an insoluble matrix, such as cellulose. They are then incubated with the patient's serum. Antibodies present in the serum bind to the allergens. Unbound antibodies are then flushed away, leaving only specific antibodies bound to the allergen matrix. The presence of bound IgE is then determined by incubating the matrix with either a very specific antiglobulin directed at epitopes on the ε heavy chains or with the IgE binding site of the α chain of FcεR1. The antiglobulin or the α chain is chemically coupled to a marker, such as an enzyme or radioisotope. After a second buffer wash, any unbound protein is flushed away, and the bound antiglobulin or α chain remaining can then be measured by either determining its radioactivity or enzyme activity. The signal intensity is proportional to the amount of IgE-specific antiglobulin or α chain bound, which in turn is proportional to the amount of specific IgE that reacted with the allergen.

The first of these assays to be developed was the radioallergosorbent test (RAST). This initially used insolubilized anti-IgE to capture serum IgE and used radiolabeled anti-IgE after washing to measure how much IgE was present in blood (Fig. 20.3). This assay was subsequently modified using an allergen coupled to cyanogen bromide-activated cellulose beads (Sephadex). When incubated in serum, antibodies of all classes bind to the allergen. However, after washing to remove any unbound serum proteins, the remaining bound IgE can be detected and quantified by the addition of radiolabeled anti-IgE antiglobulin. RASTs continue to improve and are increasingly automated. Currently, the most advanced substrate is an encapsulated hydrophobic carrier polymer (a cellulose sponge) to which the allergen is covalently coupled (Phadebas-RAST). Other available tests include the multi-allergosorbent chemiluminescence assay and an immunocheminometric assay.

Although radioisotopes were initially used as labels for primary binding tests, they have many disadvantages. Non-isotopic labels are more user friendly and have a longer shelf life, whereas isotope detection systems are expensive. This expense, combined with the hazards of radioactivity and the need to dispose of radioactive material in a safe manner, has ensured that radioimmunoassays are only used in specialized laboratories when highly sensitive assays are absolutely required. Thus, enzyme labeling is much more practical. The most popular enzymes used in ELISAs include alkaline phosphatase, horseradish peroxidase, and β-galactosidase. An alternative method is to label the reagents with biotin and then detect the biotin using its specific binding protein, streptavidin. Biotin can bind to proteins without affecting their biological

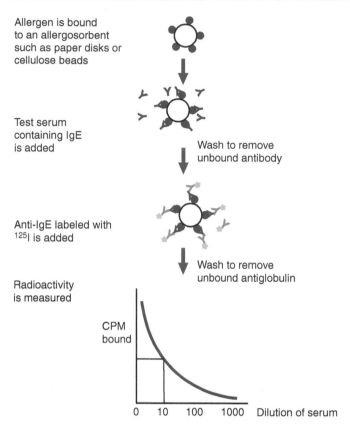

Allergen is bound
to an allergosorbent
such as paper disks or
cellulose beads

Test serum
containing IgE
is added

Wash to remove
unbound antibody

Anti-IgE labeled with
^{125}I is added

Wash to remove
unbound antiglobulin

Radioactivity
is measured

CPM
bound

0   10   100   1000   Dilution of serum

Fig. 20.3   The radioallergosorbent test. In the presence of IgE, radiolabeled anti-IgE is bound. As serum is diluted, the amount bound isotope drops.

activity. Streptavidin binds strongly and specifically to biotin. The amount of bound biotin can be readily determined if the streptavidin is conjugated with an enzyme label.

A more recent innovation has involved an adaptation of chip technology that uses microarrays of allergenic proteins attached to an activated silica chip (Fig. 20.4). Very small quantities of crude or purified allergens can be spotted on a chip using a robotic applicator. The spot size can be as small as 200 μm in diameter. This permits thousands of allergenic proteins to be spotted onto a single silica chip in a well-defined pattern. Positive reactions are then identified using miniature-scale fluorescence. For example, some microarrays use biotin-labeled anti-IgE, followed by streptavidin conjugated with the fluorescent dye Cy-3. Only positive allergen dots will fluoresce, and these can be scanned and quantified using a specially designed fluorescence microscope.

The most advanced of these microarray assays can provide quantitative antigen-specific IgE levels when fully automated, and thus deliver precise reproducible results in a short time. Because they use miniaturized chips, they require little serum, and the tests can be repeated readily. They can also be adapted to use purified native or recombinant allergens. The disadvantages of these microarrays are that they do not deliver immediate results, unlike skin testing. They may also lack sensitivity for some allergens, and some reactions may be inhibited by the presence of allergen-binding IgG.

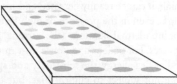

1. Multiple different allergens are spotted onto a microarray plate

2. Test serum added and then washed off

3. Biotin-labeled antiglobulin added and then washed off

4. Fluorescent strepavidin is used to detect any bound biotin

5. Fluorescence intensity of each dot is read automatically

Fig 20.4   The principle of an antibody microarray. Serum can be tested for reactivity to hundreds of different allergens at one time. Allergen spots are applied automatically to the plate in a defined pattern. For example, it is usual for the allergen spots to be applied in triplicate. Both positive and negative control spots must also be present. Either colored or fluorescent labeled antiglobulins may be used to detect any bound IgE. The plates are read automatically by a plate reader.

Microarrays have been successfully developed for testing horses with severe asthma due to the presence of serum IgE against a large diversity of allergens. The source of these allergens is the dust released by forage and bedding. The specific allergens in this case are printed onto nitrocellulose membranes. In this way, hundreds of allergens from sources such as pollens, bacteria, fungi, and arthropods can be tested. They can be used to test either horse serum or bronchoalveolar lavage fluid. However, bronchoalveolar lavage fluid must be concentrated 40-fold first. Microarrays such as these have indicated that the major allergens in these horses are molds such as *Aspergillus fumigatus*, *Alternaria alternata*, and *Aspergillus terreus*. Others include Culicoides midges, pollens, and even latex.

IMMUNOENZYME ASSAYS

Enzyme-linked Immunosorbent Assays (ELISAs)

One common assay used to detect and measure antigen-specific antibodies is the ELISA, which involves the use of enzyme-labeled antiglobulins. Microwells in polystyrene plates are normally used for this assay (the commonly used plate uses 96 wells). The wells are first filled with an allergen solution. Proteins bind firmly to polystyrene surfaces, so that after unbound allergens are removed by washing, the wells remain coated with a layer of allergen molecules. The coated plates can be stored until required. To conduct the assay, patient serum is added to the wells. Antibodies present in the serum bind to their specific allergens. After incubation and washing to remove unbound antibodies, the presence of bound antibodies can be detected by adding a solution containing an antiglobulin chemically linked to an enzyme. This labeled antiglobulin binds to the antibody and following incubation and washing, can be detected by adding a solution containing the enzyme substrate. The enzyme and substrate are selected to ensure that a colored product develops in the tube. The intensity of the color that develops is therefore proportional to the amount of enzyme-linked antiglobulin that is bound, which in turn is proportional to the amount of antibody present in the serum under test. Color intensity may be estimated visually or colorimetrically. The sensitivity of the assay depends on the affinity of the antibodies and the detection system used.

Bound IgE can be detected using an enzyme-labeled monoclonal or polyclonal antiglobulin directed against the ε heavy chain of IgE. One problem with the use of antiglobulins may be some degree of cross-reactivity between different immunoglobulin classes. An equally specific detection method is to use the labeled α chain of the high-affinity IgE receptor FcεRI. The α chain is the extracellular IgE binding chain of the receptor that binds IgE with very high specificity. In addition, this receptor-binding test is not species-specific, and the same assay can be used for both dogs and cats. IgG antibodies neither bind to the receptor nor inhibit IgE binding. This ALLERCEPT™ system works on the same basis as a conventional ELISA with wells coated with specific allergens (Fig. 20.5). Following exposure to the test serum, an enzyme-labeled α chain is added. It binds only to IgE and after washing, it can be readily detected and measured. The FcεRIα assay can detect the presence of anti-flea IgE, even in the presence of high levels of anti-flea IgG. This assay correlates well with the results of intradermal skin tests (the current "gold standard") and correctly predicts its results in over 90% of cases. For pollens and house dust mites, its sensitivity and specificity are 86% and 92%, respectively. For flea allergy, the sensitivity and specificity are 87% and 71%, respectively.

Serologic assays are not subject to clinical bias, but there is a poor correlation between the results obtained by serology or skin testing and clinical severity. There is also a poor correlation between ELISA results and intradermal testing. Serological assays are especially prone to a high level of false-positive results (low specificity). A negative ELISA generally rules out extrinsic disease. The best results are obtained by testing individual allergens rather than groups of allergens. This poor correlation between direct IgE measurements and in vivo methods, such as skin testing, probably reflects the occurrence of intrinsic atopic dermatitis (AD). Heavily parasitized dogs may also have elevated polyclonal IgE levels, which may result in false-positive serological results. The presence of cross-reactive carbohydrate determinants (CCDs) may also result in false-positive results. It is also possible that immunoglobulins of classes other than IgE may contribute to the development of AD in dogs. For these reasons, many veterinary dermatologists prefer intradermal skin testing to serological assays.

Chemiluminescence Immunoassays

Chemiluminescence assays are highly sensitive alternatives to conventional enzyme-based assays. Their basic principle is the same, but instead of a label that changes color, they use a label that emits light when exposed to its substrate. This light can be detected and measured using a luminometer. One such example is the use of a horseradish peroxidase label. Light is emitted when mixed with hydrogen peroxide and suitable chemical enhancers. Other assays use the enzyme luciferase. Luciferase assays can be used to measure total IgE levels by comparing the light emitted in the assay to a standard curve. These tests can also be used to measure specific IgE levels against a panel of multiple allergens, such as food allergens or respiratory allergens, and can be fully automated in the multiple allergen simultaneous test (MAST). Rather than being restricted to 96-well plates, these MAST assays can be applied to immunoblots or even to allergen-impregnated threads.

Western Blotting

A solution to the problem of identifying protein allergens in a complex mixture is the use of a technique called Western blotting (Fig. 20.6). This is a three-stage primary binding test. The first stage involves electrophoresis of the crude allergen solution on gels so that each protein component is resolved into a single band. The second stage involves the blotting or transfer of these protein bands to an immobilizing nitrocellulose membrane. This is accomplished by placing the membrane on top of the gel and sandwiching the two between sponges saturated with buffer.

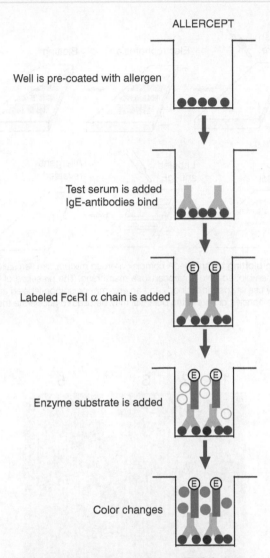

ALLERCEPT

Well is pre-coated with allergen

Test serum is added
IgE-antibodies bind

Labeled FcεRI α chain is added

Enzyme substrate is added

Color changes

Fig 20.5 The indirect enzyme-linked immunosorbent assay (ELISA). Antigen is bound to the wells in a styrene plate. The presence of bound antibody is detected by means of an enzyme-labeled FcεRI α chain. Addition of the enzyme substrate leads to a color change proportional to the amount of bound antibody. This color change can be estimated visually or read in an ELISA reader (a specially adapted spectrophotometer).

The membrane-gel sandwich is supported between rigid plastic sheets and placed in a buffer reservoir, and an electrical current is passed between the sponges. The protein bands are then transferred from the gel to the membrane without loss of resolution.

The third stage involves visualization of the transferred antigens using an enzyme immunoassay. The membrane is first incubated with a specific antiserum. After the membrane has been washed, enzyme-labeled antiglobulin solution is added. When this is removed by washing, the enzyme substrate is added, and color develops in the bands where the antibody bound to the antigen (Fig. 20.7). Western blotting can be used to identify important allergens in complex microorganisms or parasites.

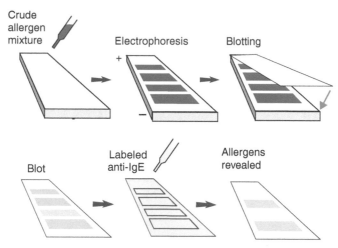

Fig 20.6 **The Western blotting technique.** A complex allergen mixture, like flea saliva, is first separated by electrophoresis. It is then blotted onto a nitrocellulose membrane. The presence of the specific protein allergens are revealed by use of specific antibody and an enzyme- or isotope-labeled antiglobulin. The blotting stage may use passive transfer, or an electric potential may be used to accelerate the process.

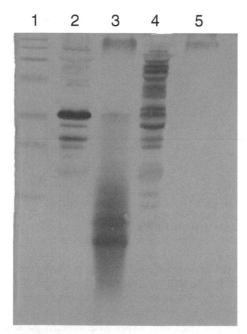

Fig 20.7 **A Western blot assay performed using serum from a sensitized dog against various fractions of soy.** Lane 1: Pre-stained markers. Lane 2: Globulin fraction of whole soy. Lane 3: Hydrolyzed globulin fraction of whole soy. Lane 4: Whey fraction of whole soy. Lane 5: Hydrolyzed whey fraction of whole soy. Stained with anti-canine IgE labeled with alkaline phosphatase. The dark bands are locations where the IgE has bound to an allergen. (Courtesy Dr. Robert Kennis)

It is important to note that a prime concern regarding all these assays is the lack of standardization of allergen extracts. Extracts from different manufacturers may have very different allergen concentrations. This is not unreasonable: How does one compare the allergen content in pollen to the allergen content in mite feces or the allergen content in a peanut? These assays work best to determine non-atopic status. The allergens are not defined and differ among laboratories. Different allergen panels are required for different species and locations.

LIVE CELL ASSAYS

While assays utilizing live cells have been widely used in research laboratories, they are not widely employed in diagnostic procedures. They are both time consuming and expensive. Additionally, reagents and assay methods have yet to be standardized.

Basophil Degranulation Assays

While rarely used as stand-alone diagnostic tests, basophil degranulation assays can be useful tools to clarify discordant results. Starting with whole blood or a purified basophil preparation, increasing concentrations of allergen are added. A small amount of IL-3 is also added to increase test sensitivity. IgE cross-linking and basophil degranulation will then occur. As a result, basophils release mediators such as histamine or cysteinyl leukotriene C_4. After incubation, the cells are centrifuged, the supernatants are collected, and their histamine or leukotriene content are assayed.

Using this basophil degranulation test and measuring histamine release, a positive result is determined if a significant fraction (up to 20%) of cellular histamine is released. The diagnostic sensitivity (false-negatives) of these tests is highly variable, ranging from 50% with β-lactams and wasp venom to 94% with inhalant allergens such as house dust mites and cat or dog dander. Likewise, the test specificity when compared to intradermal skin testing (false-positives) ranges from 45% to 90%, depending on the allergen. Not all animals release mediators from their basophils during antigen challenge. In humans, 10% to 15% of subjects are non-releasers.

A cellular antigen stimulation test (CAST), which measures basophil leukotriene release, has been commercialized in Europe and the United States. Selected allergen extracts that are known to be non-toxic to basophils are provided. Assays such as CASTs are less sensitive than skin tests and are therefore prone to false-negative results. These may range from 18% for aspirin to 85% for selected food allergens. Specificity ranges from 67% to 100%. These tests are not yet widely employed for routine diagnosis of human allergic diseases.

When activated by allergens, basophils also upregulate some of their cell surface proteins, most notably CD63 and CD203c. Cytometric basophil activation assays can then be performed to count the number of these newly positive cells using a flow cytometer. Basophils are first primed by incubation in IL-3 and then exposed to specific allergens. Some cells are also treated with anti-IgE as a positive control or with a buffer as a negative control. After activation, the cells are stained with anti-CD63 labeled with the fluorescent dye phycoerythrin and counted by flow cytometry. The percentage of activated basophils is then determined. The sensitivity of the CD63 CAST was 50% relative to that of skin testing, while its specificity was 93%.

CD203c is a protein expressed only in IgE-positive basophils and mast cells. It is also upregulated by exposure to allergens or anti-IgE antibodies. It is measured in a manner similar to that of the CD63 assay. CD203c tests are easier to interpret than CD63 because CD203c is only found on basophils; CD63 is also found in platelets and other leukocytes. CD203c tests are more sensitive than the CD63 assay (75%) but are just as specific.

These basophil activation assays require endotoxin-free whole blood to be shipped to specialized laboratories. The diversity of allergens and the toxicity of some allergens will affect the results. However, they are at an early stage of development and are gradually improving.

Lymphocyte Proliferation Assays

Lymphocytes respond to antigens that bind to their receptors by dividing. To measure cell proliferation, a suspension of purified peripheral blood lymphocytes from the animal to be tested is mixed with the allergen and cultured for 48 to 96 hours. Twelve hours before harvesting, thymidine labeled with the radioactive isotope tritium is added to the cultures. If the cells proliferate, they incorporate tritiated thymidine into their DNA. Their radioactivity provides a measure of proliferation. The greater their proliferation in response to an antigen, the greater their radioactivity. The ratio of the radioactivity in the stimulated cultures to the radioactivity in the controls is called the stimulation index. The intensity of the lymphocyte proliferative response, as measured by tritiated thymidine uptake, provides an estimate of the animal's degree of sensitization. Radioactive tritium may be replaced in proliferation assays using a simple colorimetric enzyme assay. Methylthiazoldiphenyltetrazolium bromide (MTT) is a pale yellow compound that serves as a substrate for active mitochondrial enzymes. These enzymes change the MTT color to dark blue. The intensity of this color change is a measure of the number of living cells in a culture. In proliferation assays, the number of living cells increases, and this can be measured colorimetrically. The test is sufficiently sensitive to quantify the increase in T cell numbers triggered by allergens.

In Vivo Assays

DIAGNOSIS

The term "hypersensitivity" denotes inflammation that occurs in response to a normally harmless material. For example, unsensitized animals normally do not react to the intradermal injection of antigens. However, if an animal is given an intradermal injection of an allergen to which it is sensitized, it will provoke local inflammation. Vasoactive molecules are released to produce redness (erythema) as a result of capillary dilation, as well as circumscribed edema (a wheal) due to increased vascular permeability. The reaction may also generate an erythematous flare due to arteriolar dilation caused by a local axon reflex. This wheal-and-flare response to an allergen reaches maximal intensity within 30 minutes and then disappears within a few hours. A late-phase reaction sometimes occurs 6 to 12 hours later.

Intradermal skin testing using very dilute aqueous solutions of allergens has been widely used for the diagnosis of allergies, especially canine AD. Following injection, the site is examined for an inflammatory response. The results obtained must be interpreted carefully, as false-negative and false-positive responses may occur. For example, the concentration of antigens in commercial skin testing solutions may be too low. Dogs may be up to 10 times less sensitive than humans to intradermal allergens, such as pollens, fungi, or dander. Other false-negative responses may be due to steroid treatment. False-positive reactions may be due to the presence of irritants, such as preservatives, in allergen solutions. The allergens used for intradermal skin testing commonly include extracts from trees, grasses, fungi, weeds, dander, feathers, house dust mites, and insects.

It has proven difficult to develop reliable in vivo or in vitro tests for food allergies. Test procedures that have been described include intradermal testing with food antigens, lymphocyte proliferation assays, fecal food-specific IgE assays, patch testing, or gastroscopic or colonoscopic testing. A critical analysis of these tests has indicated that IgE testing of serum has low repeatability, and lymphocyte proliferation assays are accurate but overly complex. Food allergens generally do not provide satisfactory skin test responses because they have a sensitivity of only 10% to 33%. The patch test has a high negative predictability for protein allergens (a negative result suggests that the antigen is well tolerated) and, as a result, might be useful in formulating the protein content of an elimination diet. It is not a useful diagnostic test for canine food allergies. Neither colonoscopy nor gastroscopy were useful, nor were fecal IgE assays. Elimination diet trials remain the best diagnostic procedure for food allergies.

Intradermal Skin Testing

The traditional wheal-and-flare skin test has excellent sensitivity and has been used for many years in both human and veterinary medicine (Fig. 20.8). As with other in vitro tests, the most significant drawback is the lack of standard allergen extracts. There is also a lack of consensus on how to quantify the results obtained. Intradermal tests are semiquantitative and may be affected by drug treatment. There is also an element of risk and discomfort to animals. Since 1990, many important allergens from dust mites, pollens, dander, insects, molds, and foods have been cloned and sequenced, and recombinant proteins have been expressed. This has raised the issue of whether crude and complex natural extracts have any advantages over recombinant allergens in diagnostic tests or immunotherapy. Thus, while recombinant allergens can be very pure, patients may react differently to complex mixtures. A single recombinant protein may not contain all the determinants recognized by allergen-specific IgE.

In humans, it is customary to test children using skin prick tests. These tests are simple to perform, induce minimal irritation, have good specificity, and have a low risk of severe adverse reactions. A drop of the allergen solution is placed on the skin. It is then introduced into the epidermis by means of needle puncture through the drop. Following the skin prick, excess allergens are blotted off. Any resulting inflammation is read at 15 to 20 minutes when the wheal reaches its maximum diameter. The test may yield variable results, mainly as a consequence of variations in the skill of the tester and cooperation from the subject. However, it has a lower sensitivity compared to intradermal tests. Prick testing is not performed on dogs because of the difficulty in controlling an animal for the required period. Intradermal skin testing requires about a 1000-fold lower dose of allergen than a prick test to produce a positive skin reaction of the same size.

Allergen Solutions

Intradermal skin testing is the method of choice for dogs and horses. Aqueous extracts of allergens are routinely used. Allergens are also available in concentrated solutions for use in immunotherapy, but they must be diluted before intradermal testing. Conversely, allergens can also be

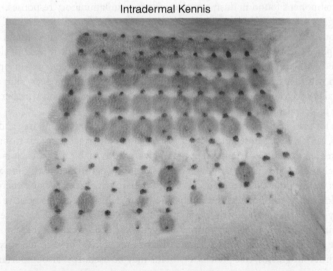

Intradermal Kennis

Fig. 20.8 A panel of intradermal skin tests performed on a dog. Each spot denotes a position where a small volume of dilute allergen was injected intradermally. If the dog is allergic to that allergen, a local reaction characterized by redness and swelling occurs around the injection site. (Courtesy Dr. Robert Kennis)

purchased for skin test strength, but these are unsuitable for immunotherapy. Allergen solutions have a limited shelf life, especially after dilution, and they should not be used after their expiration date. Allergen solutions also lose potency over time. Undiluted allergen solutions can be stored for up to 8 weeks when refrigerated, and diluted allergen solutions for no more than 2 weeks. However, they must not be frozen. They must be allowed to warm to room temperature before administration and returned to the refrigerator immediately after use.

It is important that only high-quality allergen preparations be used in diagnosis and for allergen-specific immunotherapy (ASIT). Dried pollens are treated with ether to remove lipids before extraction in a buffered saline solution. Fungal antigens are aqueous extracts of cultured fungi or, in some cases, fungi collected from wild sources. Like pollen grains, these are defatted and extracted in buffered aqueous solutions. Screened house dust is extracted using a buffered aqueous solution and dialyzed to remove low-molecular-weight toxic molecules. The extract is then concentrated to a standard protein concentration. Other potential allergens, such as epidermal extracts, are prepared in the same way by aqueous extraction of defatted extracts. Insect allergens are generally produced from the whole bodies of these insects, either trapped in the wild or grown in laboratory colonies, such as house dust mites.

Allergen solutions are standardized based on their protein content, as determined by protein nitrogen units (PNU). It is usual to employ these solutions at a concentration of 1000 PNU/mL; however, some allergen solutions may give more consistent results at lower concentrations.

Biological standardization of these extracts is often difficult. Clearly, much depends on the use of high-quality, well-characterized raw materials. This may be difficult. For example, house dust mite allergens prepared in the same way in different countries show different degrees of reactivity with IgE. Traditionally, PNUs were determined because most allergens were found to be proteins. One PNU represents approximately 0.06 µg of protein. More recently, human allergens have been quantified as histamine equivalents in prick testing (HEP) or bioequivalent allergen units (BAU). In vitro testing by ELISA may prove to be a better method of standardization.

One persistent problem in standardizing allergens is the presence of toxic substances, such as endotoxins and proteases in allergen solutions. For example, endotoxins are readily detected in house dust extracts, and may be sufficient to influence skin test responses. β-glucan, a common fungal wall component found in dust, can also influence inflammatory responses.

The allergens selected for skin testing depend on the specifics of each animal. These include marked regional and seasonal differences observed in AD. Veterinarians should be aware that allergens employed for prick testing in humans may not be relevant to AD in dogs. Likewise, there may be major differences in exposure to environmental allergens based on location and lifestyle, even within a small geographic area. It is prudent practice to review skin testing results, at least annually, and to determine which allergens are never positive and whether any responses are changing in prevalence.

Allergens for testing are obtained from several major sources, including tree and grass pollens, weed pollens, molds, house dust mites, other insects, and epidermal allergens from other species. Allergen mixes are sometimes employed because, given the available skin area, it is rarely possible to test all likely candidate allergens. This mixing should be performed with caution and consideration. It serves little purpose to randomly mix unrelated allergens because there is no way of knowing which of the components in the mixture is the culprit if a test is positive. Likewise, the mixtures may not correlate well with individual allergen results and even produce contradictory results. In principle, if it is necessary to mix allergens, seek to mix those that are closely related and would be expected to show a high degree of cross-reactivity. For example, mixtures containing to eight different grasses, tree pollens, or molds may be used. It is also important to note that allergens reactive in one species may not be significant in others. For example, the house dust mite allergens Der p 1 and Der p 2 are important in humans but not in dogs. There is also limited cross-reactivity between the allergens of the two house dust mite species. Mold proteases have been reported to destroy certain grass and weed pollen allergens in a mixture during storage. In general, it is preferable to use only individual allergen extracts whenever possible. It should also be pointed out that one of the reasons for performing intradermal testing is to identify the specific allergens required for immunotherapy.

Allergen extracts, as their name implies, are complex mixtures, not all of which act as allergens. Therefore, it is essential to use standardized extracts whenever possible. Thus, they should have a standard composition and contain all important allergens from the source. The allergens should, as far as possible, be in a constant ratio, and contents should not vary significantly between batches. There should be some form of quantitation of allergenic activity so that they have consistent potency. No standardized extracts are available for animals. Extracts are often standardized based on weight/volume or protein nitrogen units, neither of which directly measures allergen content. Therefore, it is inevitable that there may be significant between-batch variation despite the manufacturer's best intentions. Allergens extracted from biological sources contain many non-allergenic proteins, in addition to potent allergens and possible contaminants. It is a good rule to recognize that allergen reagents from different manufacturers will detect slightly different IgE populations and are not interchangeable.

In principle, allergens should be administered at the highest concentration of an extract that does not induce a reaction that can be interpreted as a false-positive. Thus, it is desirable to identify a "threshold concentration" by which reactions may be judged, but this has proven difficult. How does one differentiate a false-positive from a true positive? One possible mechanism is to test serial dilutions of an allergen solution, but this may not be possible or appropriate in client-owned animals.

Before skin testing, it is important to ensure that the animal has not received medications that could interfere with the test results. For example, the antihistamine hydroxyzine effectively suppressed skin test responses to fleas and histamine for 9 days. Its withdrawal period should therefore be 10 days. Antihistamines with longer half-lives should have an even longer withdrawal period. The tricyclic antidepressant doxepin also suppresses skin responses for several weeks. Oral glucocorticoids should also be withdrawn for a minimum of 3 weeks and injectable glucocorticoids for 8 weeks. However, each case should be assessed individually. Dogs with inflamed or infected skin should not be tested at that time. If there are skin lesions present, make sure that the injection sites are as far away as possible to avoid confusion.

While skin testing can be performed in non-sedated tranquil dogs, most veterinarians prefer to minimize stress. Animals under stress can release corticosteroids, which may affect the test results. Sedation makes the task easier and more convenient for all concerned. Sedatives that do not appear to influence skin reactivity include xylazine hydrochloride, medetomidine, thiamylal, halothane, isoflurane, and methoxyflurane. Oxymorphone, ketamine/diazepam, acepromazine, and propofol should be avoided.

By convention and convenience, the skin of the lateral thorax is commonly chosen for testing. The site is gently shaved but should not be washed or scrubbed. The individual injection sites should be marked with a waterproof marker and placed at least 3 cm apart, with approximately 60 sites injected. In horses, the neck above the jugular groove is preferred.

Positive and negative control injections should be used. The most common positive control substance is histamine phosphate solution 0.001% (1:100,000). The negative control should be the allergen diluent solution, which is commonly 0.9% phosphate-buffered saline.

The allergen is inoculated using a tuberculin or 1-mL syringe using a 26- or 27-gauge needle. Different syringes and needles should be used for each allergen. It is usual to inject 0.05 mL of each allergen intradermally. A well-defined bleb shows that the injection was placed correctly. The injection of air bubbles should be avoided because this may damage the skin and may interfere with reading the test. If the injection site is too deep, a bleb will not develop, and a false-negative result may be obtained. The needle should be gently withdrawn to avoid hemorrhage.

It is usual to read intradermal skin tests 15 to 30 minutes after injection when the wheal and flare have reached their greatest intensity. They may be read subjectively or preferably objectively by measuring and recording wheal diameter in millimeters. Some clinicians also measure the flare diameter. There are no standardized criteria for determining positivity or negativity. One suggested measure is that positive reactions should have a diameter at least 3 mm greater than the negative control. It is also conventional to score each lesion on a scale from 0 to 4, where 0 is equal to the negative control and 4 is equal to the positive control. Any reaction scored >2 should be regarded as positive. In humans, increasing dilutions of allergens are commonly tested, but this is uncommon in animal testing. With the ready availability of cell phones, a photograph should be taken of the test results. Thermal imaging is increasingly being used in human medicine. Late-phase reactions are well recognized in humans. They have also been reported in dogs. However, their clinical significance remains unclear.

Allergy testing in cats is more difficult because their reactions to intradermal testing may be indistinct, short lived, and difficult to evaluate. Cat skin is remarkably elastic. As a result, it can readily accommodate the edema fluid released in a positive skin test reaction without developing a large or obvious wheal.

Intradermal skin testing in atopic horses appears to yield inconsistent results. Thus, there may be little or no correlation between skin test responses on each side of the neck for many allergens. Likewise, there is a poor correlation between intradermal test results and serum allergen-specific IgE, except for potent allergens such as house dust mites.

False-negative intradermal skin test results can result from improper technique, poor quality allergen solution (or the wrong allergen), drug interference, some host factors, and seasonality. Prior therapy may have suppressed IgE levels to below detection values, lesions may not be induced by allergens, or IgE may simply not be involved in the process. The causes of false-positive intradermal skin tests include not only poor technique and needle trauma, but also the presence of irritants in the test antigen solutions, irritated skin with injection sites spaced too closely, and cross-reactivity. Some concentrated allergens for human use are preserved in dilute glycerin. These may sting when injected into dogs and are best avoided.

Prausnitz-Küstner Test

The Prausnitz-Küstner (PK) test was originally developed in 1921 when Otto Prausnitz injected Heinz Küstner's serum into his own skin. Küstner was allergic to fish. When Prausnitz ate some fish, his skin at the site of the serum injection became red and inflamed. This test was subsequently used to detect specific antigen responsiveness in human patients. The PK test involves taking serum from a suspected allergic animal and injecting it intradermally into a normal recipient. The recipient animal is challenged with the suspect antigen at the same site 24 to 48 hours later. If antibodies are present, there will be an immediate reaction at the injection site. This test is no longer used in clinical practice.

Passive cutaneous anaphylaxis is an experimental technique used to detect IgE antibodies. In this test, dilutions of test serum are injected at different sites into the skin of a normal animal. After 24 to 48 hours, an antigen solution is administered intravenously. Each positive injection site will show an immediate inflammatory response. The injected antibodies may remain fixed in the skin for a very long period. In the case of calves, this may be as long as 8 weeks. Because it is sometimes difficult to detect very mild inflammatory responses, the reactions can be made more visible by injecting the test animal intravenously with Evans blue dye. The dye binds to serum albumin and does not normally leave the bloodstream. At injection sites where vascular permeability is increased, dye-labeled albumin enters the tissue fluid and forms a striking blue patch (Fig. 20.9).

Patch Tests. The offending allergens in allergic contact dermatitis cases may be confirmed by the use of a patch test after removal of the suspected antigen and by patch testing. These are described in Chapter 19.

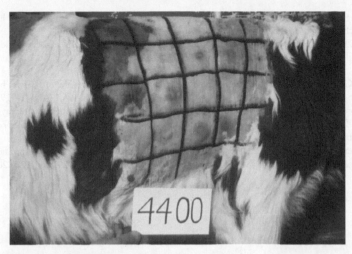

Fig 20.9   Passive cutaneous anaphylaxis (PCA) reactions in a calf. Several different sera were tested for PCA activity on the flank of a normal calf. The blue color of the reactions is due to the presence of Evans blue dye. This dye binds to serum albumin and makes the inflammatory reactions easier to see. (Courtesy Dr. P. Eyre).

Suggested Reading

Belova S, Wilhelm S, Linek M, et al. Factors affecting allergen-specific IgE levels in cats. *Can J Vet Res*. 2012;76(1):45-51.

Bethlehem S, Bexley J, Mueller RS. Patch testing and allergen-specific serum IgE and IgG antibodies in the diagnosis of canine adverse food reactions. *Vet Immunol Immunopathol*. 2012;145(3-4):582-589. doi: 10.1016/j.vetimm.2012.01.003

Buckley L, Schmidt V, McEwan N, Nuttall T. Cross-reaction and co-sensitization among related and unrelated allergens in canine intradermal tests. *Vet Dermatol*. 2013;24(4):422-e92. doi: 10.1111/vde.12044

Delgado C, Lee-Fowler TM, DeClue AE, Reinero CR. Feline-specific serum total IgE quantitation in normal, asthmatic, and parasitized cats. *J Feline Med Surg*. 2010;12(12):991-994. doi: 10.1016/j.jfms.2010.08.006

Halliwell R, Kovalik M. Performing and interpreting allergy tests: their value and pitfalls. In: Torres SMF, Roudebush P, eds. *Advances in Veterinary Dermatology*. Wiley Blackwell; 2017;235-240. doi: 10.1002/978119278368.ch7.10

Hamilton RG, MacGlashan DW Jr, Saini SS. IgE antibody specific activity in human allergic disease. *Immunol Res*. 2010;47(1-3):273-284. doi: 10.1007/s12026-009-8160-3

Hensel P, Santoro D, Favrot C, Hill P, Griffin C. Canine atopic dermatitis: detailed guidelines for diagnosis and allergen identification. *BMC Vet Res*. 2015;11;196. doi: 10.1186/s12917-015-0515-5

Hillier A, DeBoer DJ. The ACVD task force on canine atopic dermatitis (XVII): Intradermal testing. *Vet Immunol Immunopathol*. 2001;81(3-4):289-304. doi: 10.1016/s0165-2427(01)00313-0

Lauber B, Molitor V, Meury S, et al. Total IgE and allergen-specific IgE and IgG antibody levels in sera of atopic dermatitis affected and non-affected Labrador and Golden retrievers. *Vet Immunol Immunopathol*. 2012;149(1-2):112-118. doi: 10.1016/j.vetimm.2012.05.018

Layne EA, De Boer DJ. Allergen-specific IgE in nonatopic dogs. *Vet Dermatol*. 2019;30(1):78-79. doi: 10.1111/vde.12704

MacGlashan DW Jr. Basophil activation testing. *J Allergy Clin Immunol*. 2013;132(4):777-787. doi: 10.1016/j.jaci.2013.06.038

Okayama T, Matsuno Y, Yasuda N, et al. Establishment of a quantitative ELISA for the measurement of allergen-specific IgE in dogs using anti-IgE antibody cross-reactive to mouse and dog IgE. *Vet Immunol Immunopathol*. 2011;139(2-4):99-106. doi: 10.1016/j.vetimm.2010.09.002

Shade K-TC, Conroy ME, Washburn N, et al. Sialylation of immunoglobulin E is a determinant of allergic pathogenicity. *Nature*. 2020;582(7811):265-270. doi: 10.1038/s41586-020-2311-z.

Tsukui T, Sakaguchi M, Kurata K, et al. Measurement for canine IgE using canine recombinant high affinity receptor α chain. *J Vet Med Sci.* 2012;74(7):851-856. doi: 10.1292/jvms.10-0520

van Damme CMM, van den Broek J, Sloet van Oldruitenborgh-Oosterbaan MM. Discrepancies in the bilateral intradermal test and serum tests in atopic horses. *Vet Dermatol.* 2020;31(5):390-e104. doi:10.1111/vde.12871

Wassom DL, Grieve RB. In vitro measurement of canine and feline IgE: a review of FcεRIα-based assays for detection of allergen-reactive IgE. *Vet Dermatol.* 1998;9:173-178. doi:10.1046/j.1365-3164.1998.00121.x

White S, Moore-Colyer M, Marti E, et al. Development of a comprehensive protein microarray for immunoglobulin E profiling in horses with severe asthma. *J Vet Intern Med.* 2019;33(5):2327-2335. doi: 10.1111/jvim.15564

Zhou Z, Pieper JB, Campbell K. Intralaboratory reliability and variability for allergen-specific immunoglobulin type E serology testing. *J Amer Anim Hosp Assoc.* 2019;55(3):124-129. doi: 10.5326/JAAHA-MS-6761

CHAPTER 21

Allergies in Veterinarians

After pollen and house dust mites, furred animals are the most common source of respiratory allergens affecting humans. Animal allergens are ubiquitous. Not only are they found in homes where pets are present, but they are also inadvertently transported to distant sites. Widespread pet ownership, as well as changes in intensive animal agriculture, have the potential to spread animal allergens across many human environments. The use of animals in research also represents a significant source of allergen exposure in animal care workers. A Polish study published in 2006 indicated that 44% of laboratory animal veterinarians were skin prick test-positive in response to rat, mouse, hamster, guinea pig, or rabbit allergens. Pruritus, rhinitis, chronic throat irritation, irritated eyes, coughing and sneezing, asthma, and rashes were common results. The development of allergic dermatitis on the hands, with dry and cracked skin, scaling, blistering, redness, and swelling, is also very common. An Australian survey in 2009 indicated that hand dermatitis was a problem in approximately 16% of practicing veterinarians. Surveys have also indicated that depending on the country, the rate of allergic sensitization to cats in a population of patients suffering from allergies ranged from 1.2% to 22.4%, with a mean of 8.8%. In Sweden, between 1994 and 2009, there was an increase in sensitization to cats from 16% to 26%, to dogs from 13% to 25%, and to horses from 8% to 10%.

Allergens

Mammalian allergens are predominantly derived from the skin, saliva, and urine. Because these allergen molecules stick to fur, they can be dispersed throughout the environment as hair and dander are shed. They are also dispersed by urination. Allergens bind to small dust particles that may remain airborne for long periods of time. Allergens can also stick to human clothing and hair and are thus easily transported to locations where animals have never been present. Indoors, allergen particles adhere to textile surfaces such as carpets, upholstered furniture, mattresses, and pillows. As expected, their concentration may be up to 200 times higher in homes with pets than in homes without pets. Nevertheless, non-residential sites, such as offices, schools, and daycare centers, are also places where allergic individuals may encounter animal allergens. The level of exposure to animal allergens can be reduced by pet removal or thorough cleaning, but this may not be possible outside homes.

Allergens must be identified and classified; they are then officially recognized by a subcommittee of the World Health Organization and the International Union of Immunological Societies (IUIS). This subcommittee maintains an allergen database at www.allergen.org. As described previously, the name of each allergen is derived from the scientific name of its source using the first three letters of the genus, the first letter of the species, and then followed by a number in order of their characterization. Thus, Can d 1 was the first dog allergen to be fully characterized. Major allergens are those recognized by more than 50% of the affected patients. The major mammalian allergens fall into four protein families: lipocalins, secretoglobins, kallikreins, and latherins (Fig. 21.1). Serum albumins are also important allergens.

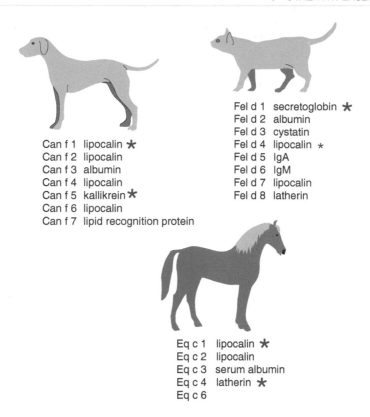

Can f 1 lipocalin ✱
Can f 2 lipocalin
Can f 3 albumin
Can f 4 lipocalin
Can f 5 kallikrein ✱
Can f 6 lipocalin
Can f 7 lipid recognition protein

Fel d 1 secretoglobin ✱
Fel d 2 albumin
Fel d 3 cystatin
Fel d 4 lipocalin ✱
Fel d 5 IgA
Fel d 6 IgM
Fel d 7 lipocalin
Fel d 8 latherin

Eq c 1 lipocalin ✱
Eq c 2 lipocalin
Eq c 3 serum albumin
Eq c 4 latherin ✱
Eq c 6

Fig. 21.1 The major allergens produced by domestic mammals. The asterisks denote the most signifi-cant allergens.

LIPOCALINS

Lipocalins are small extracellular proteins that account for more than half of mammalian-derived respiratory allergens. At least 50 members of the family have been identified so far, and at least one major lipocalin allergen is produced by each species. Examples include Can d 1 in dogs, Fel d 4 in cats, Equ c 1 in horses, Bos d 2 in cattle, Rat n 1 in rats, and Mus m 1 in mice. These are relatively small proteins about 200 amino acids in length. Their sequence homology is low, but they all appear to have a common structural feature: a hydrophobic binding pocket. In this pocket, they carry small hydrophobic molecules, such as lipids, steroids, retinoids, or pheromones. Lipocalins are synthesized in the liver as well as in some exocrine glands. As a result, they are found in body fluids, skin, sebum, sweat, and saliva.

SECRETOGLOBINS

Two major mammalian allergens, Fel d 1 and rabbit Ory c 3, are members of the secretoglobin family. Fel d 1 has been extensively studied because of its importance in allergies to cats. It is a tetrameric protein formed by two 18-kDa heterodimers. It is produced in the sebaceous, salivary, and anal glands. As a result, it is predominantly found in the skin and fur. Interestingly, its biological function remains unknown. It is a dominant allergen, and as a result, 60% to 90% of people with cat dander allergy react to it. Rabbit secretoglobin is found in rabbit fur, and approximately 77% of rabbit-allergic patients react to it.

KALLIKREINS

The only mammalian allergen that belongs to the kallikrein family is Can f 5. It is a major urinary allergen produced by male dogs since it originates in the prostate. It is also detectable in dog dander. Up to 70% of patients with dog allergies have been reported to react to recombinant Can f 5, while 38% of these patients react to this allergen alone.

LATHERINS

Latherin, or Equ c 4, is a potent surfactant found in horse sweat and saliva. In horses, it probably acts as a wetting agent that serves to cool the skin. It is this protein that causes lathering when horses become hot. Approximately 77% of subjects with horse allergy react to latherin. Fel d 8 is a minor allergen from cat saliva that is related to latherin.

SERUM ALBUMINS

Albumins are the major proteins found in blood serum. They are relatively small, with a molecular weight of 65–70 kDa. They are present in animal dander, milk, and other secretions. They are classified as minor allergens because they are only recognized by approximately 30% of patients. However, albumins have a conserved structure and sequences, and as a result, cross-react extensively between species.

Specific Environments

Laboratory animal facilities housing rats and mice may also contain high levels of specific allergens. Obviously, the level of these allergens will differ between rooms, depending upon their functions and the type of caging system employed. Rodent allergens can be readily transferred from animal housing facilities to public areas and homes. While clothes may be changed, hair caps may not be in routine use, and hair is likely to be the main method of allergen spread. Airborne rodent allergens occur in a wide range of particle sizes and can be carried over relatively long distances. They can remain floating in air for at least 60 minutes after the animals have been disturbed.

Farms, especially dairy barns, may contain high levels of the major bovine allergens. In practice, these vary greatly between premises. Passive transfer of these allergens, such as Bos d 2, on work clothing and overalls results in the presence of allergens in farmhouses. As expected, it is found at 5000 times lower concentrations in homes than in dairy barns. A concentration gradient of Bos d 2 allergens has been found to extend from animal barns to a radius of at least 3 miles. A similar situation occurs in horse stables, but allergen concentrations decline rapidly with distance from the stable doors.

Veterinarians

Veterinarians face several hazards as a part of their professional responsibilities. Some are obvious, such as bites and scratches. There are also many zoonotic diseases that they may contract. However, one of the most common hazards is the development of allergic disease. Veterinarians work in environments where animal dander and bird feathers are abundant. They may be required to work in dusty barns. It is unsurprising that they can mount Th2 responses that develop into clinical allergies. It has been estimated that at least one-third of veterinary professionals develop allergies to animal dander. In most cases, personal circumstances preclude leaving the profession, and as a result, avoidance is not a solution.

The obvious clinical signs of allergy include itchy eyes resulting in lacrimation, chronic rhinitis, or bronchitis with dyspnea, malaise, and urticarial skin rashes. While veterinarians might tend to "soldier on", it is important for them to consult with an allergist regarding treatment and allergen-specific immunotherapy (ASIT). The situation is complicated because many veterinarians and technicians have pets of their own, and it may be almost impossible to move to a dander-free environment.

While avoidance may be difficult, these allergies also have a significant psychological impact. Therefore, efforts should be made to minimize excessive allergen exposure. Thus, affected individuals should try to avoid personally clipping or grooming patients. They should assign these tasks to non-allergic team members. When work is finished, workers should change their clothes and wash thoroughly. It is also possible to identify trigger factors. Thus, there may be a specific breed or procedure that triggers allergic attacks. It is also important to note that veterinary professionals, like everyone else, can become allergic to environmental allergens, such as house dust mites, pollens, and molds.

PREVALENCE

A recent survey of veterinarians working in western Canada reported that 39% of them developed an allergy during their careers. Of those affected, 41% reported that they were obliged to change the way they practiced. In addition to avoiding the allergens, some were also obliged to avoid working with certain animal species or to use gloves and masks. Common sources of allergens include contact with vaginal secretions, amniotic fluid, and latex gloves, or exposure to blood proteins, parasites, and animal saliva, hair, fur, and dander. Despite the high prevalence of allergies, few veterinarians reported taking time off work as a result.

Common symptoms of animal allergies include rhinitis, asthma, and conjunctivitis. These factors may have a significant effect on the quality of life. It is estimated that pets are the third leading cause of IgE-mediated allergic asthma. In one study, more than 500,000 emergency room visits were attributed to cat allergen-induced asthma attacks in the United States.

While it is easy to recommend avoidance, many patients or parents of allergic children fail to comply with avoidance recommendations, especially where there are significant emotional consequences related to a household pet. Conversely, allergy is a commonly reported reason why animals are relinquished to shelters and has adverse impacts on cat adoption and ownership.

In a clinical survey conducted among animal workers in Tehran, 36% of the animal workers had at least one positive skin prick test for animal allergens. Of these, 43% of veterinarians and 41% of final-year veterinary students were positive, suggesting that the allergies developed even before the individuals entered practice. In this survey, the common sensitivities were horse (16%), canary (16%), cattle (13%), cats (12%), and dogs (10%). Affected workers reported respiratory, skin, and eye symptoms including cough, wheezing, dyspnea, nasal discharge, sneezing, nasal congestion, pruritus, and urticaria. The high prevalence of horse allergies is likely a local phenomenon in Iran, where contact with horses is uncommon. Urine is the main source of allergens in individuals working with laboratory rodents, such as rats, mice, and rabbits. Bird allergens, such as feather dust, serum, or droppings, can also cause occupational allergies.

VETERINARY CLINICS

Only one published study has characterized allergen concentrations in a veterinary clinic. As expected, the allergen levels differed according to the function of each room. This specific practice had many more dogs than cat patients, and as a result, Can f 1 was detected more frequently and at higher levels than Fel d 1. The highest levels were detected in the intensive care unit and the lowest in the operating room. This may simply reflect a much higher level of cleanliness in the operating room. In floor dust samples, the highest levels were found in the examination and waiting rooms. Other surfaces that had detectable levels of allergens included examination tables, computer desks, and equipment tables.

Pathogenesis

CANINE ALLERGIES

Five to ten percent of the population in affluent Western countries are allergic to dogs. Seven dog allergens have been identified. The most important dog allergens are Can f 1 and Can f 2. Both are present in saliva, but Can f 1 is also found in hair. Can f 1 is a 25-kDa cysteine protease inhibitor. The major canine allergens Can f 1-4 and Can f 6, belonging to the lipocalin and albumin families respectively, are found in dog dander and saliva. Can f 5 is a prostatic kallikrein that is homologous to human prostate-specific antigen. Therefore, it is only found in the urine of male dogs, and up to 70% of patients with dog allergy may react to it. Can f 6 has sequence similarity with Fel d 4 and Equ c 1. Thus, IgE against Can f 6 can also bind Fel d 4 and Equ c 1. Can f 1, Can f 2, Can f 4, and Can f 6 are members of the lipocalin family. Can f 5 is urinary kallikrein, and Can f 7 is the epidermal secretory protein E1. The prevalence of sensitization to Can f 7 is approximately 10% to 20%. Dog albumin (Can f 3) is allergenic, and in one study, approximately 25% of allergic individuals were sensitive to it. Interestingly, in another study of patients with dog allergy, 20% were negative for dander but positive for saliva. Dog allergens may be found on airborne particles ranging from 1–20 µm in size. At least 15% of these allergens are found on smaller particles under 5 µm. High levels of IgE to Can f 1 in young infants have been proposed to be the most important predictor of developing dog allergy in later life. As described elsewhere in this book, different dog commercial allergen extracts may have widely varying compositions (especially Can f 3) and thus give different reaction patterns on prick tests.

Hypoallergenic Dog Breeds

There are enormous differences between individual dogs in their tendency to shed allergens, but there are no consistent differences between animals of different breeds. Older dogs with drier skin may produce more dander than younger dogs. The length of the dog's coat does not influence its allergenicity. Animal sex was only significant for Can f 5. Similar results have been obtained for hypoallergenic cats and horses.

FELINE ALLERGIES

Sensitization to cats has risen to 7% to 30% among the general population and is increasing. This is by far the most common animal allergy worldwide. In atopic individuals alone, 20% to 40% are sensitized to cats. Thus, cat allergies are a major risk factor for allergic rhinitis and asthma. To date, 12 major cat allergens have been identified, with the most important and dominant being Fel d 1. It accounts for 96% of human allergic cat sensitization and 60% to 90% of the overall antigenicity of cats and cat dander. Fel d 1 is a 35- to 38-kDa tetrameric glycoprotein; it is not a lipocalin but a secretoglobin. Its function is unknown, but it may act as a pheromone. It has also been suggested that it is a skin protectant or lipid transport protein. Fel d 1 is produced in cat sebaceous glands and, as a result, is secreted onto fur. It is also produced in salivary glands and to a lesser extent in the lacrimal and anal glands, and so it is also smeared across the cat's fur during grooming. Fel d 1 production appears to be under hormonal control since males produce much more of it than females. Much more is also produced on the head of a cat than on its chest. Washing a cat removes some Fel d 1, but levels return to normal within two days. It is spread through the fur by licking and grooming, and is shed into the environment together with dander. Surveys in the United States have found Fel d 1 in 99% of homes. It is ubiquitous and found in homes with and without cats. Approximately 2% of people with cat allergy are sensitive to Fel d 2 (cat serum albumin) and it may be the primary allergen in some cases. Fel d 4 is a lipocalin. Individuals sensitized to Fel d 2 and Fel d 4 are usually also sensitized to Fel d 1. All cats generate Fel d 1 irrespective of their age, sex, breed, hair length, or housing. There is no hypoallergenic cat breed. On the other hand, the amount of Fel d 1 produced varies widely among individuals. Male cats produce 3-5 times less Fel d 1 after neutering. Fel d 1 is a sticky allergen, so it may take many months for symptoms to improve after removal of a cat from a household. This is especially the case if the rooms are carpeted. Cat allergens appear to be spread in a manner similar to dogs, with most being carried by large airborne particles. While Fel d 1 is mainly associated with particles larger than 9 μm in diameter, approximately 23% of Fel d 1 is found on very small particles <5 μm in diameter. Thus, Fel d 1 can remain airborne for several days and is readily inhaled. Multisensitization to multiple cat allergens is associated with more severe asthma. Diagnosis is based on the clinical history and results of skin prick tests. Serologic assays for detecting cat-specific IgE are also useful.

A method of treating cat food has the potential to significantly reduce the production of environmental Fel d 1. In this procedure, dry cat food pellets are coated with an egg yolk preparation containing chicken IgY against Fel d 1. When hens are immunized, they mount a strong antibody response, and these IgY antibodies are concentrated in egg yolk. Thus, immunizing chickens and harvesting their egg yolks is an economical method for obtaining antibodies. When eaten by a cat, the antibodies bind and neutralize salivary Fel d 1. The amount of Fel d 1 in hair and dander drops. As a result, environmental levels of this allergen drop significantly and have the potential to reduce the severity of the disease in people with cat allergy.

EQUINE ALLERGIES

As pointed out above, the prevalence of sensitization to horses depends directly on the degree of contact with horses. One survey showed a skin-prick positivity rate of 7% to 10% in a population in northern Sweden. A study conducted in horses to determine if there were differences in allergen shedding in dander and saliva between breeds failed to show a difference using Equ c 4. However, there were major differences between individual animals. Equ c 4 is also found in saliva, where it functions as a wetting agent. It has also been found in horse urine. It is found at higher levels in stallions than in mares or geldings.

The major horse allergen is Equ c 1, which is a 25-kDa lipocalin. About 78% of equine-sensitive individuals react to it. Equ c 2 is a 17-kDa lipocalin. Equ c 3 is 67-kDa equine serum albumin. Equ c 4 is a 17-kDa latherin; (Equ c 5 was later found to be Eq c 4!). Eq c 6 is a 15-kDa lysozyme.

CATTLE ALLERGIES

Cattle allergy (except for milk allergies) usually results from occupational exposure to cattle. Bos d 2, a lipocalin, is the major respiratory allergen in cow dander. It is produced in sweat glands, where it acts as a carrier of pheromones.

LABORATORY ANIMAL ALLERGIES

It has been estimated that approximately 20% of individuals working with laboratory animals develop allergies. This is probably because these animals are handled frequently since they do not appear to be more allergenic than other species. One survey indicated that symptoms occurred in 24% of those working with mice, 25% for rats, 31% for guinea pigs, 30% for rabbits, 26% for hamsters, 30% for cats, 25% for dogs, and 24% for those working with monkeys. As with other species, many of these allergens are lipocalins. Mus m 1, the major mouse allergen, is a 19-kDa molecule produced in the liver and found in urine, hair follicles, and dander. Interestingly, male mice produce four times as much Mus m 1 than female mice because its expression is testosterone dependent. Mus m 2 is a 16-kDa glycoprotein found in hair and dander, but not in urine.

The major rat allergens, Rat n 1A and Rat n 1 B, are variants of α2-globulin. Rat n 1B is produced in the liver and is androgen-dependent. It is also produced in saliva, milk, and other exocrine secretions.

LATEX ALLERGY

Natural rubber latex is a major constituent of many medical devices, such as surgical gloves and catheters. During the 1980s and 1990s when latex gloves began to be used as a routine precaution against infections such as human immunodeficiency virus (HIV) and hepatitis, it was belatedly recognized that latex can act as a powerful allergen. Before the advent of HIV, approximately 300 million latex gloves were sold annually in the United States. By 1999, this figure had risen to 36 billion units. (It is speculated that prior to this growth in demand, latex was stored for up to 6 months prior to use under conditions where the allergens were degraded. Once demand increased, the latex was processed much more promptly, and as a result, the level of allergens increased significantly). The prevalence of latex sensitization is estimated to be about 1% to 6% of the general population, but it may be as high as 12% in healthcare workers. Most clinical cases were found to develop hand dermatitis when they wore latex gloves. Many patients also developed respiratory asthma due to exposure to gloves at work. Some individuals developed symptoms simply by entering rooms where latex gloves were in use. Many patients also develop disease upon exposure to latex in catheters. Its prevalence declined significantly once latex hazards were recognized. Most of these studies were performed in a medical context, but there is no reason to suppose that veterinarians are different.

Natural rubber latex is obtained by tapping rubber trees (*Hevea brasiliensis*). It is treated with ammonia to prevent coagulation, and the latex is then separated from the rubber. Liquid latex is mixed with additives such as antioxidants and preservatives. It is then poured into porcelain molds and heated to solidify it. Raw latex contains up to 2% plant-derived proteins. More than 250 latex peptides have been identified, but only 15 (Hev b 1-15) have been formally recognized as allergens. Many allergens in rubber tree latex can cross-react with similar molecules found in other plants, such as avocados, kiwi fruit, chestnuts, peaches, tomatoes, and bananas, which may have to be avoided by sensitized individuals. These allergies are best detected by serological methods in order to avoid the risk of anaphylaxis resulting from intradermal skin testing.

Another possible predisposing cause of latex allergy is the switch from the use of talc to cornstarch as a glove lubricant. Latex allergens adsorbed on corn starch appear to be the primary source of sensitization. In recent years, latex glove manufacturers have gradually reduced their allergen content and eliminated the use of corn starch. In 2017, the US Food and Drug Administration banned the use of powdered medical gloves as well as the absorbable powder designed to lubricate them. Because many chemicals are added to the latex solution during its production, allergic contact dermatitis to latex has also been recorded.

Because of the use of latex gloves, hand dermatitis is the most common presenting sign of latex allergy. However, other signs of latex allergy, including anaphylaxis, have been documented. Serology is generally required to confirm diagnosis. High specific IgE titers are confirmatory of latex allergy, but there is a high prevalence of false-negative results. Avoidance of natural rubber latex is the primary method of control.

As described in Chapter 13, IgE antibodies against latex allergens have been identified in horses with severe asthma syndrome. Horses are commonly exposed to rubber products, and some synthetic track surfaces may contain recycled tires.

Specific Immunotherapy

If allergen avoidance and drug treatments fail to control animal allergies, consideration should be given to specific immunotherapies based on the use of standardized allergen extracts. These are made by suspending raw materials such as defatted animal dander in water at a neutral pH to allow the soluble allergens to dissolve. The unwanted residue is removed by centrifugation and dialysis. The extracts are then standardized for composition and potency. Unfortunately, each manufacturer often has its own standards, so it is often difficult to compare allergen extracts between different manufacturers.

Two modes of immunotherapy are used to control respiratory allergies: subcutaneous immunotherapy (SCIT) and sublingual immunotherapy (SLIT). Each has a similar mechanism of action. Conventional SCIT is performed by subcutaneously administering a series of allergen preparations by trained medical staff (because of the ever-present risks of anaphylaxis). However, SLIT has grown in popularity because it does not require injections. The allergens are administered by liquid drops or dissolving tablets for 1–2 minutes under the tongue. This can be done at home. Treatment may continue for 3–5 years.

Both SCIT and SLIT pose a risk of adverse reactions. Local reactions are particularly prevalent. With SCIT, redness, pruritus, and swelling develop at the injection site. With SLIT, oropharyngeal pruritus and swelling may develop. Systemic reactions may also occur, up to and including anaphylaxis. Adverse reactions from SCIT occur at a rate of 0.2% per injection.

Specific immunotherapy appears to work well in individuals with allergic rhinitis and reduces both nasal and ocular symptoms. It also effectively reduces the need for medication. It is less effective in controlling asthma, probably because of the diversity of asthma endotypes.

Suggested Reading

References available online at expertconsult.com.

Chan SK, Leung DYM. Dog and cat allergies: current state of diagnostic approaches and challenges. *Allergy Asthma Immunol Res.* 2018;10(2):97-105. doi: 10.4168/aair.2018.10.2.97

Chen C-M, Tischer C, Schnappinger M, Heinrich J. The role of cats and dogs in asthma and allergy—a systematic review. *Int J Hyg Environ Health.* 2010;213(1):1-31. doi: 10.1016/j.ijeh.2009.12.003

Díaz-Perales A, González-de-Olano D, Pérez-Gordo M, Pastor-Vargas C. Allergy to uncommon pets: new allergies but the same allergens. *Front Immunol.* 2013;4:1-6. doi: 10.3389/fimmu.2013.00492

Elbers AR, Blaauw PJ, de Vries M, et al. Veterinary practice and occupational health. An epidemiological study of several professional groups of Dutch veterinarians. I. General physical examination and prevalence of allergy, lung function disorders and bronchial hyperreactivity. *Vet Q.* 1996;18(4):127-131. doi: 10.1080/01652176.1996.9694711

Harrison DJ. Controlling exposure to laboratory animal allergens. *ILAR J.* 2001;42(1):17-35. doi: 10.1093/ilar.42.1.17

Kelly KJ, Sussman G. Latex allergy: Where are we now and how did we get there? *J Allergy Clin Immunol Pract.* 2017;5(5):1212-1216. doi: 10.1016/j.jaip.2017.05.029

Krakowiak A, Wiszniewska M, Krawczyk P, et al. Risk factors associated with airway allergic diseases from exposure to laboratory animal allergens among veterinarians. *Int Arch Occup Environ Health.* 2007;80(6):465-475. doi: 10.1007/s00420-006-0153-0

Leggat PA, Smith DR, Speare R. Hand dermatitis among veterinarians from Queensland, Australia. *Contact Derm.* 2009;60(6):336-338. doi: 10.1111/j.1600-0536.2009.01562.x

Moghtaderi M, Farjadian S, Abbaszadeh Hasiri M. Animal allergen sensitization in veterinarians and laboratory animal workers. *Occup Med.* 2014;64(7):516-520. doi: 10.1093/occmed/kqu097

Samadi S, Heederik DJJ, Krop EJM, Jamshidifard A-R, Willemse T, Wouters IM. Allergen and endotoxin exposure in a companion animal hospital. *Occup Environ Med.* 2010;67(7):486-492. doi: 10.1136/oem.2009.051342

Satyaraj E, Wedner HJ, Bousquet J. Keep the cat, change the care pathway: a transformational approach to managing Fel d 1, the major cat allergen. *Allergy.* 2019;74 Suppl 107(Suppl 107):5-17. doi: 10.1111/all.14013

Virtanen T. Immunotherapy for pet allergies. *Hum Vaccin Immunother.* 2018;14(4):807-814. doi: 10.1080/21645515.2017.1409315

Wintersand A, Asplund K, Binnmyr J, et al. Allergens in dog extracts: Implications for diagnosis and treatment. *Allergy.* 2019;74(8):1472-1479. doi: 10.1111/all.13785

Wood RA. Laboratory animal allergens. *ILAR J.* 2001;42(1):12-16. doi: 10.1093/ilar.42.1.12

Zahradnik E, Raulf M. Respiratory allergens from furred mammals: environmental and occupational exposure. *Vet Sci.* 2017;4(3):38-55. doi:10.3390/vetsci4030038

Zahradnik E, Raulf M. Animal allergens and their presence in the environment. *Front Immunol.* 2014;5:76. doi: 3389/fimmu.2014.00076

ABBREVIATIONS AND ACRONYMS

ACD	ALLERGIC CONTACT DERMATITIS	GWAS	GENOME-WIDE ASSOCIATION STUDY
AD	ATOPIC DERMATITIS		
AFR	ADVERSE FOOD REACTION	HDM	HOUSE DUST MITE
AhR	ARYL HYDROCARBON RECEPTOR	HDN	HEMOLYTIC DISEASE OF THE NEWBORN
APRIL	ACTIVATION AND PROLIFERATION-INDUCED LIGAND	HMGB-1	HIGH MOBILITY GROUP BOX (PROTEIN)-1
ASA	ACETYLSALICYLIC ACID	HR	HISTAMINE RECEPTOR
ASIT	ALLERGEN-SPECIFIC IMMUNOTHERAPY	5-HT	5-HYDROXYTRYPTAMINE (SEROTONIN)
CAST	CELLULAR ANTIGEN STIMULATION TEST	HSC	HEMATOPOIETIC STEM CELL
CBH	CUTANEOUS BASOPHIL HYPERSENSITIVITY	IAD	INFLAMMATORY AIRWAY DISEASE
		IDO	INDOLEAMINE DIOXYGENASE
CCL/CXCL	CHEMOKINES	IBH	INSECT BITE HYPERSENSITIVITY
CCR/CXCR	CHEMOKINE RECEPTORS	IFN	INTERFERON
CGRP	CALCITONIN GENE-RELATED PEPTIDE	IL-	INTERLEUKIN-
		ILC	INNATE LYMPHOID CELL
COPD	CHRONIC OBSTRUCTIVE PULMONARY DISEASE	ITAM	IMMUNORECEPTOR TYROSINE-BASED, ACTIVATION MOTIF
COX	CYCLOOXYGENASE	JAK	JANUS KINASE
DAMP	DAMAGE-ASSOCIATED MOLECULAR PATTERN	KIT	THIS IS NOT AN ACRONYM. THE ORIGINAL GENE WAS FOUND IN THE FELINE SARCOMA VIRUS.
DC	DENDRITIC CELL		
DIC	DISSEMINATED INTRAVASCULAR COAGULATION	LT	LEUKOTRIENE
		MBP	MAJOR BASIC PROTEIN (IN EOSINOPHILS)
ECP	EOSINOPHIL CATIONIC PROTEIN		
EDN	EOSINOPHIL-DERIVED NEUROTOXIN	MHC	MAJOR HISTOCOMPATIBILITY COMPLEX
ELISA	ENZYME-LINKED IMMUNOSORBENT ASSAY	MRGPR	MAS-RELATED G-PROTEIN RECEPTOR
EPO	EOSINOPHIL PEROXIDASE	NET	NEUTROPHIL EXTRACELLULAR TRAP
FAD	FLEA ALLERGY DERMATITIS	NOD	NUCLEOTIDE OLIGOMERIZATION DOMAIN (PATTERN RECOGNITION RECEPTORS)
FcR	Fc (IMMUNOGLOBULIN) RECEPTOR		
FDA	FOOD AND DRUG ADMINISTRATION (USA)	NOS	NITRIC OXIDE SYNTHASE
		NGF	NERVE GROWTH FACTOR
GM-CSF	GRANULOCYTE/MONOCYTE COLONY-STIMULATING FACTOR	NK cells	NATURAL KILLER CELLS

NKT cells	NATURAL KILLER T CELLS	SLIT	SUBLINGUAL IMMUNOTHERAPY
NLR	NOD-LIKE RECEPTOR	SP	SUBSTANCE P (A NEUROPEPTIDE)
NSAID	NON-STEROIDAL ANTI-INFLAMMATORY DRUG	SRS-A	SLOW-REACTING SUBSTANCE OF ANAPHYLAXIS
PAF	PLATELET ACTIVATING FACTOR	STAT	SIGNAL TRANSDUCER AND ACTIVATOR OF TRANSCRIPTION
PAMP	PATHOGEN-ASSOCIATED MOLECULAR PATTERN	TCS	TOPICAL CORTICOSTEROID
PAR	PROTEASE-ACTIVATED RECEPTOR	TEWL	TRANSEPIDERMAL WATER LOSS
PCA	PASSIVE CUTANEOUS ANAPHYLAXIS	TGF	TRANSFORMING GROWTH FACTOR
		Tfh	FOLLICULAR HELPER T CELL
PRR	PATTERN RECOGNITION RECEPTOR	Th1	TYPE 1 HELPER T CELL
RAO	RECURRENT AIRWAY OBSTRUCTION	Th2	TYPE 2 HELPER T CELL
		Th17	T CELL THAT SECRETES INTERLEUKIN 17
RAST	RADIOALLERGOSORBENT TEST	TLR	TOLL-LIKE RECEPTOR
SCAR	SEVERE CUTANEOUS ADVERSE REACTION	TNF	TUMOR NECROSIS FACTOR
		Treg	REGULATORY T CELL
SCF	STEM CELL FACTOR (KIT LIGAND)	TSLP	THYMIC STROMAL LYMPHOPOIETIN
SCFA	SHORT CHAIN FATTY ACID	VEGF	VASCULAR ENDOTHELIAL GROWTH FACTOR
SJS	STEVENS-JOHNSTON SYNDROME		

INDEX